ARTERIAL CONDUITS IN MYOCARDIAL REVASCULARIZATION

ARTERIAL CONDUITS IN MYOCARDIAL REVASCULARIZATION

EDITED BY

Gianni D. Angelini

MD, MCh, FRCS

British Heart Foundation, Professor of Cardiac Surgery
University of Bristol, Bristol Heart Institute
Bristol, UK

Alan J. Bryan

DM, FRCS

Consultant Senior Lecturer
Bristol Heart Institute
University of Bristol, Bristol Royal Infirmary
Bristol, UK

Robert Dion

MD

Professor of Surgery and Head, Department of Thoracic and Cardiovascular Surgery
Cliniques Universitaires Saint-Luc, Université Catholique de Louvain,
Brussels, Belgium

ARNOLD

A member of the Hodder Headline Group
LONDON • SYDNEY • AUCKLAND
Co-published in the USA by Oxford University Press, Inc., New York

First published in Great Britain 1996, by
Arnold, a member of the Hodder Headline group,
338 Euston Road, London NW1 3BH

Co-published in the United States of America by
Oxford University Press, Inc.,
198 Madison Avenue, New York, NY 10016
Oxford is a registered trademark of Oxford University Press

Whilst the advice and information in this book is believed to be true and accurate at the date of going to press, neither the author[s] nor the publisher can accept any legal responsibility or liability for any errors or omissions that may be made. In particular (but without limiting the generality of the preceding disclaimer) every effort has been made to check drug dosages; however it is still possible that errors have been missed. Furthermore, dosage schedules are constantly being revised and new side-effects recognized. For these reasons the reader is strongly urged to consult the drug companies' printed instructions before administering any of the drugs recommended in this book.

British Library Cataloguing in Publication Data
A catalogue record for this book is available from the British Library

Library of Congress Cataloging-in-Publication Data
A catalog record for this book is available from the Library of Congress

ISBN 0 340 610247

Typeset in 10/11pt Plantin by
Phoenix Photosetting, Chatham, Kent
Printed and bound in Great Britain by
The Bath Press, Avon

Contents

Part III Right Gastroepiploic Artery

Part IV Inferior Epigastric Artery

Part V Other arterial conduits

Part VI Postoperative Management and Reoperation

Contributors

Christophe Acar, MD, PhD, Associate Professor of Cardiovascular Surgery, Hôpital Bichat, Paris, France

Gianni D Angelini MD, MCh, FRCS, British Heart Foundation Professor of Cardiac Surgery, Bristol Heart Institute, University of Bristol, Bristol Royal Infirmary, Bristol, UK

Philippe L Baele MD, Professor of Anaesthesiology, Cliniques Universitaires Saint-Luc, Université Catholique de Louvain, Brussels, Belgium

Hendrick B Barner MD, Professor of Surgery, Washington University School of Medicine, St Louis, Missouri, USA

John R Breaux MD, Mills Cardiovascular, New Orleans, LA, USA

Alan J Bryan DM, FRCS, Consultant Cardiac Surgeon, Bristol Heart Institute, University of Bristol, Department of Cardiovascular Surgery, Bristol Royal Infirmary, Bristol, UK

Michel Buche MD, Consultant Cardiac Surgeon, Service de Chirurgie Cardiovasculaire et Thoracique, Cliniques Universitaires UCL de Mont-Godinne, Yvoir, Belgium

Alain Carpentier MD, PhD, Professor and Chief of Cardiovascular Surgery, Hôpital Broussais, Paris, France

Adrian H Chester PhD, Lecturer, Department of Cardiothoracic Surgery, National Heart and Lung Institute, Harefield Hospital, Harefield, UK

Graham J Cooper MD, FRCS (Ed), Senior Registrar, Department of Cardiac Surgery, Guy's Hospital, London, UK

Patrick Chenu MD, Consultant Cardiologist, Service de Cardiologie, Cliniques Universitaires UCL de Mont-Godinne, Yvoir, Belgium

Alain Deloche MD, Professor of Cardiovascular Surgery, Hôpital Broussais, Paris, France

Robert Dion MD, Professor of Thoracic and Cardiovascular Surgery, Cliniques Universitaires Saint-Luc, Universite Catholique de Louvain, Brussels, Belgium

Jean-Noël Fabiani MD, Professor of Cardiac Surgery, Hôpital Broussais, Paris, France

Andrew C Fiore MD, Associate Professor of Surgery, St Louis University Medical School, St Louis, Missouri, USA

Sheila E Francis BSc, PhD, Lecturer, University Section of Cardiology, Northern General Hospital, Sheffield, UK

Martin Goenen Professor, Department of Intensive Care Medicine, Cliniques Universitaires Saint-Luc, Université Catholique de Louvain, Brussels, Belgium

George E Green MD, Professor of Clinical Surgery (retired), Columbia University, Attending Surgeon (retired), Columbia-Presbyterian Medical Center, New York, NY, USA

Oliver Gurné MD, Consultant Cardiologist, Service Cardiologie, Cliniques Universitaires UCL de Mont-Godinne, Yvoir, Belgium

Claude Hanet MD, Consultant Cardiologist, Cliniques Universitaires Saint-Luc, Université Catholique de Louvain, Brussels, Belgium

Cathy M Holt BSc, PhD, Lecturer, University Section of Cardiac Surgery, Northern General Hospital, Sheffield, UK

Takaaki Isshiki MD, FACC, Associate Professor, Division of Cardiology, Teikyo University Medical School, Tokyo, Japan

Luc Jacquet MD, Consultant Cardiologist, Cardiothoracic Intensive Care Unit, Cliniques Universitaires Saint-Luc, Université Catholique de Louvain, Brussels, Belgium

Victor Jebara MD, Associate Professor of Cardiovascular Surgery, Hôtel Dieu de France, Beirut, Lebanon

Nicholas T Kouchoukos MD, Professor, Division of Cardiothoracic Surgery, Washington University Medical Center, St Louis, MO, USA

Cody L Leger RNFA, CNOR, Consultant Cardiologist, Mills Cardiovascular, New Orleans, LA, USA

Thomas F Lüscher MD, Professor of Cardiology, University Hospital, Inselspital Bern, Switzerland

Bruce W Lytle MD, Senior Lecturer, Department of Thoracic and Cardiovascular Surgery, The Cleveland Clinic Foundation, Cleveland, OH, USA

Noel L Mills MD, Director, Mills Cardiovascular, New Orleans, LA, USA

Erwin Schroeder MD, Consultant Cardiologist, Service Cardiologie, Cliniques Universitaires UCL de Mont-Godinne, Yvoir, Belgium

Frank M M Smedts MD, PhD, Consultant Pathologist, Department of Pathology, Canisius-Wilhelmina Hospital, Nijmegen, The Netherlands

Hisayoshi Suma Professor, Department of Cardiac Surgery, Catholic University of Sacred Heart, Rome, Italy and Department of Cardiovascular Surgery, Mitsui Memorial Hospital, Tokyo, Japan

Jacques A M Van Son MD, PhD, Consultant Cardiologist, Division of Cardiothoracic Surgery, University of California at San Francisco, San Francisco, CA, USA

Peter Wilde MRCP, FRCR, Consultant Cardiac Radiologist, Department of Clinical Radiology, Bristol Royal Infirmary, Bristol, UK

Magdi H Yacoub KBE, FRCS, Professor of Cardiac Surgery, National Heart and Lung Institute, Harefield Hospital, Harefield, UK

Zhihong Yang MD, Lecturer, Cardiology, Cardiovascular Research, University Hospital, Inselspital Bern, Switzerland

Foreword

Few problems have proved as vexing to cardiologists, cardiac surgeons and patients as the high long-term failure rate of saphenous vein grafts used as conduits between the aorta and the coronary vascular system. A combination of intimal hyperplasia and accelerated atherosclerosis result in long-term patency rates of about 50% after 10 years. This, of course, means that for some patients critical graft failure will occur remarkably close to the time of the original operation while other patients may experience 20 years of benefit and have vein grafts in place that appear pristine at the time of reoperation. There appears to be little sense of predictability to the failure of vein grafts. Veins from the same leg in the same person have differing long-term patencies and the full spectrum of patency is inadequately understood as is the distribution curve for time-based graft failure. This is because of the limited numbers of studies in which cardiac catheterization and graft injection are performed. Considering the relatively short length of saphenous vein grafts used to bypass the coronary circulation as compared with the great length of saphenous vein grafts when used for peripheral revascularization, the fundamental biology that impedes long-term patency remains even more of a mystery.

The earliest pioneers in the use of arterial conduits for myocardial revascularization deserve great credit for the intuitive utilization of arteries to replace diseased arteries. The functional benefit of arterial grafts has withstood the test of time and now represents the mainstay of strategies for long-term preservation of coronary blood flow. The past 10 years has seen great interest in expanding the use of arterial grafts to the coronary circulation. With the expanded use of arterial grafts, more fundamental appreciation of the biology of medium-sized arteries has evolved. It has become clear that all such arteries are not the same. The relative thicknesses of the intima, media and adventitia vary from arteries from one location to the next. The same is true for the thickness of the basement membrane, innervation, and the distribution of the *vasa vasorum*. More recent studies have demonstrated that the inherent biological properties of the endothelium also differ in their capacity to generate important biological vasodilators and vasoconstrictors, sensitivity to growth factors and proclivity for development of hyperplastic or injury responses to the combination of arterial flow and the modulation of circulating lipids.

In parallel with the enhanced use of arterial conduits for myocardial revascularization has been an accelerated interest in the biology of the vascular endothelium. Fifteen years ago the vascular endothelium was regarded as a relatively passive 'barrier' between the blood and the arterial media. Today, vascular endothelium is regarded as one of the most important regulatory organs in human biology, playing a critical role in hypertension, angiogenesis, atherosclerosis, and organ perfusion. Since use of arterial conduits and enhanced understanding of vascular biology have evolved in parallel, literature has tended to accumulate in sporadic form and for the general reader it has been difficult to acquire this information in a comprehensive and focused manner.

In this textbook, Angelini, Bryan and Dion present the subject in a structured fashion that will be of great interest to all practising cardiac surgeons. Many of the elusive details surrounding the use of arterial conduits are presented in a comprehensive manner so that this book serves as an important primer for its readers. The authors are authoritative and experienced, the art work is of help, and the advantages and disadvantages for each of the graft types are well elaborated. The material presented is more detailed than in most textbooks of cardiac surgery and explores the biology of vascular conduits in a manner that is meaningful to clinicians. The subject is of great importance and the future should show further evolution in our understanding of the factors that optimize utilization of arterial conduits for myocardial revascularization.

Professor Andrew S. Wechsler
Medical College of Virginia
Virginia Commonwealth University
Richmond
1995

Preface

Coronary artery surgery has been in a continuous state of evolution since its earliest days, more than thirty years ago. One of the most profound changes in practice was the adoption of the left internal thoracic artery graft in the mid 1980s, following the demonstration of improved outcome with its use compared to venous grafts. Since this time there have been major developments, with the introduction of bilateral and complex internal thoracic artery grafting and the use of other conduits such as the gastroepiploic, inferior epigastric and radial arteries.

While we still await confirmatory evidence of improvements in late survival associated with the use of multiple arterial conduits, we have little doubt that in time these benefits will become obvious, particularly in younger patients. As with other areas in cardiac surgery, we believe that while the use of multiple arterial grafts is more time consuming and technically demanding, this will be justified by improved late outcomes.

Our aim in this international multi-author text has been to draw together contributions from a range of cardiac surgeons, cardiologists and scientists to provide comprehensive coverage of the use of arterial conduits in myocardial revascularization. These include history, basic science and clinical aspects, as well as practical surgical guidelines to the user and limitations of the range of arterial conduits now available.

For our own part in this, close links have developed between the Bristol Heart Institute at the University of Bristol and the Department of Cardiovascular and Thoracic Surgery of the Cliniques Universitaires Saint-Luc (Catholic University of Louvain) in Brussels, not only in terms of friendship, but also in allowing the interchange of clinical skills and research ideas. We are indebted to our expert colleagues in both institutions for their contributions. However, we must also particularly thank our friends and mentors across the globe for their endeavours, many of whom are widely recognized as experts in their field and who have facilitated our task by the excellence of their contributions.

Finally, we must thank those people who have provided us with so much practical help, including N. Merrell, J. Wild, M. Dits, E. Debecker, C. Flamand and S. Uytterhoeven for their work on the manuscripts. We would also like to thank Gary James and Michèle Lemaire for the technical illustrations and the cover of the book.

We hope that those who read this text will learn as much as we have during the editing process, and we encourage the reader to adopt the practical guidelines within the text since they should provide a sound basis for clinical practice.

G.D. Angelini
A.J. Bryan
R. Dion
August 1995

Part I
Introduction

1 History of arterial grafts in myocardial revascularization

George E. Green

Atherosclerotic obstruction of coronary arteries has affected humans for at least three thousand years as it has been documented in Egyptian Mummies,[1] but it has been less than three hundred years since the syndrome of angina pectoris was recorded, and its cause correlated with coronary arterial obstruction. (The study by John Hunter may have been particularly focused because he suffered from angina and prophetically remarked that his life was at the mercy of any rogue who provoked him. A consortium of rogues, the Board of St George's Hospital did provoke him and his prophecy was fulfilled: in the midst of heated controversy at a board meeting Hunter collapsed and died.)[2,3] Less than one hundred years ago the first clinical diagnoses of myocardial infarction were made.[4,5] Electrocardiographic diagnosis was described in the 1920s and recognition and diagnosis was widespread in the 1930s. During that time the histopathology of myocardial ischaemia was studied in detail and soon after the development of collateral circulation to ischaemic myocardium was described.[6] During the 1930s surgeons made experimental attempts to bring new blood flow to ischaemic myocardium with pedicled grafts of various organs (muscle, cutaneous tissues, spleen, intestine, lung) applied to the epicardium.

Experimental grafting

Gordon Murray in 1937 may have been the first surgeon to conceive of and to perform the experimental grafting of an artery (internal thoracic artery (ITA)) into the heart muscle in the attempt to augment collateral flow, but it was undoubtedly Arthur Vineberg (Fig. 1.1) who, during the course of his long career, explored and established the validity of this concept. Vineberg's first publication in 1946 described three experimental approaches to grafting the internal thoracic artery into heart muscle.[7] One of these approaches was associated

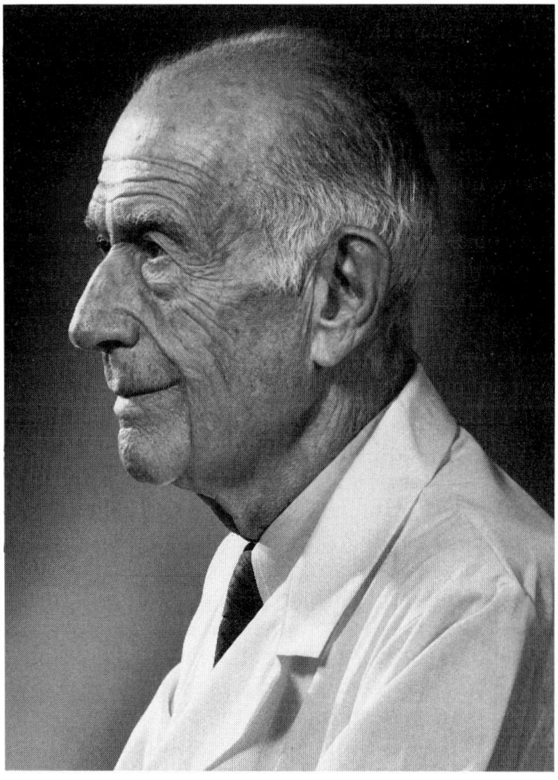

Fig. 1.1 Arthur M. Vineberg (1903–88) pioneered indirect revascularization by experimentally and clinically grafting the internal thoracic artery into the myocardium.

with closure of the grafted artery. Vineberg concentrated his study on the technique that resulted in a patent graft. His work was viewed with bemusement by those surgeons who were aware of it. Nonetheless in 1950, four years after publication of his first experimental work, he began clinical application of his operation.[8] In patients with angina decubitus, mortality was forbidding but in those with lesser degrees of ischaemia it was acceptable. In some patients clinical results were gratifying. Confirmatory studies were only possible by postmortem examination. Vineberg described several instances in which not only the grafted arteries maintained patency but material injected into them filled the native coronary arteries. The audacity of clinical application caught the attention of the surgical world. Vineberg's constancy of purpose kept a segment of the surgical world thinking about the possibility of surgical treatment of ischaemic heart disease.

Notable work was done by many surgeons to evaluate Vineberg's contentions. It was startling that implantation of a bleeding artery into the myocardium did not result in the formation of haematoma. David Sabiston showed that haematoma did not occur because there was no net forward flow in newly placed myocardial arterial implants.[9] Systolic contraction of heart muscle emptied the blood that filled the implant in diastole. Rhythmic to and fro motion of blood in the implant mitigated against thrombosis. Sabiston's evaluations extended to measuring flow through canine implants and showed that even long after operation the flow was of very small magnitude, in the range of 5 ml per minute. Vineberg supported the significance of this flow by developing models of canine coronary occlusion and showing the protective effects of his implants.[10]

Other surgical approaches were tried. Among them was that of distal ITA ligation, proposed by Robert Glover to increase flow into mediastinal branches of the ITA and thereby to increase flow to ischaemic myocardium.[11] The procedure was based on anatomical studies which had delineated coronary collateral flow from the ITA that developed in response to coronary occlusion.[6] The source of these collaterals was mediastinal branches of the ITA reaching the myocardium in the pericardial investments around the pulmonary veins draining to the heart. The surgical procedure made little sense because of the miniscule size of the collateral branches compared to the total network of ITA branches. Widespread application of it was aborted by conspicuous early clinical failure.

Experimental coronary endarterectomy and ITA – coronary artery grafting were reported in 1956.[12] In 1957 Charles Bailey performed clinical coronary endarterectomy but overwhelming problems were soon apparent.[13]

The intensity of the gathering interest in the possibilities of surgical intervention for ischaemic heart disease led to Emerick Szilagyi's study of the feasibility of direct arterial surgery in coronary disease.[14] He concluded that surgery would rarely be feasible because atherosclerosis usually affected coronary vessels down to the 2 mm level. Despite this caution, reports of experimental anastomoses to larger proximal coronary canine segments continued to be published as late as 1964.[15] Oddly, Julius Jacobson's report of consistent success in anastomosing arteries as small as 1 mm by using a surgical microscope for high magnification went almost unnoticed.[16]

Coronary arteriography

Surgical ferment added urgency to the search for a means of definitive coronary arteriography. It was discovered by Mason Sones in 1958 and he had perfected it to an art by 1962.[17]

In 1962 Vineberg, visiting Sones' laboratory, was greatly impressed by the quality of the arteriograms, and asked if Sones could selectively opacify ITA implants. Sones said 'sure'. Vineberg asked if he would study patients who had been helped by ITA implants. Sones said 'I can do it. But you won't like it.' Vineberg responded by referring three patients. The first study showed no coronary disease and an occluded implant. The second study showed no coronary disease, a patent ITA implant but no flow from it to the coronary circulation. The third study showed severe occlusive coronary disease, a patent implant and flow from the implant to the coronary circulation. Vineberg's reaction is not remembered but Sones was galvanized (as related by Dr Julio Sosa who worked as Sones' fellow 1960–4). Sones urged Donald Effler (Fig. 1.2), Chief of the Cardiac Surgical Section of the Cleveland Clinic, to visit Montreal and study Vineberg's operation. Sones was determined that the procedure be done with the scrutiny of pre- and postoperative coronary arteriography, and be applied on a meaningfully large scale.

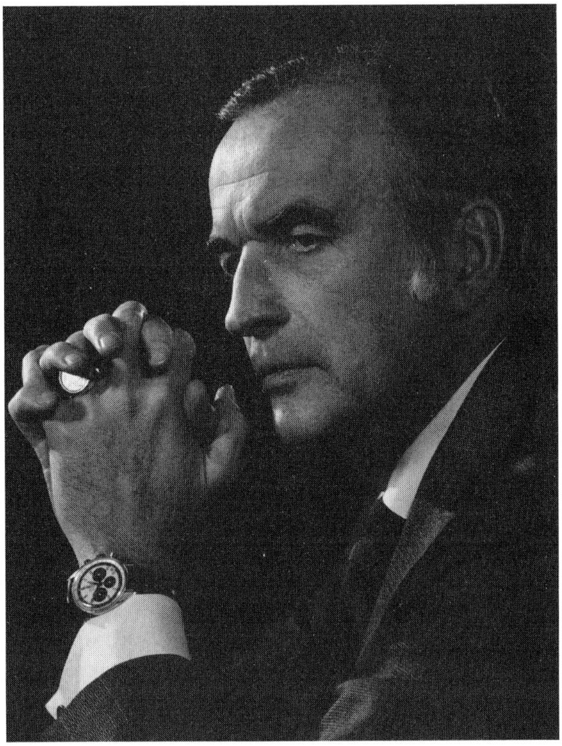

Fig. 1.2 Donald B. Effler (1915–) established surgical treatment of ischaemic heart disease as an accepted practice, refining and validating Vineberg's procedure in large clinical trials.

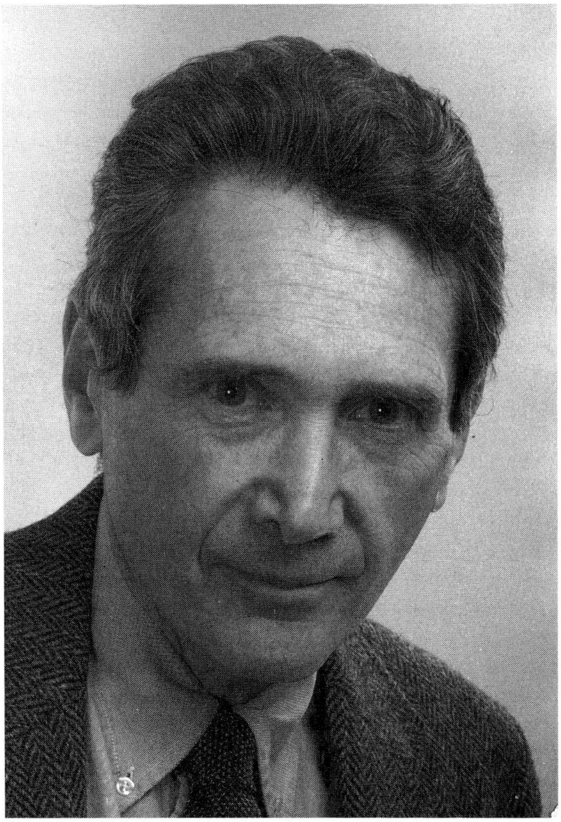

Fig. 1.3 George E. Green (1932–) pioneered direct arterial revascularization by using microsuture technique to sew the internal thoracic artery to distal coronary segments.

ITA anastomosis

By 1965 Effler was able to describe the frequency with which and the mechanism by which ITA implants augmented myocardial blood flow in patients with ischaemic heart disease.[18] He was invited to present the data at the 1965 Convention of The American Heart Association in Miami, Florida. I was attending that meeting to present data confirming Jacobson's contention that with high magnification blood vessels of 1 mm in diameter could be anastomosed with consistent success.[19] My surgical interest at that time was using the technique to revascularize free grafts of jejunum transposed to the neck to replace segments of cervical oesophagus,[20] but listening to Effler describe the arteriolar communications which could develop between the implanted ITA and distal coronary branches I thought of anastomosing the ITA directly to a distal coronary vessel (Fig. 1.3). The large clinical experience presented by Effler left no doubt that arteriolar connections could alleviate ischaemic heart disease. The drawback to the procedure was the prolonged time required for development of the connections. Because of my experimental experience I was sure the ITA could be anastomosed to a distal coronary segment 1 mm in diameter. Such an anastomosis would be ten times the size of an arteriole and would be effective from the moment of surgical completion.

Internal thoracic–coronary artery anastomosis was first reported from the experimental laboratory in 1956.[12] It was repeated by many surgeons in many laboratories with many techniques and in 1964 was reported in conjunction with the use of the heart/lung machine.[15] All these demonstrations were anastomoses of the ITA to proximal coronary segments, approximately 3 mm in diameter. A misunderstanding of statements about the proximal location of coronary occlusions may have led to this perseverative work. The major occlusions usually were proximal, but atherosclerotic thickening extended well beyond them. These thickenings were the basis of Szilagyi's warning that bypass surgery would rarely be feasible to vessels more than 2 mm in diameter.

In 1965 I began a project of ITA anastomosis to 1 mm distal LAD segments. The project included proximal LAD ligation, blood flow measurement early and late after anastomosis, and late postoperative (18 months) cineangiography.[21] The success of these experiments brought me to grips with clinical application. Despite the fact that I had conducted the work in the surgical laboratory of New York University, permission for clinical application at New York University was denied in September of 1967. The story of the search for a place for clinical application illuminates surgical thinking of the time. ITA implantation had become accepted and was performed in most university centres. It was so firmly established that extensions of it were achieved with implants of the intercostal artery,[22] the right gastroepiploic artery[23] and the splenic artery.[24] By contrast, direct microsuture anastomosis despite impressive experimental data, was considered not clinically feasible. Most of my letters of inquiry went unanswered, but there were some respondents. C. Walton Lilehei, the dynamic pioneer of cardiac surgery was encouraging but was in the process of leaving the University of Minnesota to become Chairman of the Department of Surgery at the New York Hospital, the Cornell Medical Center, and could not sponsor any new projects. Adrian Kantrowitz thought the data interesting but wanted the experiments repeated in his laboratory. Donald Effler invited me to show him the postoperative cineangiograms, was much impressed by them, favoured clinical application at the Cleveland Clinic, but wanted me to do it as his resident. Michael DeBakey did not reply to the letter but during one of his visits to New York City an introduction was arranged. He listened closely to my proposal. His reply was definitive: clinical application was impossible, coronary bypass surgery was not feasible.

Many years later DeBakey claimed precedence in coronary bypass surgery contending that he had performed the first successful coronary bypass operation in 1964.[25] In 1964 Dr Edward Garrett was Dr DeBakey's associate. As related by Dr Garrett:

> A patient with intractable angina had been referred to Dr DeBakey for ITA implant surgery. Angiography showed a severe left main coronary stenosis. He instructed me to discharge the patient from the surgical service. He left Houston for a scheduled trip. While he was away the patient was readmitted to the hospital with unstable angina. The cardiologist urged me to undertake surgical intervention. I explained that no benefit would accrue from an ITA implant for many weeks and the procedure was inappropriate for the patient. The cardiologist then suggested endarterectomy. Angiography had shown the left main coronary stenosis to be of short extent. I replied that the surgical risk of endarterectomy would be 50 per cent. The cardiologist thought that acceptable and so did the patient. Surgery was scheduled. In those days we used a formidable incision – bilateral anterior thoracotomy. It did give good exposure. Through that big incision it was quickly apparent that what seemed like a short left main coronary stenosis by angiography was in fact severe atherosclerotic change well into both the anterior descending and circumflex arteries. I knew successful endarterectomy could not be done, but something now *had* to be done. I had done saphenous vein bypasses to distal tibial arteries. I prepared a saphenous vein segment, sewed one end to the aorta, made an incision in a soft section of the anterior descending artery and sewed the saphenous vein graft to it. The patient did well. When Dr DeBakey returned the patient was ready for discharge from the hospital. I explained the situation to him. He became very excited and told me to schedule patients for him to operate. I did so. We knew very little about perioperative care for ischemic heart disease in those days. The patients operated died. Dr DeBakey forbade any further such surgery.

Two random events suddenly opened the way for clinical application of ITA to coronary anastomosis. The explosive impact of heart transplantation reported in December of 1967 made other cardiac procedures seem minor by comparison. Moreover, in December of 1967 The *Journal of Thoracic and Cardiovascular Surgery* published a report by the Russian surgeon Kolessov of ITA–LAD anastomosis in six patients.[26] Although the procedure had been prohibited at the New York University Hospital, Dr David Tice, Director of Surgery at the New York Veterans Administration Hospital, invited me to do it there. The first ITA–LAD anastomosis in the United States was done there in February of

1968.[21] During that same month Bailey and Hirose did the first ITA suture anastomosis to right coronary using the right internal thoracic artery.[27]

Although Sones had discovered coronary arteriography in 1958 and by 1968 had brought it to a very high point, few laboratories could match his capability. In New York, coronary arteriography could define proximal areas of obstruction but rarely defined the status of the distal circulation. Postmortem dissection had made it clear to me that although isolated areas of proximal atherosclerosis did occur, other areas extended well beyond the proximal obstruction in skip-like fashion. Placing a graft between two areas of stenosis seemed less sensible than placement far distally beyond the last atherosclerotic stenosis. My choice was placement of the ITA graft to the distal third of the LAD, usually a normal thin walled segment about 1.5 mm in diameter. My expectation was not to achieve normal myocardial perfusion but to augment flow to the ischaemic myocardium. In 1968 I operated on eighteen patients. Although all were desperately ill no operating room fatalities occurred. Nevertheless, there were six early postoperative deaths. Postmortem examination showed patent ITA anastomoses but severe triple vessel disease.

In June of 1968 saphenous vein graft to the right coronary artery, which had been introduced by Rene Favaloro, was combined with ITA anastomosis to the LAD. Although Bailey and Hirose described right ITA artery to right coronary anastomosis in 1968, I was reluctant to use this procedure because so often the main right coronary artery is markedly thickened and dilated. Tissue mismatch of ITA to RCA would be a technical problem. More importantly the size mismatch of small ITA to large RCA would cause turbulence of flow at the anastomosis. I feared this would make anastomotic stenosis likely. Skill in routing the ITA parallel to the phrenic nerve so that it could reach the PDA was to come later, as was the use of free ITA grafts arising from the aorta.

In 1969 I began to perform anastomoses to the circumflex artery, and with the advent of triple bypasses the problem of early postoperative mortality was resolved. By 1969 several centres were performing coronary bypass surgery. Most used only saphenous vein grafts. I was considered odd for persisting in the use of the ITA. I persisted because in my practice when angina recurred, angiography almost invariably showed saphenous vein graft stenosis or occlusion to be the cause of the recurrent angina. Therefore, despite criticism I continued to use the ITA on a routine basis for anastomosis to the LAD. Several other surgeons felt that ITA grafts would prove to be preferable to saphenous vein grafts. Earle Kay felt so strongly that he initiated the use of both ITAs as grafts and reported a large series in 1974.[28]

Sterling Edwards (Fig. 1.4), a vigorous proponent of ITA grafts and of use of the surgical microscope initiated the additional use of the splenic artery pedicled graft in 1973 in order to achieve triple bypass using arteries only.[29] Between 1972 and 1975 Edwards performed fifteen splenic artery anastomoses. In 1973 while mobilizing the splenic artery he encountered an aneurysmal segment of the splenic artery. In its stead he mobilized and used the right gastroepiploic artery as a graft to the right coronary. He found the right gastroepiploic much easier to mobilize than the splenic and he found it to be of adequate size. He did not report the use of it. In 1974 he accepted the Chairmanship of the Department of Surgery at the University of New Mexico. In this capacity he found he could no longer practice both cardiac and vascular surgery and discontinued cardiac surgical practice in 1975.

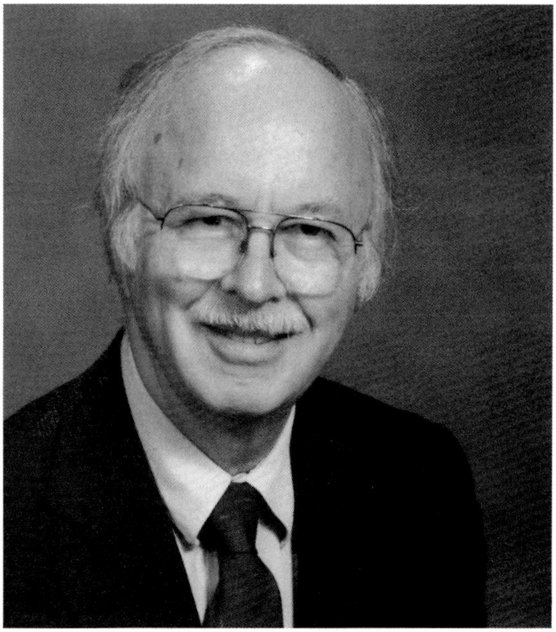

Fig. 1.4 W. Sterling Edwards (1920–) was the earliest and most influential advocate of Green's work and a pioneer of total direct arterial revascularization, using both internal thoracic arteries, splenic and gastroepiploic arteries.

Edwards commanded great respect in the cardiac surgical community. Because of his early enthusiasm and support I was allowed to extend my work to the New York University Hospital. His prestige was such that had he continued in cardiac surgical practice I believe the microscope would have come into general use. He joked that I had seriously interfered with the work of his vascular surgery laboratory by introducing him to the microscope. His standard model for creating and studying arterial thrombosis had been endarterectomy of the canine superficial femoral artery. He told me that performing endarterectomy with a microscope ruined the model by eliminating thrombosis.

Floyd Loop was another early enthusiast of ITA anastomosis. In order to extend its use he introduced the free ITA graft, detached from its subclavian origin and anastomosed to the ascending aorta.[30] This anastomosis was demanding because of the marked difference in thickness of the aorta and the ITA. To resolve this problem Hendrick Barner recommended anastomosing it to the hood of a vein graft[31] and George Schimert recommended anastomosing it to a vein patch in the aorta.[32] Because of the difficulty of handling the thin walled and friable ITA, Alain Carpentier introduced the radial artery free graft in 1973.[33] He hoped it would have the haemodynamic advantage of the ITA graft and the further advantage of being much easier to handle because of its thicker wall. It soon appeared that radial artery grafts were subject to a prohibitive incidence of fibrosis and occlusion – 75 per cent within a year.[34] They were universally abandoned until 1990. Renewed use and re-evaluation was based on the possible protective affect of calcium blocking agents.

Even enthusiasts of arterial grafting acknowledged that the ITA was a far more demanding graft than the saphenous vein. As skilled a surgeon as Favaloro wrote in 1970: 'It is highly doubtful that full clinical application of this procedure will reach a large scale: the anastomosis is extremely difficult to perform mostly because of the fragile wall of the internal mammary artery rather than of the coronary artery itself, and the limitation of the size of the anastomosis by the caliber of the internal mammary artery in its distal portion.'[35]

Favaloro's statement highlights the difference in technique required for ITA grafts as compared to the saphenous vein graft technique which he and Effler developed at the Cleveland Clinic. That technique, using no magnification was based on placement of interrupted sutures deep into the vascular graft, shallowly into the coronary artery and deeply into surrounding epicardium. Placement of sutures deep into the ITA will result in anastomotic stricture. The ITA does not have sufficient size to spatulate over a cuff of epicardium. The most consistently successful mode of anastomosis is precise wall-to-wall approximation. The precision of approximation increases with increasing magnification. The difficulty of this anastomosis led to a damping of enthusiasm for it. In 1975 Claude Grondin expressed these reservations because in his hands ITA patency was no better than saphenous vein graft patency one year after operation.[36] Issues of surgical technique were not considered. Between 1976 and 1983 few surgeons used the ITA.

Restudies

In 1970, when I left New York University to initiate the coronary surgery program at St Luke's Hospital, a clinical follow-up program was initiated by Dr Airlie Cameron of the Division of Cardiology. Soon thereafter, Dr Julio Sosa who had worked with Sones during the development of coronary angiography, and who had participated in the first angiographic studies of ITA implants expressed interest in referring patients for and restudying them after ITA anastomosis. The restudies were not done arbitrarily. They were strongly advocated to evaluate recurrence of angina, recurrent myocardial infarction, or signs of ischaemia on electrocardiographic stress tests. Few restudies were performed prior to 1975. During the latter part of the decade restudies became more frequent. By 1981 Sosa had restudied thirty-seven patients who had both ITA and saphenous vein grafts. The mean time following operation was seven years. Analysis of the data was striking: 94 per cent of the ITA grafts were widely patent; 50 per cent of the saphenous vein grafts were occluded and 50 per cent of those patent showed atherosclerotic stenosis within the body of the graft. In 1981 the data was abstracted and submitted for presentation at the annual meeting of the American Association for Thoracic Surgery. It was not selected for presentation. I was puzzled but persistent and resubmitted the data in 1982. The resubmission was selected, presented in the spring of 1983 and published later that year.[37] By then similar angiographic studies had come from Montreal.[38] In 1984 Grondin, whose 1975 publication dampened enthusiasm for ITA grafts, reversed his position and became a champion of the procedure.[39] The use of sequential ITA grafts was described,[40] and John

Pym described the use of the right gastroepiploic artery for anastomosis to the distal right coronary artery.[41]

In 1985 Cameron collated the fifteen year follow-up data of the 748 patients operated at St Luke's Hospital between 1970 and 1973. There was a highly significant advantage conferred to those patients who had single ITA anastomosis in combination with saphenous vein grafts as compared to those having saphenous vein grafts alone. There was even further advantage to those patients who had double ITA anastomosis.[42] The number of patients having double ITA anastomoses was too small to reach statistical significance but I found the trend compelling. I was eager to understand why ITA grafts fared so much better than saphenous vein grafts.

ITA histological properties

I had taken particular care to try at the time of surgery to match the size of saphenous vein grafts closely to coronary size so they could approximate the haemodynamic advantages of ITAs.[43] One obvious difference between the vein graft and the ITA graft was that of nutrient vessels. All *vasa vasorum* were disrupted in the process of removing a saphenous vein graft from the leg. It was known to take many weeks before nutrition of the wall of the vein graft was reconstituted.[44] This seemed a plausible explanation for the 10 per cent of saphenous grafts that suffered early fibrotic occlusion, but the explanation for late atherosclerosis which affected the majority of saphenous vein grafts was not apparent, until the publication of the work of Frank Sims.

Sims, a pathologist, accepted the resistance of the ITA to atherosclerosis as a known fact. Wanting to study the incidence and severity of coronary atherosclerosis in residents of the Fiji Islands he used each subject's ITA as a standard of normality and then compared the intimal thickness of the coronary to that of the ITA, in age groups ranging from the first to the eighth decade. In so doing he noticed that the defining boundary between the intima and the media, the internal elastic lamina (IEL), was radically different in ITAs from that in the coronaries.[45] The IEL of the ITA was usually dense and unbroken. The IEL of the coronary was usually fragmented. Smooth muscle cells migrated through gaps in the IEL and changed from a synthetic to a hyperplastic mode in their new locale. He later discovered that endothelium of ITAs was stable but large patches of coronary endothelium sloughed continually. Endothelium anchored to the IEL; when IEL was deficient endothelial slough ensued. He showed that all the arteries of domestic animals are similar to the ITA. Human arteries are similar to the coronary. Human veins have even more deficiencies of IEL than human arteries.[46]

Free ITA grafts

I had avoided using free grafts of the ITA because I feared that the disruption of the *vasa vasorum* would make them no better than saphenous vein grafts. Sims' emphasis on the internal structure of the vessel caused me to think again.

Loop had introduced the use of the free ITA graft in 1973. In 1985 I was eager to know if there had been late studies of these grafts. Did they become atherosclerotic? Loop, then in the process of evaluating the late studies, assured me there were no signs of atherosclerotic change. He confided that anastomotic stricture at the aorta had been a problem, but that was a technical matter and subject to solution. He had seen no fibrous strictures such as typically occurred in radial artery grafts. The absence of early stricture (subintimal fibrosis) in free ITA grafts was striking. I had thought such strictures in saphenous vein grafts as well as in radial artery grafts were a consequence of disruption of *vasa vasorum*. I undertook a small study of *vasa vasorum* of ITAs in comparison to radial arteries. Injection of barium gel into ITAs revealed multiple prominent branches throughout their length. Histologic study of these same vessels revealed the *vasa vasorum* of the adventitia of ITAs to be filled with the barium. Clearly the *vasa vasorum* of the ITA originated from its own branches. As soon as an ITA graft was anastomosed to the aorta the nutrition of its wall would be restored. In contrast, radial arteries showed no prominent branches and *vasa vasorum* were not filled by injection of the artery. Moreover, the IEL of the radial artery did not have the integrity of the ITA. Cameron's clinical follow-up studies of pedicled ITA grafts, Loop's angiographic follow-up studies of free ITA grafts,[47] and the logic of Sims' studies compelled me to resolve to evaluate the use of ITAs for as many grafts as feasible in all patients, using free grafts when pedicle grafts were not feasible, and including the use of sequential techniques.

Putting that resolution into practice was relatively easy in 1985 because enthusiasm for arterial grafting in both the cardiological and cardiac surgical communities was growing. Synchronous with Cameron's study a similar study from Cleveland was published.[48] Robert Dion's pioneering work in the broad application of bilateral and sequential ITA grafts was well underway and beginning to be recognized.[49] Similar work was being done by Rankin.[50]

Problems with ITA use

Acknowledgement of the superiority of the ITA graft had created such a demand for its performance that it quickly became the standard graft to the LAD in the majority of surgical practices. Scrutiny of the results may not have been optimal, but there was frequent comment and sporadic publication concerning the danger of 'ITA spasm'[51] and 'hypoperfusion' due to the use of ITA.[52] Documentation of the dynamics of 'spasm' and/or 'hypoperfusion' left much to be desired. 'Spasm' may well have been the consequence of disruption of the wall of the ITA during mobilization, and 'hypoperfusion' may have been the consequence of suturing technique. Review of the literature of 1986–7 on ITA surgery showed seven reports from four different countries of *successful* balloon angioplasty of stenotic ITA anastomoses.[53] Unsuccessful attempts at dilatation and many unreported anastomotic stenoses were matters of concerned conversation. Clearly a technical problem was abroad. It had been presaged by Szilagyi in 1958[14] and defined by Favaloro in 1970.[35] In contrast to surgeons of other disciplines most cardiac surgeons shunned the high magnification afforded by the surgical microscope. Some persisted in the use of no magnification, most used the low magnification of optical loupes. Occasionally the problem posed by the small size of the ITA was addressed but instead of optical magnification physical stretching of the graft – by hydrostatic or mechanical dilatation – was recommended.[54,55]

Aside from anastomotic problems, the small size of the ITA posed problems of mobilization. An easy solution was taking a wide swath of chest wall with the arterial pedicle. This may well have been the cause of high rates of infection reported from some surgical centres when single ITA grafts were used, and even higher rates when bilateral ITA grafts were used.[56]

Respiratory dysfunction due to phrenic nerve palsy or paralysis was occurring but was rarely studied in detail.[57] It constituted a significant problem when unilateral and a grave problem when bilateral. Its cause was occasionally mechanical – trauma to the phrenic nerve as it entered the chest behind and immediately adjacent to the ITA. More often it was the result of cold injury to the phrenic nerve imposed by the use of iced saline slush in the pericardium. The nerve may have been made more vulnerable to surgical cold injury by mobilization of the ITA where the phrenic branches do contribute to the vascularity of the phrenic nerve. Its occurrence was exceedingly rare when iced saline slush was not used.

These very real problems, the resolution of which required diligent care, deterred most surgeons from widespread use of bilateral, free or sequential grafts. It did not deter all. Dion established Brussels as a centre for multiple ITA grafts using bilateral and sequential techniques. He recognized early on the significance of Hisayoshi Suma's work with the right gastroepiploic artery[58] and made it a centrepiece of the symposium held in Brussels in 1991. He endorsed and explored use of the inferior epigastric artery, described by Luiz Puig[59] and Michel Buche and Jean-Claude Schoevardts.[60]

The first long-term follow-up study to demonstrate statistically the clinical advantage of bilateral ITA grafts was that of Keith Naunheim and Hendrick Barner.[61] It was based on surgery performed in 1972, when skill in routing pedicle grafts to the right coronary artery was unevolved and free grafts were not yet being used. More dramatic advantage of multiple ITA grafts in reducing the incidence of recurrent angina and myocardial infarction during five years after operation was published in 1994.[62] Proof of preferential reduction of mortality by multiple ITA grafts will require further years of clinical follow-up, as will determining the fate of right gastroepiploic and inferior epigastric artery grafts. Meanwhile, the studies of Gianni Angelini and others on the biochemical properties of arterial grafts serve as a beacon.

References

1. Long AR. Cardiovascular renal disease report of three thousand years ago. *Arch Path* 1931; **12:** 92–4.
2. Heberden W. Some account of a disorder in the breast. *Med Trans Coll Physns Lond* 1772; **2:** 59–67.
3. Leibowitz Jo. *The History of Coronary Heart Disease.* Berkley and Los Angeles: University of California Press, 1970: 102.
4. Obrastzow WP, Straschesko ND. Zur kenntnis der thrombose der koronararterien des hertzens. *Z Klin Med* 1910; **71:** 116–32.

5. Herrick JB. Clinical features of sudden obstructions of the coronary arteries. *J Am Med Ass* 1912; **59:** 2015–20.
6. Hudson CL, Moritz AR, Wearn JT. Extracardiac anastomoses of coronary arteries. *J Exp Med* 1932; **56:** 919–26.
7. Vineberg AM. Development of anastomosis between coronary vessels and transplanted internal mammary artery. *Can Med Ass J* 1946; **55:** 117–19.
8. Vineberg AM. Coronary vascular anastomoses by internal mammary artery implantation. *Can Med Ass J* 1958; **78:** 871–9.
9. Sabiston DC, Fauteux JP, Blalock A. An experimental study of the fate of arterial implants in the left ventricular myocardium with comparison with other organs. *Ann Surg* 1957; **145:** 927–42.
10. Vineberg A, Mahanti B, Litvak J. Experimental gradual coronary artery constriction by ameroid constrictors. *Surgery* 1960; **47:** 765–71.
11. Glover RP, Davila JC, Kyle RH *et al.* Ligation of the internal mammary arteries as a means of increasing blood supply to the myocardium. *J Thorac Surg* 1957; **34:** 661–78.
12. Absolon KG, Aust JB, Varco RL and Lillehei CW. Surgical treatment of occlusive coronary disease by endarterectomy or anastomotic replacement. *Surgery Gynec Obstet* 1956; **103:** 180–5.
13. Cannon JA, Longmire WP, Kaltus AA. Considerations of the rationale and technique of coronary endarterectomy for angina pectoris. *Surgery* 1959; **46:** 197–211.
14. Szilaqyi DE, McDonald RT, France LT. The applicability of angioplastic procedures in coronary atherosclerosis. An estimate through postmortem injection studies. *Ann Surg* 1958; **148:** 447–61.
15. Spencer FC, Young NK, Prachusbmoh K. Internal mammary–coronary artery anastomosis performed during cardiopulmonary bypass. *J Cardiovasc Surg* 1964; **5:** 292–7.
16. Jacobson JH, Suarez EL. Microsurgery in anastomosis of small vessels. *Surg Forum* 1960; **11:** 243–5.
17. Sones FM Jr, Shirey EK. Cine coronary arteriography: *Mod Conc Cardiovasc Dis* 1962; **31:** 735–8.
18. Effler DB, Sones FM, Groves LK and Suarez E. Myocardial revascularization by Vineberg's internal mammary artery implant: evaluation of postoperative results: *J Thorac Cardiovasc Surg* 1965; **50:** 527–33.
19. Green GE, Som ML, Wolff WI: Experimental microvascular suture anastomosis. *Circulation* 1965: **33 (Suppl. 1):** 199–203.
20. Green GE, Som ML: Free grafting and revascularization of the intestine. I. Replacement of the cervical esophagus. *Surgery* 1966; **60:** 1012–16.
21. Green GE, Reppert EH, Stertzer SH. Coronary arterial bypass grafts. *Ann Thor Surg* 1968; **5:** 443–50.
22. Pearce CW, Hyman AL, Brewer P, Smith PE, Creech O. Myocardial revascularization: Implantation of intercostal artery. *J Thorac Cardiovasc Surg* 1966; **52:** 809–28.
23. Bailey CW, Hirose T, Brancato R, Aventura A, Yamamoto N. Revascularization of the posterior (diaphragmatic) portion of the heart: *Ann Thorac Surg* 1966; **2:** 791–805.
24. Bloomer WD, Beland AJ, Cope J. Clinical use of the splenic artery for myocardial revascularization. Technical considerations. *Ann Thorac Surg* 1968; **5:** 419–28.
25. Garrett HE, Diethrich EB, DeBakey ME. Aortocoronary bypass with saphenous vein graft. Seven year followup. *J AM Med Ass* 1973; **223:** 792–4.
26. Kolessov VI. Mammary artery–coronary artery anastomosis as method of treatment for angina pectoris. *J Thorac Cardiovasc Surg* 1967; **54:** 535–44.
27. Bailey CP, Hirose T: Successful internal mammary–coronary arterial anastomosis using a 'minivascular' suturing technic. *Int Surg* 1968; **49:** 416–27.
28. Kay EB, Naraghipour H, Beg Ra, Demaney M, Tambe A, Zimmerman HA. Internal mammary artery bypass graft – long term patency rate and follow-up: *Ann Thorac Surg* 1974; **18:** 269–79.
29. Edwards WS, Lewis CE, Blakely WR. Coronary artery bypass with internal mammary and splenic artery grafts. *Ann Thorac Surg* 1973; **15:** 35–40.
30. Loop FD, Spampinato N, Cheanvechai C, Effler DB. The free internal mammary artery bypass graft. Use of the IMA in the aorta-to-coronary artery position. *Ann Thorac Surg* 1975; **70:** 278–1.
31. Barner HB. The internal mammary artery as a free graft. *J Thorac Cardiovasc Surg* 1973; **66:** 219–21.
32. Schimert G, Vidne BA, Lee AB Jr. Free internal mammary artery graft. An improved surgical technique. *Ann Thorac Surg* 1975; **19:** 474–7.
33. Carpentier A, Guermonprez JL, Deloche A *et al.* The aorta-to-coronary radial artery bypass graft. *Ann Thorac Surg* 1973; **16:** 111–21.
34. Curtis JJ, Stoney WS, Alfred WCJ. Intimal hyperplasia: a cause of radial artery aorto-coronary bypass graft failure. *Ann Thorac Surg* 1975; **20:** 628–35.
35. Favaloro RD *Surgical treatment of coronary arteriosclerosis*. Baltimore: Williams & Wilkins, 1970; 6.
36. Grondin CM, Lesperance J, Bourassa MG, Campeau L. Coronary artery grafting with the saphenous vein or internal mammary artery. *Ann Thorac Surg* 1975; **20:** 605–15.
37. Singh RN, Sosa JA, Green GE. Long term fate of the internal mammary artery and saphenous vein grafts. *J Thorac Cardiovasc Surg* 1983; **86:** 359–63.
38. Campeau L, Enjalbert M, Lesperance J *et al.* Atherosclerosis and late closure of aorto-coronary saphenous vein grafts: sequential angiographic studies at 2 weeks, 1 year, 5 to 7 years, and 10 to 12 years after surgery. *Circulation* 1983; **68** (Suppl.2): 1–7.
39. Grondin CM: Late results of coronary artery graft-

ing. Is there a flag on the field? (editorial). *J Thorac Cardiovasc Surg* 1984; **87**: 161–6.
40. Tector AJ, Schmahl TM, Canino VR *et al.* The role of the sequential internal mammary artery grafts in coronary surgery. *Circulation* 1984; **70** (Suppl.1): 222–5.
41. Pym J, Brown PM, Charette EJ. Gastroepiploic-coronary anastomosis. *J Thorac Cardiovasc Surg* 1987; **94**: 256–9.
42. Cameron A, Kemp HG, Green GE. Bypass surgery with the internal mammary artery graft: 15 year followup. *Circulation* 1986; **74** (Suppl.III): 30–6.
43. Green GE, Hutchinson JE, McCord CW. Choice of saphenous vein segments for aortocoronary grafts. *Surgery* 1971; **69**: 924–7.
44. Wyatt AP, Rothnie BG, Taylor GW. The vascularization of vein grafts. *Br J Surg* 1964; **51**: 378–81.
45. Sims FH. A comparison of coronary and internal mammary arteries, and implications of the results in the etiology of atherosclerosis. *Am Heart J* 1983; **105**: 560–6.
46. Sims F. The pathology of the internal thoracic artery. In: Green GE, Singh RN, Sosa JA. *Surgical revascularization of the heart: The internal thoracic arteries.* New York:Igaku-Shoin 1991: 18–62.
47. Loop FD, Lytle BW, Cosgrove DM: Golding LAR, Taylor PC, Stewart RW. Free aorta-coronary internal mammary artery graft. Late results. *J Thorac Cardiovasc Surg* 1986; **92**: 827–31.
48. Loop FD, Lytle BW, Cosgrove DM *et al.* Influence of the internal mammary artery graft on 10-year survival and other cardiac events. *New Engl J Med* 1986; **314**: 1–6.
49. Dion R, Verhelst R, Rousseau M *et al.* Sequential mammary grafting. *J Thorac Cardiovasc Surg* 1989; **98**: 80–9.
50. Rankin JS, Newman GE, Bashore TM *et al.* Clinical and angiographic assessment of complex mammary artery bypass grafting. *J Thorac Cardiovasc Surg* 1986; **92**: 832–46.
51. Sarabu MR, McClung JA, Fass A *et al.* Early post-operative spasm in left internal mammary artery bypass grafts. *Ann Thorac Surg* 1987; **44**: 199–200.
52. Jones EL, Lattouf OM, Weintraub WS. Catastrophic consequences of internal mammary artery hypoperfusion. *J Thorac Cardiovasc Surg* 1989; **98**: 902–7.
53. Green GE. Expanded role of the internal mammary artery: *Current Opin Cardiol* 1987; **2**: 987–9.
54. Mills NL, Bringaze WL. Preparation of the internal mammary artery graft. Which is the best method? *J Thorac Cardiovasc Surg* 1989; **98**: 73–7.
55. Fogarty TJ. Discussion of preparation of the internal mammary artery graft. Which is the best method? *J Thorac Cardiovasc Surg* 1989; **98**: 79.
56. Green GE, Swistel DG, Castro J, Hillel Z, Thornton J. Sternal blood flow during mobilization of the internal thoracic arteries. *Ann Thorac Surg* 1993; **55**: 967–70.
57. Abd AG, Braun NT, Baskin MI *et al.* Diaphragmatic dysfunction after open heart surgery: treatment with a rocking bed. *Archs Intern Med* 1989; **111**: 881–6.
58. Suma H, Fukumoto H, Atsuro T. Coronary artery bypass grafting by utilizing *in situ* right gastroepiploic artery. Basic study and clinical application. *Ann Thorac Surg* 1987; **44**: 394–7.
59. Puig LB, Ciongolli W, Cividanes GV *et al.* Inferior epigastric artery as a free graft for myocardial revascularization. *J Thorac Cardiovasc Surg* 1990; **99**: 251–5.
60. Buche M, Schoevardts JC, Chalant CH. Multiple vessel coronary revascularization using both *in situ* mammary arteries and a free inferior epigastric artery. *J Thorac Cardiovasc Surg* 1990; **4**: 754–5.
61. Naunheim K, Barner H, Fiore A: Update. Results of internal thoracic artery grafting over 15 years: single versus double grafts. *Ann Thorac Surg* 1992; **53**: 716–8.
62. Green GE, Cameron AC, Goyal A, WongC–S, Schwanede J. Five year followup of microsurgical multiple internal thoracic artery grafts. *Ann Thorac Surg* 1994; **58**: 74–79.

2 Surgical anatomy and histological characteristics

Jacques A.M. Van Son and Frank M.M. Smedts

The primary consideration that has led to the use of the internal thoracic artery (ITA) as the conduit of choice for coronary artery bypass surgery is its relative freedom from atherosclerosis and superior clinical performance compared to saphenous vein in the long term.[1–3] To extend the role of arterial conduits further, selected use of multiple ITA grafts, the right gastroepiploic (GEA) and the inferior epigastric artery (IEA) has been advocated in young patients or when more conventional conduits are unsuitable or unavailable.[4–11] The radial artery which had been used in the past and abandoned because of its high failure rate[12–14] is currently being re-evaluated.[15]

During the last 5 years we have investigated the histological properties of the ITA, the GEA, IEA and radial arteries. This chapter summarizes our findings.

Internal thoracic artery

Surgical anatomy

The ITA originates from the first part of the subclavian artery, on its concavity, opposite to the thyrocervical trunk (Fig. 2.1). It follows a parasternal course, bilaterally, lying on the posterior aspect of the costal cartilages approximately 1–2 cm from the lateral border of the sternum. Each ITA is accompanied by a pair of veins that unite to form a single vessel, which ascends medial to the artery and drains into the corresponding brachiocephalic vein. This vascular bundle is covered by the parietal pleura. Between the artery and the pleura is a deep fascial plane as far as the third costal cartilage. Inferior to this, the transversus thoracis muscle is interposed between the vessels and the pleura.

With one exception, there is no major difference between right and left ITA. On the left, proximally, the artery runs very close to the chest wall, whereas on the right there can be up to 1 cm of connective tissue between the proximal ITA and the costal

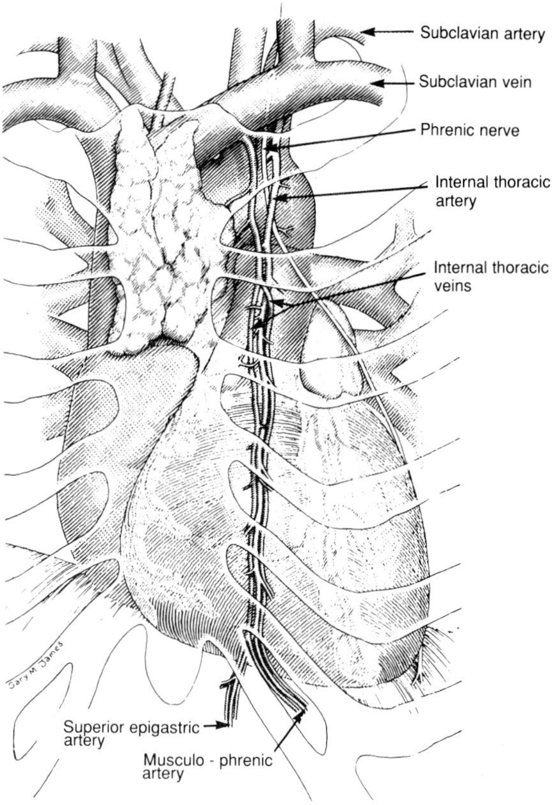

Fig. 2.1 Anatomical relations of the ITA.

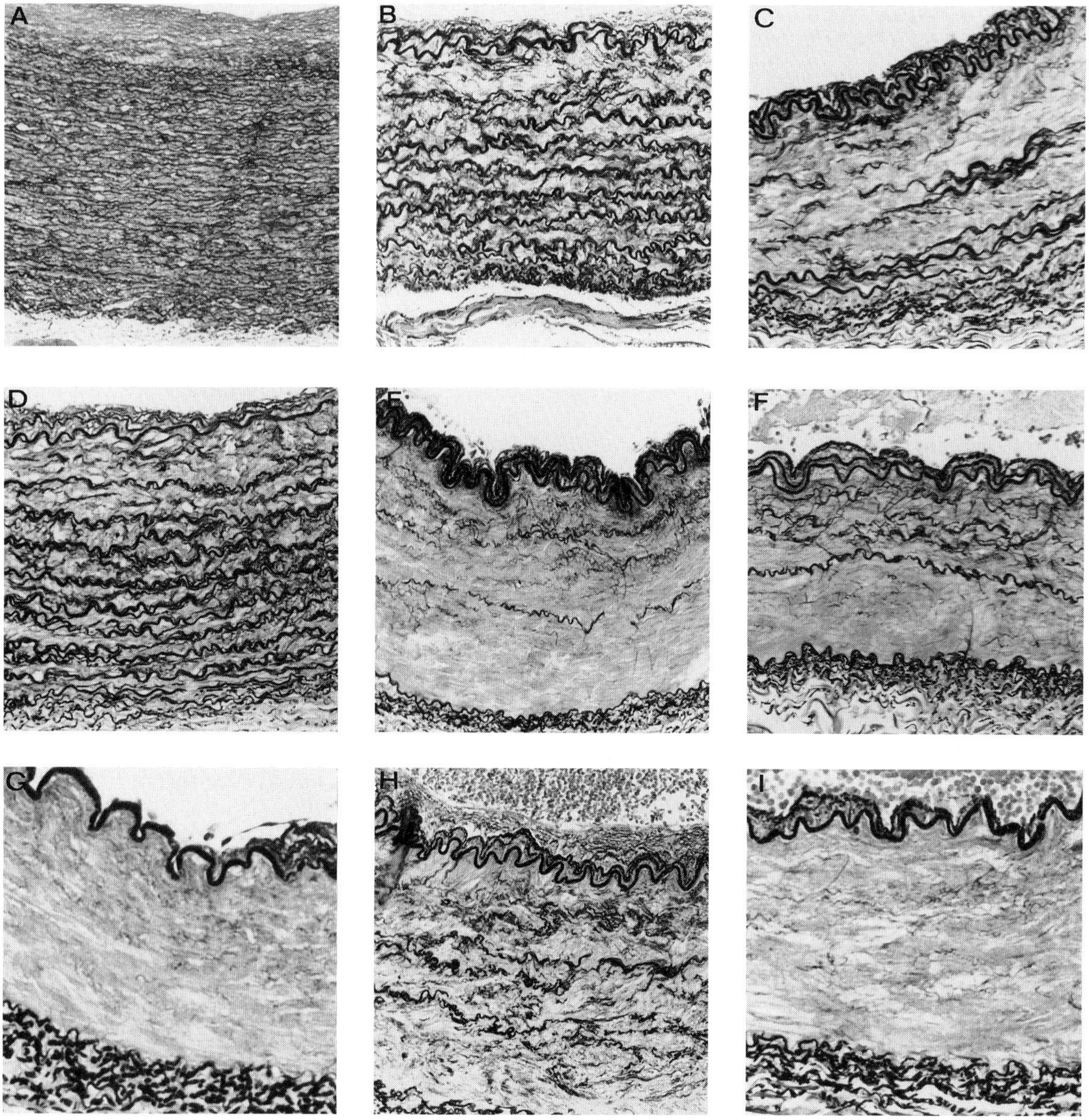

Fig. 2.2 Documentation of the varying histological pattern of the ITA along its downstream course in a 56-year-old man: (a) subclavian artery in direct proximity to the origin of the ITA, its media containing 30–40 elastic lamellae; (b) the origin of the ITA with a mean number of ten elastic lamellae in its media; (c) proximal segment of the ITA with an elastomuscular media, containing a mean number of five elastic lamellae; (d) mid segment of the ITA with an almost purely elastic media containing a mean number of nine elastic lamellae; (e) distal segment of the ITA with a predominantly muscular media and a limited number of elastic lamellae; (f) proximal 1 cm of musculophrenic artery with rare elastic lamellae in a predominantly muscular media; (g) distal musculophrenic artery with a muscular media containing rare elastic fibers; (h) proximal 1 cm of superior epigastric artery with few incomplete elastic lamellae in a predominantly muscular media; (i) distal superior epigastric artery with a muscular medial containing rare elastic fibres. Elastin-trichrome after Masson stain; (a) × 80, (b)–(h) × 140. Reproduced with permission from Van Son *et al.*[16]

cartilages. This may be the result of the difference in the anatomy of the subclavian arteries, the left originating from the aorta and the right from the innominate artery.

The ITA may give origin to a number of branches to mediastinal structures: a medial thymic branch is most common. The pericardiacphrenic artery arises from the posterior surface and accompanies the phrenic nerve. Two anterior intercostal arteries originate in each of the upper five intercostal spaces and perforating branches accompany the branches of the intercostal nerves. In the sixth intercostal space, the ITA divides into two terminal branches, the superior epigastric and musculophrenic arteries. The craniocaudal branch, the superior epigastric artery, enters the sheath of the rectus abdominis muscle through the interval between the costal and sternal attachments of the diaphragm. At first the superior epigastric artery lies posterior to the rectus muscle, but then perforates and supplies the muscle, its terminal branches anastomosing with the terminal branches of the IEA which originates from the external iliac artery. The musculophrenic artery is directed obliquely downward and laterally, posterior to the cartilages of the eighth, ninth, and tenth ribs. It perforates the diaphragm near the eighth or ninth costal cartilage, and ends, considerably reduced in size, opposite the last intercostal space. It gives off anterior intercostal branches to the seventh, eighth and ninth intercostal spaces. Some other branches of the musculophrenic artery course to the lower part of the pericardium, dorsally to the diaphragm, and down to the abdominal muscles.

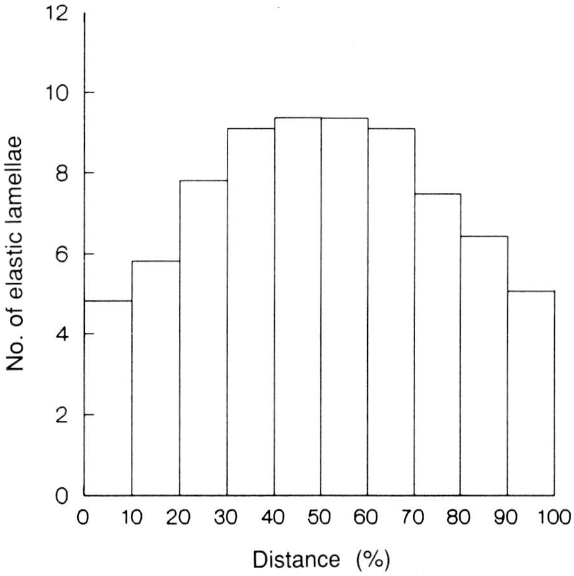

Fig. 2.3 Distribution of the mean number of elastic lamellae in the media of the ITA along its downstream course.

Histological characteristics

The ITA was harvested in eleven individuals and examined histologically at 1 cm intervals.[16] At its origin from the subclavian artery (Fig. 2.2a) the media of the ITA was invariably elastic, containing eight to eighteen (mean, ten) elastic lamellae (Fig. 2.2b). In two of the eleven individuals studied, the media of the entire ITA was elastic. In the remaining nine an alternating histological pattern was observed: the first 20–30 per cent of the artery was elastomuscular (Fig. 2.2c) and the smooth muscle content was greater with only five to seven (mean six) elastic lamellae (Fig. 2.3). More distally there was a rather abrupt transition into an elastic pattern which continued for 70–80 per cent of the total length of the artery (Figs 2.2d and 2.3). Beyond this point, in all nine individuals, a second elastomuscular segment analogous to the proximal one was observed. In five of these the elastomuscular segment extended up to the terminal bifurcation whereas in the remaining four it abruptly converted into a muscular pattern with infrequent elastic lamellae (Fig. 2.2e).

In seven individuals the elastomuscular pattern in the distal part of the artery continued in the proximal 1–2 cm of the musculophrenic artery (Fig. 2.2f); more distally the media became muscular (Fig. 2.2g). In the remaining four individuals with a muscular pattern in the distal part of the ITA, the latter continued into the musculophrenic artery. In all eleven individuals the media of the superior epigastric artery was predominantly muscular (Figs 2.2h and 2.2i).

The absence of elastic lamellae in the media had a profound effect on the degree of intimal hyperplasia: the intima was significantly thicker in the purely muscular segment (25.6 per cent) compared to the elastic (16.7 per cent), elastomuscular (15.3 per cent), and muscular (17.5 per cent) segments. ($P < 0.01$). Although the degree of intimal hyperplasia was slightly greater in the proximal and distal elastomuscular segments than in the elastic segments, these differences were not significant. These data are in agreement with the fact that the number of discontinuities in the circumferential internal elastic lamina increases from the elastic (median, 21; interquartile range, 7) to the elastomuscular (median, 41; interquartile range, 11) and muscular (median, 89; interquartile range, 12) segments.[17] In a further morphometric study of the ITA and other arterial conduits the combined intimal/medial thickness in the flaccid state was 350 ± 92 μm (Table 2.1).[18] All the *vasa vasorum* were confined to the adventitia.

The mean cross-sectional luminal area of the proximal elastomuscular and elastic segments of the ITA (both 1.9 mm^2) was significantly greater than that of the distal elastomuscular segment of the ITA (1.2 mm^2) and that of the muscular segments of the musculophrenic artery (0.9 mm^2) and superior epigastric artery (0.7 mm^2).

Table 2.1 Combined width of intima and media in various arterial conduits and left anterior descending coronary artery[a]

	Width of intima and media (μm)	
Arteries (n = 17)	*Fixation in flaccid state*	*Fixation at 100 mmHg pressure*
LAD	320 ± 63	
ITA	350 ± 92	313 ± 209
GEA	291 ± 109	303 ± 100
IEA	249 ± 87	284 ± 136
RA	529 ± 52	

LAD, left anterior descending coronary artery; ITA, internal thoracic artery; GEA, right gastroepiploic artery; IEA, inferior epigastric artery; RA, radial artery. Data are shown as the mean ± standard deviation.

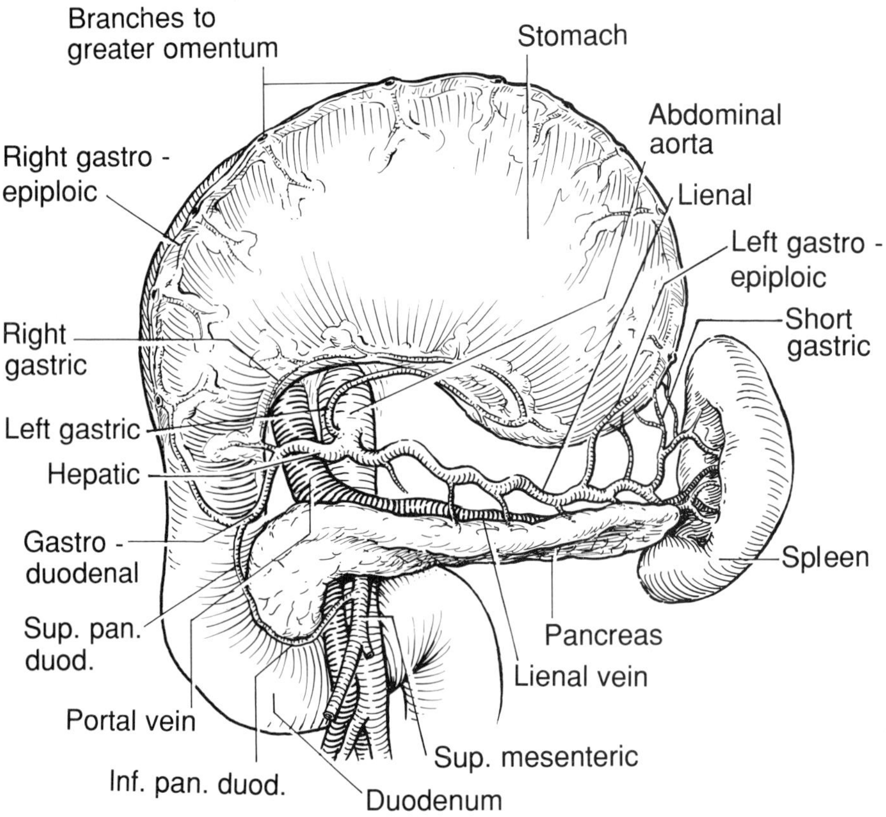

Fig. 2.4 Anatomical relations of the right GEA.

Right gastroepiploic artery

Surgical anatomy

The right GEA is the larger of the two terminal branches of the gastroduodenal artery, the other being the superior pancreaticoduodenal artery (Fig. 2.4). The GEA follows a course from right to left along the greater curvature of the stomach at a somewhat variable distance. It lies between the two layers of the gastrocolic ligament or the ventral two layers of the greater omentum when these are not adherent to the colon. It gives off a large ascending pyloric branch near its origin and terminally it anastomoses with the left gastroepiploic branch of the splenic artery. It supplies a number of ascending gastric branches to the stomach and descending branches to the greater omentum.

Histological characteristics

The GEA was harvested in eleven individuals; the media consisted primarily of smooth muscle cells, with rare elastic fibres. (Fig. 2.5).[19] The width of intima and media in the proximal, mid, and distal segments of the artery is listed in Table 2.2. The mean number of discontinuities in the circumferential internal elastic lamina of the GEA (42 ± 27) was similar to that observed in the elastomuscular segments of the ITA.

In another histological study the mean combined width of the intima and media in the flaccid GEA was 291 ± 109 μm (Table 2.1).[18] The *vasa vasorum* were confined to the adventitia.

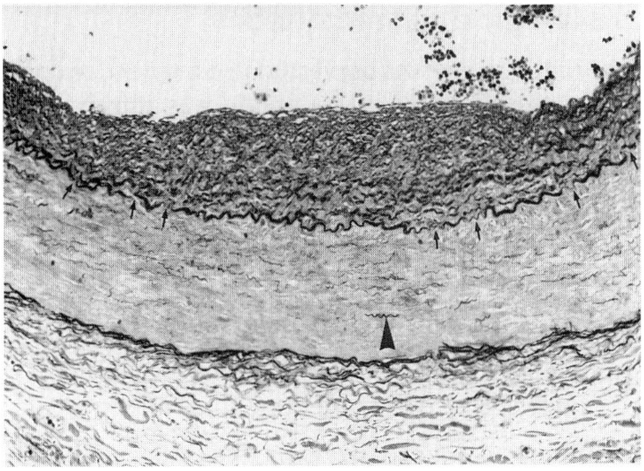

Fig. 2.5 Proximal right GEA. Note the muscular media with rare elastic fibers (arrowhead) and the discontinuities in the internal elastic lamina (arrows). Elastin-trichrome after Masson stain, × 140.

Table 2.2 Combined width of intima and media of the right gastroepiploic artery at its proximal, mid, and distal segments

	Width (μm)[a]			
Layer	*Proximal*	*Mid*	*Distal*	*P Value*[b]
Intima	58.9 ± 41	37.3 ± 22	40.8 ± 33	NS
Media	245.9 ± 107	253.7 ± 103	187.1 ± 38	NS

[a] Data are shown as the mean ± standard deviation.
[b] Student's t test.
NS = not significant.

Inferior epigastric artery

Surgical anatomy

The IEA arises from the medial aspect of the external iliac artery just proximal to the inguinal ligament (Fig. 2.6). At first it lies in the extraperitoneal tissue at the medial side of the deep inguinal ring, in close

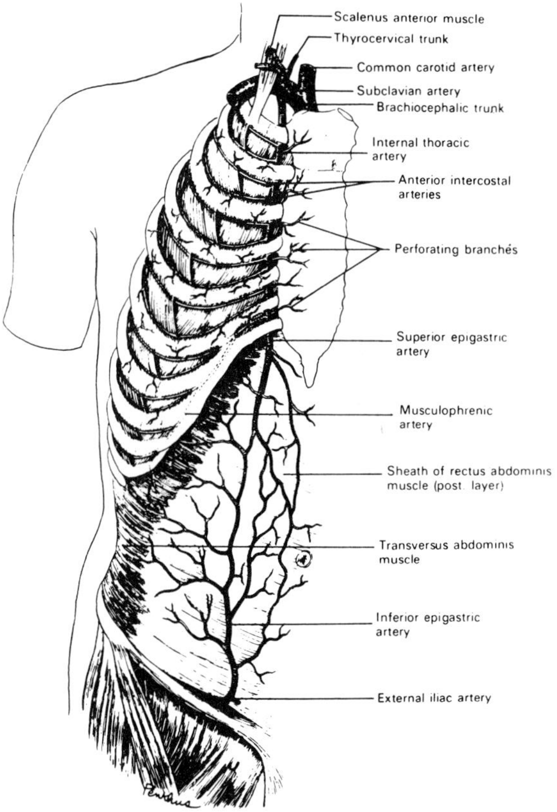

Fig. 2.6 Anatomical relations of the right IEA.

posterior relation to the inguinal canal. The ductus deferens, as it enters the abdomen, hooks around the lateral side of the artery. Accompanied in its course by its two satellite veins, the IEA ascends obliquely and medially towards the umbilicus; after piercing the transversalis fascia, it enters the rectus sheath at the linea semilunaris (semilunar fold of Douglas). It then follows a cephalad vertical course. Direct arterial communications between the superior and inferior epigastric arteries may exist in the region of the umbilicus in approximately 40 per cent of cases.[20]

Histological characteristics

The IEA was harvested in eleven individuals (mean age 64 years). The media was purely muscular, with rare elastic lamellae in the proximal part of the artery up to 2–3 cm from its origin (Fig 2.7).[18] A mild to moderate degree of intimal hyperplasia was observed. The mean number of discontinuities in the circumferential internal elastic lamina of the IEA (39 ± 17) was similar to that observed in elastomuscular segments of the ITA.

The mean width of the intima and media of the IEA was 249 ± 87 μm (Table 2.1). In all instances, the *vasa vasorum* were confined to the adventitia.

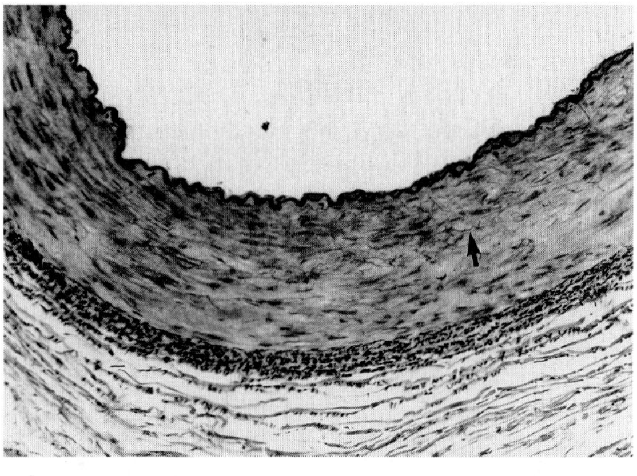

Fig. 2.7 Proximal IEA. Note the muscular media with rare elastic fibers (arrow). Elastin-trichrome after Masson stain, × 140.

Radial artery

Surgical anatomy

Opposite the neck of the radius, approximately 1 cm below the elbow joint, the brachial artery terminates as the radial and ulnar arteries (see Fig. 17.2). The radial artery is smaller in calibre than the ulnar artery. The radial artery passes along the radial aspect of the forearm to the wrist. The proximal part of the artery is covered by the belly of the brachioradialis muscle. The rest of the artery is superficial, being covered only by skin and the superficial and deep fasciae and lying directly on the radius in the more distal part of its course. The radial artery has numerous collateral branches, particularly in its distal segment. The artery passes around the lateral aspect of the wrist joint, to the dorsum of the hand where it passes between the first and second metacarpals to continue as the deep palmar arch.

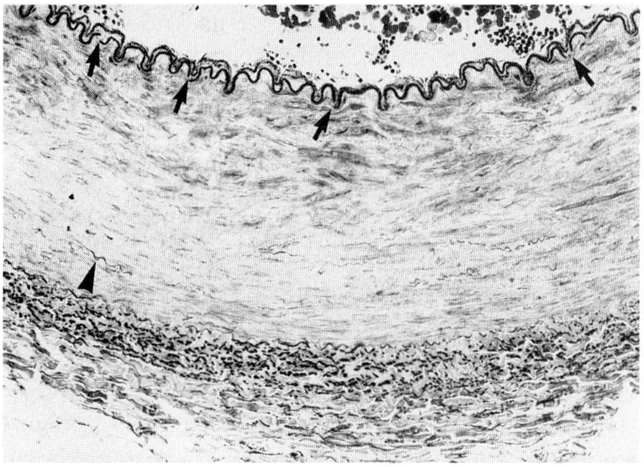

Fig. 2.8 Proximal radial artery. Note the relatively thick muscular media with rare elastic fibers (arrowhead) and the discontinuities in the internal elastic lamina (arrows). Elastin-trichrome after Masson stain, × 140.

Histological characteristics

The radial artery was harvested in eleven individuals (mean age 64 years). The media was purely muscular (Figure 2.8)[18] and a mild to moderate degree of intimal hyperplasia was observed. The mean number of discontinuities in the circumferential internal elastic lamina of the radial artery (45 ± 28) was similar to that found in the elastomuscular segments of the ITA. The mean width of the intima and media of the flaccid radial artery was 529 ± 52 μm (Table 2.1). The *vasa vasorum* were confined to the adventitia and the outer one third of the media.

Comment

Although the cause of the apparent protection of the ITA from intimal thickening and atherosclerosis remains obscure, a few inferences can be drawn on the basis of our studies and accumulated evidence from research in vascular pathology.

Histological research has established that the first stage of intimal thickening is caused by invasion of smooth muscle cells from the media through the fenestrated internal elastic lamina.[21] In the first decade of life this intimal thickening can already be observed. Sims[22,23] has suggested that the occurrence of discontinuities in the internal elastic lamina provokes early and progressive intimal hyperplasia. Stimuli that trigger proliferation may include the influence of blood constituents and haemodynamic forces on smooth muscle cells.[24]

It is therefore possible that elastic arteries may be less prone to intimal hyperplasia than muscular arteries. In the former, intimal hyperplasia develops at a considerably delayed rate because of the fewer smooth muscle cells present in the media. In addition, the multiple elastic lamellae and the internal elastic lamina form barriers to their invasion. Moreover, elastin, the basic component of the elastic tissue of the media, is a bradytrophic, relatively inert tissue with a low metabolic rate. The media of the elastic artery therefore has a lower intrinsic demand for oxygen and substrates than the media of the muscular artery.

In our histological studies a correlation has been shown between the absence of elastic lamellae in the media and an increased number of discontinuities in the internal elastic lamina and, as a potential result of this, increased intimal thickening.[16,18] The intima was significantly thicker in the purely muscular segments of the musculophrenic and superior epigastric arteries compared to the ITA. Similar findings were reported by Sims and Gavin[25] in a comparative histological study between the muscular coronary artery and the primarily elastic ITA, in which the number of discontinuities in the internal elastic lamina and the degree of intimal thickening were significantly greater in the former vessel. Based on these observations it was concluded that elastic lamellae in the media may protect against the occurrence of discontinuities in the internal elastic lamina and against intimal thickening, even if the number of lamellae is small. The study by Sims and Gavin[25] also suggests that gaps in the internal elastic lamina allow smooth muscle cells of the media to migrate into the intima and proliferate. The rate of this growth reflects the response of medial smooth muscle cells to wall tension. Other studies[26,27] confirm the structural importance of the internal elastic lamina and its relationship to intimal thickening. Research in vascular pathology has shown that medial smooth muscle cells are mesenchymal cells capable of changing from a contractile to a synthetic phenotype in response to damage to the internal elastic lamina and increasing tangential tension on the vessel wall.[28] This process leads to active cell division and synthesis of collagen, elastin, and proteoglycan matrix.[29,30] After penetration from the media into the intima, the proliferating smooth muscle cells produce elastin, often as a coherent reduplicated internal elastic lamina, which can be seen as single or multiple thin sealing layers on the luminal aspect of the defective internal elastic lamina. This phenomenon was frequently observed in our specimens, especially in arteries with a purely muscular media. Almost invariably such repair is imperfect, and with the passage of time, breakdown of the reduplicated internal elastic lamina occurs, leading to serious impairment of attachment of enthothelial cells, cell loss and the development of bare areas. Such bare areas may enhance the infiltration of macromolecules of all sizes, including lipoproteins and cells of the circulating blood, thus accelerating the development of atherosclerotic lesions.[31,32]

Due to the effect of shear stress on the proliferation of smooth muscle cells from the media into the intima, the rate of intimal thickening may be enhanced in the central aorta and its branches in comparison with the ITA, in which the haemodynamics are less vigorous.[33,34] Such a proliferative smooth muscle cell response has been observed in systemic and pulmonary hypertension and in the culture of medial cells from hypertensive animals and from experimental atherosclerosis.[35–38] A considerably greater degree of intimal thickening was observed in the subclavian artery and the first centimetre of the ITA than in the remainder of it.

The findings as presented in these studies may have implications for the selection of the anastomotic site in the ITA. A considerable interindividual variability in the extent of a primarily elastic media in the ITA was observed. In seven patients the distal segment of the ITA was either elastic or elastomuscular, whereas in four it was muscular with rare elastic lamellae. These observations suggest that it may be beneficial not to use the distal part of the ITA. This strategy has the additional advantage that the cross-sectional luminal diameter of the artery may better match the diameter of the coronary artery to be grafted better. Selection of the anastomotic site in the musculophrenic or superior epigastric arteries is not encouraged because of the potentially increased risk of intimal thickening and the significantly smaller luminal diameter of these vessels and the greater tendency to vasospasm.

To maximize the benefits of the elastic and elastomuscular ITA the shortest possible route to the heart should be established.[39–42] For the same reason bilateral and sequential grafting may be advantageous.[43–45] To gain additional length, when required, a number of techniques have been described.[46] However, we do not favour complete or partial skeletonization of the ITA, as advocated by some investigators[43,44,47] in the belief that this technique carries an increased risk of iatrogenic distruption of the internal elastic lamina. This may be especially deleterious in segments with a high muscular content because it may provoke enhanced intimal thickening.[48] Any discrepancy in early patency rate between *in situ* and free ITA grafts has been attributed primarily to technical problems associated with the proximal aortic anastomosis.[49] After the early phase, late patency rates of free ITA grafts approximate those of *in situ* grafts, consistent with the hypothesis that the intima and media of the non-diseased ITA are nourished entirely from the lumen.

The number of discontinuities in the internal elastic lamina in the muscular GEA is greater than that in the elastic segment of the ITA.[19] This probably reflects the absence of elastic lamellae in the media capable of exerting a protective effect against the development of discontinuities in the internal elastic lamina. Therefore, we believe that some scepticism towards the long-term patency of the GEA is warranted, especially if this conduit is used as a free graft. The muscular character of the media of the GEA may result in increased vulnerability to intimal thickening and ultimately atherosclerosis once the artery wall is exposed to the forceful shear stress. Thus, although a number of investigators[50,51] have found only a mild to moderate degree of intimal thickening in the GEA, this finding must be interpreted with caution, because it reflects the situation at the time of harvesting of the GEA but not necessarily following grafting. Future clinical studies with regard to the long-term patency rate of the GEA as a coronary artery bypass graft will prove whether our scepticism is justified or not.

The number of discontinuities in the internal elastic lamina of the IEA is similar to that of the GEA and elastomuscular segments of the ITA. Based on the lower elastic content of the media of the IEA as compared to the ITA, we hypothesize that the former may have an increased tendency toward intimal thickening. Although early patency rates of the IEA ranging from 88 to 97 per cent have been reported[10,11] based on our observations, we predict less satisfactory long-term patency rates of this arterial conduit.

Reports from the 1970s unanimously condemned the use of the radial artery as a conduit for myocardial revascularization on the basis of an alarmingly high early occlusion rate.[12–14] It may be true that the observed discrepancy in early patency between the previous and current experience[15] may partially have been caused by accelerated intimal hyperplasia as a result of dilatation of the vessel with graduated probes and by stripping the vessel of the surrounding tissue. Such focal damage, which is more likely to occur in thick muscular conduits such as the radial artery than in elastic segments of the ITA, may trigger a cascade of events and may ultimately enhance progressive intimal thickening.[17]

In our studies we measured a mean width in the media of the radial artery of approximately 500 μm, as opposed to 330 μm for the ITA, 280 μm for the GEA and 240 μm for the IEA. In addition, nutrition of the thick media of the radial artery is mainly, but not only, through diffusion from the lumen, as we did observe penetration of *vasa vasorum* into the outer media. Although the thick media of the radial artery may be advantageous with regard to ease of performance of the proximal anastomosis, it also may predispose the conduit to a greater degree of ischaemia and potentially fibrosis in the outer layer of the media. Because the GEA and IEA have a considerably thinner media, a less critical relationship exists between metabolic demand and supply of the media, and therefore the potential for ischaemia in these vessels may be less. In addition, we have found a considerable number of discontinuities in the internal elastic lamina of the radial artery harvested in its natural environment, with mild to moderate intimal hyperplasia. Based on these findings we speculate that the potential for intimal hyperplasia may be considerably more pronounced in the radial artery than in the ITA.

Future perspectives

In a recent study the potential suitability of the intercostal artery as a conduit in myocardial revascularization was assessed.[52] Three combinations of histological pattern were observed along the course of the fourth to ninth intercostal arteries (n = 11): a proximal elastic segment followed by subsequent elastomuscular and muscular segments (n = 3), a proximal elastomuscular segment with the remainder of the artery being muscular (n = 6), and a completely muscular pattern (n = 2). The mean luminal diameter of the fifth intercostal artery varied from 1.4 ± 0.3 mm at the origin to 0.9 ± 0.2 mm at 30 cm. The mean intimal thickness at these locations was 54 ± 38 μm and 25 ± 16 μ, respectively, and the mean medial thickness was 205 ± 38 μm and 70 ± 45 μm, respectively. These histological findings, mean luminal diameter and mean diameter of the intima and media were similar in all the intercostal arteries other than the fifth.

A recent anatomical study concluded that it is feasible to use the intercostal artery as an *in situ* graft in myocardial revascularization.[53]

In summary, the intercostal artery may potentially be suitable as a coronary artery bypass graft (both *in situ* and as a free graft) based on its favourable properties in terms of thickness of intima and media, the latter being elastic or elastomuscular in the proximal segment in the majority of the investigated arteries.

References

1. Lytle BW, Loop FD, Cosgrove DM, Ratliff NB, Easley K, Taylor PC. Long-term (5 to 12 years) serial studies of internal mammary artery and saphenous vein coronary bypass grafts. *J Thorac Cardiovas Surg* 1985; **89:** 248–58.
2. Loop FD, Lytle BW, Cosgrove DM *et al.* Influence of the internal mammary artery graft on 10-year survival and other cardiac events. *New Engl J Med* 1986; **314:** 1–6.
3. Grondin CM, Campeau L, Lesperance J, Enjalbert M, Bourassa MG. Comparison of late changes in internal mammary artery and saphenous vein grafts in two consecutive series of patients 10 years after operation. *Circulation* 1984; **70 (Suppl 1):** 207–12.
4. Dion R, Verhelst R, Rousseau M *et al.* Sequential mammary grafting. *J Thorac Cardiovasc Surg* 1989; **98:** 80–9.
5. Pym J, Brown PM, Charrette EJP, Parker JO, West RO. Gastroepiploic–coronary anastomosis: a viable alternative bypass graft. *J Thorac Cardiovasc Surg* 1987; **94:** 256–9.
6. Suma H, Fukumoto H, Takeuchi A. Coronary artery bypass grafting by utilizing *in situ* right gastroepiploic artery: basic study and clinical application. *Ann Thorac Surg* 1987; **44:** 394–7.
7. Mills NL, Everson CT. Right gastroepiploic artery: a third arterial conduit for coronary artery bypass. *Ann Thorac Surg* 1989; **47:** 706–11.
8. Lytle BW, Cosgrove DM, Ratliff NB, Loop FD. Coronary artery bypass grafting with the right gastroepiploic artery. *J Thorac Cardiovasc Surg* 1989; **97:** 826–31.
9. Vincent JG, van Son JAM, Skotnicki SH. Inferior epigastric artery as a conduit in myocardial revascularization: the alternative free arterial graft. *Ann Thorac Surg* 1990; **49:** 323–5.
10. Barner HB, Naunheim KS, Fiore AC, Fischer VW, Harris HH. Use of the inferior epigastric artery as a free graft for myocardial revascularization. *Ann Thorac Surg* 1991; **52:** 429–37.
11. Buche M, Schoevaerdts JC, Louagie Y *et al.* Use of the inferior epigastric artery for coronary bypass. *J Thorac Cardiovasc Surg* 1992; **103:** 665–70.
12. Curtis JJ, Stoney WS, Alford WC Jr, Burrus GR, Thomas CS Jr. Intimal hyperplasia. A cause of radial artery aortocoronary bypass graft failure. *Ann Thorac Surg* 1975; **20:** 628–35.
13. Carpentier A. Discussion of: Geha AS, Krone RJ, McCormick JR, Baue AE. Selection of coronary bypass: anatomic, physiological, and angiographic considerations of vein and mammary artery grafts. *J Thorac Cardiovasc Surg* 1975; **70:** 429–31.
14. Chiu R. Why do radial artery grafts for aortocoronary bypass fail? A reappraisal. *Ann Thorac Surg* 1976; **22:** 520–3.
15. Acar C, Jebara VA, Portoghese M *et al.* Revival of the radial artery for coronary artery bypass grafting. *Ann Thorac Surg* 1992; **54:** 652–60.
16. Van Son JAM, Smedts F, de Wilde PCM *et al.* Histological study of the internal mammary artery with emphasis on its suitability as a coronary artery bypass graft. *Ann Thorac Surg* 1993; **55:** 106–13.
17. Van Son JAM, Tavilla G, Noyez L. Detrimental sequelae on the wall of the internal mammary artery by hydrostatic dilation with diluted papaverine solution. *J Thorac Cardiovasc Surg* 1992; **104:** 972–76.
18. Van Son JAM, Smedts F, Vincent JG, van Lier HJJ, Kubat K. Comparative anatomic studies of various arterial conduits for myocardial revascularization. *J Thorac Cardiovasc Surg* 1990; **99:** 703–707.
19. Tavilla G, van Son JAM, Verhagen AF, Smedts F. Retrogastric versus antegastric routing and histology of the right gastroepiploic artery. *Ann Thorac Surg* 1992; **53:** 1057–61.
20. Millroy FJ, Anson BJ, McAfee DK. The rectus abdominis muscle and the epigastric arteries. *Surg Gynecol Obstet* 1960; **110:** 293–302.
21. Ross R, Glomset JA. The pathogenesis of atherosclerosis. *New Engl J Med* 1976; **295:** 369–76, 420–5.
22. Sims FH. A comparison of coronary and internal mammary arteries and implications of the results in the etiology of atherosclerosis. *Am Heart J* 1983; **105:** 560–6.
23. Sims FH. Discontinuities in the internal elastic lamina: a comparison of coronary and internal mammary arteries. *Artery* 1985; **13:** 237–43.

24. Chamley-Campbell J, Campbell GR, Ross R. The smooth muscle cell in culture. *Physiol Rev* 1979; **59:** 1–61.
25. Sims FH, Gavin JB. The early development of intimal thickening of human coronary arteries. *Coronary Artery Dis* 1990; **1:** 205–13.
26. Sims FH. The internal elastic lamina in normal and abnormal human arteries. A barrier to the diffusion of macromolecules from the lumen. *Artery* 1989; **16:** 159–73.
27. Sims FH. A comparison of structural features of the walls of coronary arteries from 10 different species. *Pathology* 1989; **21:** 115–24.
28. Campbell GR, Campbell JH, Manderson JA, Horrigan S, Rennick RE. Arterial smooth muscle. A multifunctional mesenchymal cell. *Archs Pathol Lab Med* 1988 ;**112:** 977–86.
29. Ross R. The pathogenesis of atherosclerosis: an update. *New Engl J Med* 1986; **314:** 488–500.
30. Schwartz SM, Campbell GR, Campbell JH. Replication of smooth muscle cells in vascular disease. *Circulation Res* 1986; **58:** 427–41.
31. Bocan TMA, Schifani TA, Guyton JR. Ultrastructure of the human aortic fibrolipid lesion. Formation of the atherosclerotic lipid-rich core. *Am J Pathol* 1986; **123:** 413–24.
32. Bylock AL, Gerrity RG. Visualization of monocyte recruitment into atherosclerotic arteries using fluorescent labelling. *Atherosclerosis* 1988; **71:** 17–25.
33. Sottiurai VS, Kollros P, Glagov S, Zarins CK, Mathews MB. Morphologic alteration of cultured arterial smooth muscle cells by cyclic stretching. *J Surg Res* 1983; **35:** 490–7.
34. Dartsch PC, Hammerle H, Betz E. Orientation of cultured arterial smooth muscle cells growing on cyclically stretched substrates. *Acta Anat* 1986; **125:** 108–13.
35. Folkow B. Structure and function of the arteries in hypertension. *Am Heart J* 1987; **114:** 938–48.
36. Schwartz SM, Reidy MA. Common mechanisms of proliferation of smooth muscle cells in atherosclerosis and hypertension. *Hum Path* 1987; **18:** 240–7.
37. Esterly JA, Glagov S, Ferguson DJ. Morphogenesis of intimal obliterative hyperplasia of small arteries in experimental pulmonary hypertension. *Am J Path* 1968; **52:** 325–7.
38. Schmidt A, Grunwald J, Buddicke E. ^{35}S-Proteoglycan metabolism of arterial smooth muscle cells cultured from normotensive and hypertensive rates. *Atherosclerosis* 1982; **45:** 299–310.
39. Pacifico AD, Sears NJ, Burgos C. Harvesting, routing, and anastomosing the left internal mammary artery graft. *Ann Thorac Surg.* 1986; **42:** 708–10.
40. Jones EL, Lattouf O, Lutz JF, King SB III. Important anatomical and physiological considerations in performance of complex mammary – coronary artery operations. *Ann Thorac Surg* 1987; **43:** 469–77.
41. Vander Salm TJ, Chowdhary S, Okike ON, Pezzella AT, Pasque MK. Internal mammary artery grafts: the shortest route to the coronary arteries. *Ann Thorac Surg* 1989; **47:** 421–7.
42. Buxton B, Knight S. Retrophrenic location of the internal mammary artery graft. *Ann Thorac Surg* 1990; **49:** 1011–2.
43. Sauvage LR, Wu H, Kowalsky TE *et al.* Healing basis and surgical techniques for complete revascularization of the left ventricle using only the internal mammary arteries. *Ann Thorac Surg* 1986; **42:** 449–65.
44. Galbut DL, Traad EA, Dorman MJ *et al.* Seventeen-year experience with bilateral internal mammary artery grafts. *Ann Thorac Surg* 1990; **49:** 195–201.
45. Fiore AC, Naunheim KS, Dean P *et al.* Results of internal thoracic artery grafting over 15 years: single versus double grafts. *Ann Thorac Surg* 1990; **49:** 202–9.
46. Cosgrove DM, Loop FD. Techniques to maximize mammary artery length. *Ann Thorac Surg* 1985; **40:** 78–9.
47. Keeley SB. The skeletonized internal mammary artery. *Ann Thorac Surg* 1987; **44:** 324–5.
48. Daly RC, McCarthy PM, Orszulak TA, Schaff HV, Edwards WD. Histologic comparison of experimental coronary artery bypass grafts: similarity of in situ and free internal mammary artery grafts. *J Thorac Cardiovasc Surg* 1988; **96:** 19–29.
49. Loop FD, Lytle BW, Cosgrove DM, Golding LAR, Taylor PC, Stewart RW. Free (aorto-coronary) internal mammary artery graft: late results. *J Thorac Cardiovasc Surg* 1986; **92:** 827–31.
50. Suma H, Takanashi R. Arteriosclerosis of the gastroepiploic and internal thoracic arteries. *Ann Thorac Surg* 1990; **50:** 413–16.
51. Suma H, Wanibuchi Y, Furuta S, Isshiki T, Yamaguchi T, Takanashi R. Comparative study between the gastroepiploic and the internal thoracic artery as a coronary bypass graft. Size, flow, patency, histology. *Eur J Cardiothorac Surg* 1991; **5:** 244–7.
52. Van Son JAM, Smedts F, Korving J, Guyt A, de Kok LB. Intercostal artery: histomorphometric study to asses its suitability as a coronary bypass graft. *Ann Thorac Surg* 1993; **56:** 1078–81.
53. John LCH, Chan CLH, Anderson DR. Potential use of the intercostal artery as an in situ graft: a cadaveric study. *Ann Thorac Surg* 1995; **59:** 190–5.

3 Biological and vasomotor properties of the internal thoracic artery: role of the endothelium

Zhihong Yang and Thomas F. Lüscher

Different blood vessels have differing susceptibility to atherosclerotic change both as native vessels and as bypass grafts. Clinical observation demonstrates that in the same patients atherosclerotic change occurs often in the coronary artery, but rarely in the internal thoracic artery (ITA),[1,2] although both are exposed to the same cardiovascular risk factors. On the other hand, saphenous veins develop intimal thickening presumed to be a precursor of late atherosclerosis, as soon as they are transplanted from the venous into the arterial circulation.[3] This suggests that in addition to the environment the blood vessels are exposed to, biological properties of the blood vessel wall are crucial determinants of their function and patency.

The vascular wall of bypass grafts is composed of a monolayer of endothelial cells lining the inner surface, smooth muscle cells and matrix in the media and fibroblasts in the adventitia. Interactions of these cells as well as interactions with blood components such as platelets and monocytes determine graft function. Of particular importance are the antithrombotic properties of endothelial cells, the ability of blood vessels to adapt to the requirements of the coronary circulation as well as the propensity of the blood vessel wall to develop atherosclerotic changes (Fig. 3.1).

This chapter discusses the biological properties of the ITA focusing on the potential role of the endothelium in controlling vascular reactivity to circulating and local vasoactive hormones. The biological properties of the ITA will also be compared with other bypass grafts.

The vascular endothelium

Following the pioneering discovery by Furchgott and Zawadzki in 1980 that the vascular endothelium produces relaxing factor(s) in rabbit aorta causing vascular relaxation,[4] it has been well established that the endothelium is an important paracrine and autocrine organ regulating vascular tone and platelet–vessel wall interaction by at least three mechanisms (Fig. 3.2):[5]

1. formation of relaxing factors such as nitric oxide (NO) and prostacyclin (PGI_2);
2. production of contracting factors such as endothelin-1 and endoperoxides (prostaglandin H_2 and thromboxane A_2);
3. activation and inactivation of endogenous vasoactive substances such as big-endothelin-1, angiotensin-I and bradykinin.

Endothelium-derived relaxing factors

Vascular endothelial cells express constitutive nitric oxide synthase (cNOS) metabolizing L-arginine into nitric oxide (NO), a potent local regulator of vasomotion and platelet function.[6–8] The activity of endothelial cNOS can be specifically, competitively inhibited by a number of analogues of L-arginine

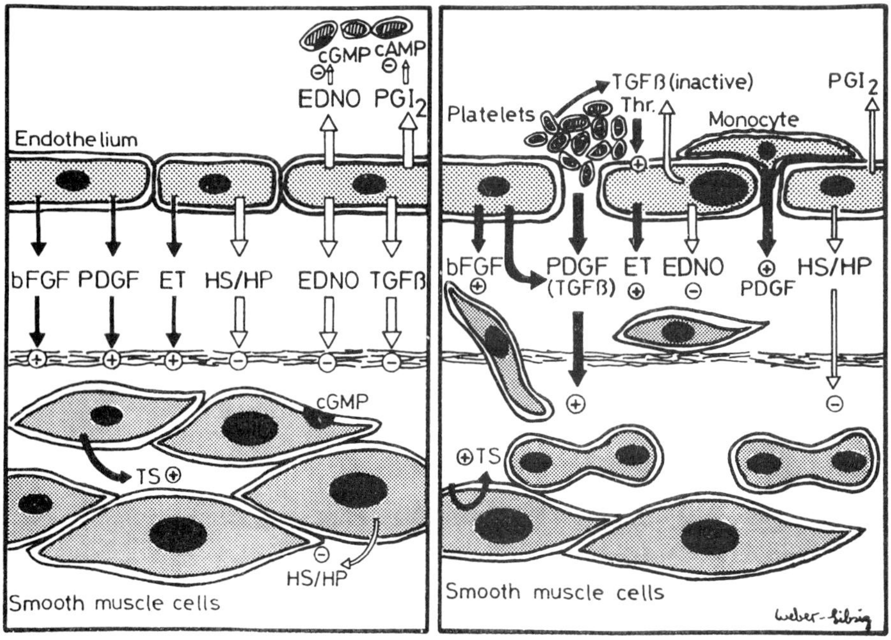

Fig. 3.1 Regulatory role of the endothelium and circulating blood cells on proliferative responses of vascular smooth muscle: The endothelium releases a variety of growth inhibitors such as heparin, heparan sulfates (HP/HS), endothelium-derived nitric oxide (EDNO) and transforming growth factor β1 (TGFβ1) (left panel) which normally keep the blood vessel wall in quiescent state, although these are able to form growth factors such as basic fibroblast growth factor (bFGF), platelet-derived growth factor (PDGF) and endothelin (ET). In diseased blood vessels, platelets and monocytes adhere (right panel) and growth factors become much more dominant leading to vascular smooth muscle proliferation and migration. PGI_2=prostacyclin; Thr=thrombin; TS=thrombospondin.

such as N^G-monomethyl-L-arginine (L-NMMA[8]). Indeed, nitric oxide is both a potent vasodilator and inhibitor of platelet adhesion and aggregation[8,9] by activating soluble guanylyl cyclase and increasing cGMP level in smooth muscle cells[10] and platelets and thereby mediates vascular relaxation and platelet inhibition.

The endothelium of the ITA spontaneously releases significant amounts of NO, which is more pronounced in comparison to saphenous vein.[11] This basal release of NO may play an important role in maintaining vascular patency, since the vasoconstriction induced by norepinephrine and serotonin are significantly reduced by the basal release of NO.[11,12] In addition, production of nitric oxide can be stimulated by a variety of vasoactive substances such as acetylcholine, histamine and thrombin.[11,13] The production of NO is much less pronounced in the saphenous vein (even in preparations without endothelial damage) than in the ITA, while the gastroepiploic artery exhibits similar endothelium-dependent relaxation in response to agonists as does the ITA.[14–16] All bypass vessels relax effectively in response to nitrovasodilators indicating that their vascular smooth muscle is capable of forming cGMP.[14–16]

Shear stress at the endothelial/blood interface also stimulates the formation of nitric oxide and mediates flow-dependent vasodilation for instance during exercise. ITA grafts, but not saphenous vein grafts, dilatate *in vivo* during atrial pacing.[17] Thus, nitric oxide importantly contributes to the ability of arterial bypass vessels to respond to the flow requirements of the myocardium.

Prostacyclin (PGI_2) is another mediator produced from arachidonic acid via the cyclo-oxygenase pathway in endothelial cells.[18] PGI_2 induces vascular relaxation and inhibits platelet activation by increasing cAMP level.[9,18] The endothelium of ITA and gastroepiploic artery (GEA) releases greater

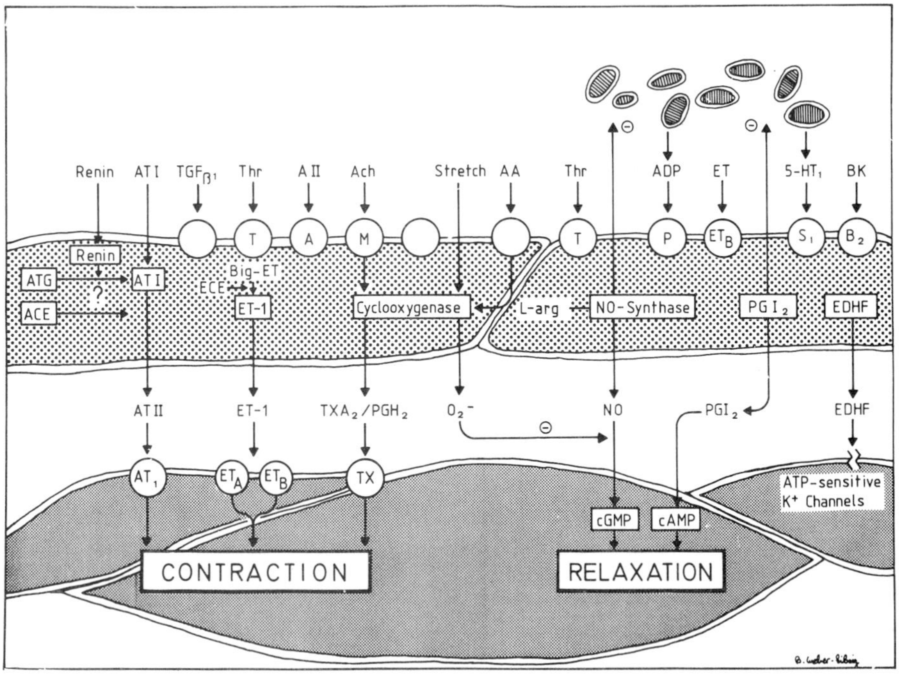

Fig. 3.2 Endothelial cells control vascular tone and platelet function by release of vasoactive substances. AA = arachidonic acid; ADP = adenosine diphosphate; AT = angiotensins; AT1 = angiotensin receptor type 1; ATG = angiotensinogen; ACE = angiotensin converting enzyme; Ach = acetylcholine; B = bradykinin receptor; BK = bradykinin; ECE = endothelin converting enzyme; EDHF = endothelium-derived hyperpolarizing factor; ET = endothelin; $ET_{A/B}$ = endothelin receptor type A/B; 5-HT = 5-hydroxytryptamine (serotonin); L-arg = L-arginine; M = muscarinic receptor; P = purinergic receptor; PGI_2 = prostacyclin; S = serotonergic receptor; T = thrombin receptor; TGFβ1 = transforming growth factor β1; Thr = thrombin; TXA_2/PGH_2 = thromboxane A_2/prostaglandin H_2; TX = thromboxane receptor.

amounts of PGI_2 than saphenous vein endothelial cells.[19–21] Of particular interest is the fact that NO and PGI_2 possess synergistic inhibitory effects on platelet function.[9] Hence, both mediators make important contributions to the antithrombotic properties of the endothelium in the ITA.

Endothelium-derived contracting factors

In addition to relaxing factors, endothelial cells also release contracting factors (Fig. 3.2). No evidence for production of endothelium-derived contracting factors in human ITA has been shown so far. In contrast, the endothelial cells of saphenous vein can release contracting factors such as thromboxane A_2 in response to acetylcholine and prostaglandin H_2 in response to histamine.[11] Both substances are able to cause vascular contraction and platelet activation. In the saphenous vein, the effects of NO are further blunted by the production of contracting factors.[11] Indeed, in patients after coronary artery bypass surgery, selective infusion of acetylcholine evokes vasodilation in ITA grafts, but contractions in saphenous vein grafts.[22]

Endothelin-1 is a 21-amino acid peptide converted from the precursor big-endothelin-1 via a endothelin converting enzyme (ECE-1) in endothelial cells (Fig 3.3).[23,24] This peptide exhibits potent vasoconstrictor effects on vascular smooth muscle, which exceed those of norepinephrine, angiotensin II and serotonin in the ITA.[25] In the ITA, smooth muscle cells express ET-A and ET-B receptors both mediating potent vasoconstriction (Fig. 3.3), which

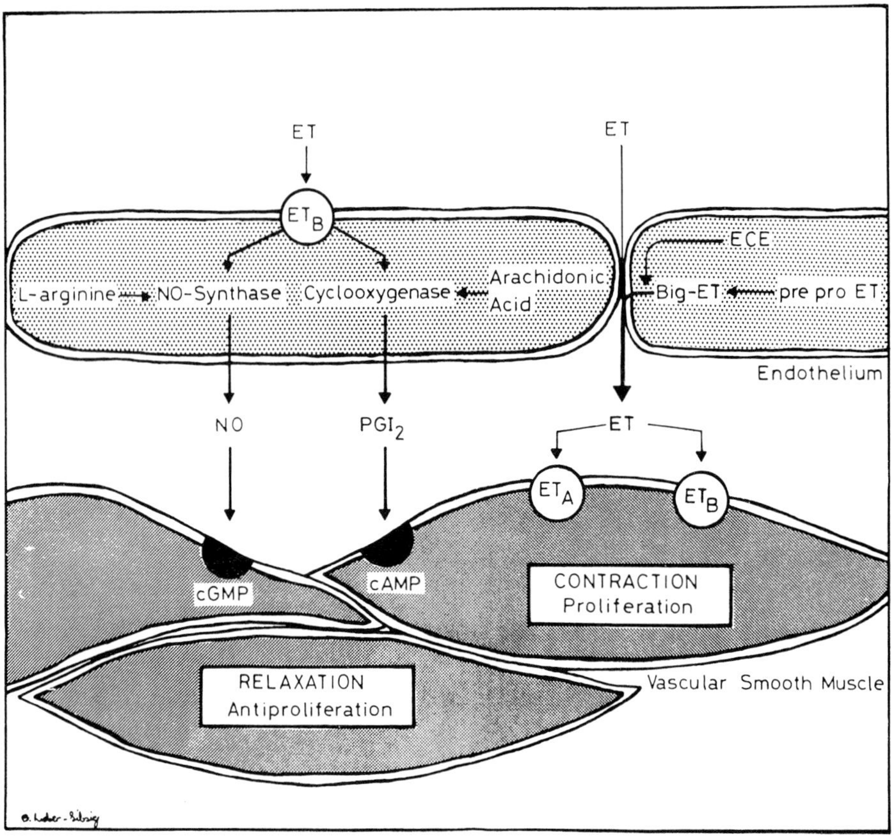

Fig. 3.3 Vascular effects of endothelin (ET) and its receptors: ET_A- and ET_B-receptors are expressed on vascular smooth muscle to mediate contraction and proliferation, while endothelial cells only express ET_B-receptors linked to the formation of nitric oxide (NO) and prostacyclin (PGI_2). These mediators are responsible for the vasodilation occurring under these conditions via increases in cyclic GMP and cyclic AMP, respectively. ECE=endothelin converting enzyme; circles=receptors.

is more pronounced in the internal thoracic veins.[26] It has been demonstrated that vascular endothelium can have ET-B receptor mediating endothelium-dependent relaxations upon stimulation by endothelin-1 via release of NO and/or PGI_2 (Fig. 3.3).[27,28] Indeed, the internal thoracic vein does exhibit a transient relaxation in response to the ET-B receptor agonist sarafotoxin S6c,[26] whereas the endothelium of ITA does not express functional ET-B receptors linked to NO and/or PGI_2 release.[26] These experiments indicate that inhibition of endothelin-1-induced vasoconstriction in patients requires the use of combined ET-A/ET-B receptor antagonists.

In both the ITA and saphenous vein, endothelium-derived nitric oxide or nitrovasodilators, but not Ca^{2+} antagonists effectively inhibit endothelin-1-induced contractions.[25,29] The amount of endothelin formed in coronary bypass vessels remains to be determined, but thrombin, angiotensin II and transforming growth factor beta (TGF-β; released from platelets) may stimulate the production of this potent peptide.[23,30]

In addition, endothelin-1 also possesses indirect vascular effects, namely it potentiates contractions of vascular smooth muscle to other vasoconstrictor agonists at low and threshold concentrations in the ITA.[31] These potentiating effects could be blocked by calcium antagonists and the mechanism involves increased calcium sensitivity of smooth muscle cells.[31] Thus, normally the endothelium protects vascular smooth cells of arterial grafts from vasoconstrictor substances; an increased formation of endothelin-1 (for instance by thrombin or TGF-β

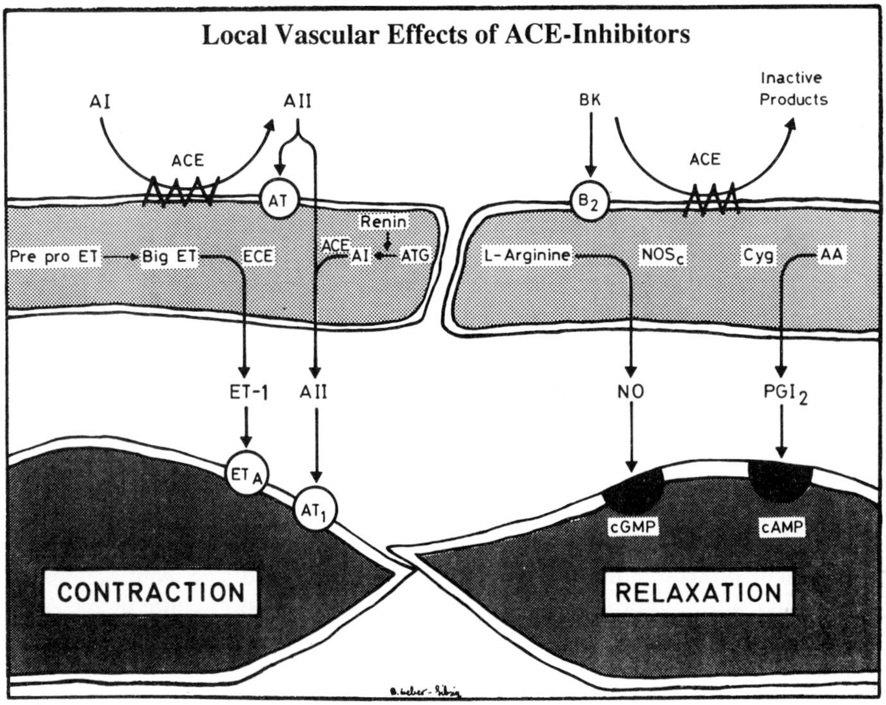

Fig. 3.4 Local vascular effects of angiotensin-converting enzyme (ACE) inhibitors on endothelium-derived vasoactive substances; ACE not only activates angiotensin (A) I into AII, but also inactivates bradykinin (Bk). Hence, in addition of inhibiting the renin angiotensin system, ACE inhibitors also stimulate the activity of the L-arginine nitric oxide (NO) pathway as well as of prostacyclin (PGI_2), particularly after stimulation with bradykinin AA-arachidonic acid; ATG=angiotensinogen; CYG=cyclo-oxygenase; ET=endothelin; NOS_C=constitutive nitric oxide synthase.

released at sites of activated coagulation and platelets) may increase vascular tone and endanger graft blood flow.

Activating and inactivating vasoactive substances

As an active organ, endothelial cells can activate or inactivate various vasoactive substances such as angiotensins and bradykinin. This is another important mechanism by which endothelial cells control vascular tone in terms of increasing or decreasing local concentrations of vasoactive hormones (Fig. 3.4). The activity of angiotensin converting enzyme (ACE) or kininase II expressed in endothelial cells, which converts angiotensin I into a more potent vasoconstrictor peptide angiotensin II and inactivates bradykinin, is more pronounced in the saphenous vein compared to the ITA.[32] Hence, inhibition of the enzyme by ACE-inhibitors augments endothelium-dependent relaxation to bradykinin and inhibits angiotensin I-induced vasoconstriction in the vein, but not in the artery. It has been demonstrated that angiotensin II stimulates intimal hyperplasia and hypertrophy in animal models, and ACE inhibitors prevent intimal thickening after mechanical injury by a balloon catheter.[33] Hence, it remains possible that these drugs are effective in the prevention of intimal proliferation of venous grafts. Indeed, at least in the rat, the ACE inhibitor cilazapril inhibits vascular wall thickening of the jugular vein implanted into the arterial circulation.[34]

Platelet–vessel wall interaction

Platelets are involved in the pathogenesis of coronary artery disease as well as coronary bypass graft disease. Platelets release a number of vasoactive substances such as adenosine diphosphate (ADP) and triphosphate (ADP), thromboxane A_2 and serotonin[35,36] which have profound effects both on platelets and vascular wall. Thrombin, a potent stimulator of platelet aggregation, is able to activate endothelial cells to release NO and/or PGI_2[37] both important inhibitors of platelet function.

Of particular interest with respect to graft function is the fact that the production of nitric oxide is stimulated by platelet-derived products such as adenosine diphosphate (ADP) and triphosphate (ADP) in the ITA, but not in the saphenous vein (even in veins in which the presence of functional endothelium has been previously confirmed by a relaxation to bradykinin.[36]) Hence, ITA grafts exhibit endothelium-dependent relaxations and inhibition of platelet function at sites where platelets are activated (Fig. 3.5);[36] this tends to flush away and disaggregate evolving platelet clots, while in the saphenous vein, this important protective mechanism is not well developed (Fig. 3.5).[36] The contractions induced by platelet-derived serotonin and thromboxane A_2 on smooth muscle cells of saphenous vein are predominant. Similar to the saphenous vein, the GEA exhibits marked contractions in response to aggregating platelets.[38]

As mentioned above, thrombin is an important amplifier of platelet–vessel wall interaction. On one hand, thrombin directly stimulates platelets to release large amount of thromboxane A_2 inducing potent vasoconstriction and platelet activation;[37] on the other hand, thrombin also simultaneously releases NO and PGI_2 from endothelial cells in the ITA,[13,37] which can prevent platelet-induced vasoconstriction in the artery with endothelium,[37] while in the arteries without endothelium, where the endothelial protective mechanisms are absent, thrombin stimulates platelets to produce large amounts of thromboxane A_2 and also serotonin causing potent vasoconstriction.[36,37] Hence, to prevent platelet-induced contractions in the human ITA without endothelium or the saphenous vein, a

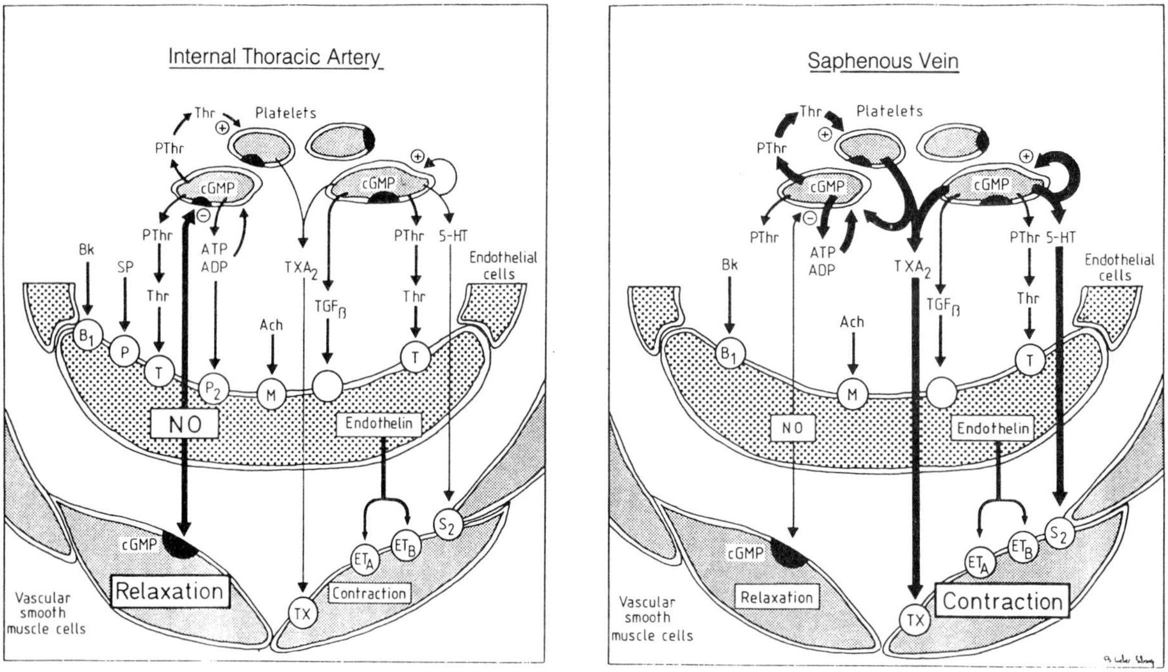

Fig. 3.5 Platelet-vessel wall interaction in arterial (left) and venous coronary bypass grafts (right): in the internal thoracic artery, platelets release adenine nucleotides activating purinergic (P) receptors and thrombin activates its receptor on endothelial cells (T) linked to the formation of EDRF or nitric oxide. This mechanism leads to vasodilation and inhibition of platelet function and thereby plays an important protective role to maintain local graft blood flow and patency. In contrast, in the vein, this pathway is less developed and the contractile effects of thromboxane A_2 (TxA_2) and serotonin (5-HT; 5-hydroxytryptamine) predominate. ADP=adenosine diphosphate; Ach=acetylcholine; cGMP=cyclic 3′5′-guanosine monophosphate; S_2=$5HT_2$-serotonergic receptor; O=receptor.

combined blockade of 5-HT_2-serotonergic receptors (by ketanserin) and of the endoperoxide/thromboxane A_2 receptors such as SQ-30741 or the thromboxane A_2 receptor/synthase inhibitor ridogrel is required (Fig. 3.5).[36,37]

Vascular smooth muscle cells

Vascular smooth muscle cells are the predominant component of the media. They are the primary regulators of vascular tone. In addition, abnormal smooth muscle cell growth is a hallmark of coronary artery disease as well as coronary bypass graft disease, in particular, venous bypass graft disease.

Venous coronary bypass grafts exhibit marked proliferative responses as soon as they are implanted into the arterial circulation due to proliferation of vascular smooth muscle cells.[3] Since in the ITA such atherosclerotic changes are much less common, differences in the behaviour of vascular smooth muscle cells of these arteries as compared to the vein must be involved. In the saphenous vein, vascular smooth muscle cell proliferation probably occurs in response to increases in transmural pressure as well as pulsatile stretch (after implantation into the coronary circulation),[39] and to injuries during surgical preparation with endothelial damage.[40] Local platelet activation and release of growth factors such as platelet-derived growth factor (PDGF) may also be involved in the pathogenesis of coronary bypass graft disease. Indeed, interestingly, cultured smooth muscle cells from saphenous vein and coronary artery exhibit profound proliferative responses to both PDGF and pulsatile stretch, while smooth muscle cells from the ITA remain unresponsive to such stimuli.[41,42]

In summary, the endothelial cells of the ITA are able to produce large amounts of NO and PGI_2 which act as vasodilators and inhibit platelet activation. In addition, the unresponsiveness of smooth muscle cells of the ITA to proliferative stimuli may also contribute to the higher late patency rate of ITA grafts compared to saphenous vein grafts.[43,44]

Acknowledgement

The authors would like to acknowledge the invaluable collaboration of Ludwig von Segesser, Erwin Bauer, Robert Siebenmann, Peter Stulz and Marko Turina in the projects. Further, we are indebted to Amanda de Sola Pinto and to Bernadette Weber-Libsig for their help in the preparation of the manuscript. Original research reported in the manuscript was supported by grants of the Swiss National Research Foundation (No. 32–36571.92), the Swiss Cardiology Foundation, the Mobiliarversicherung and the Patria Versicherung.

References

1. Singh RN. Atherosclerosis and the internal mammary arteries. *Cardivasc Intervent Radiol* 1983; **6:** 72–7.
2. Sims FH. Discontinuities in the internal elastic lamina: A comparison of coronary and internal mammary arteries. *Artery* 1985; **13:** 127–43.
3. Shelton ME, Forman MB, Bajaj A *et al.* A comparison of morphologic and angiographic findings in long-term internal mammary artery and saphenous vein bypass grafts. *J Am Coll Cardiol* 1988; **20:** 297–307.
4. Furchgott RF, Zawadzki JV. The obligatory role of endothelial cells in the relaxation of arterial smooth muscle by acetylcholine. *Nature* 1980;, **288:** 373–6.
5. Lüscher TF, Vanhoutte PM. *The endothelium modulator or cardiovascular function.* Boca Raton, Fl., USA: CRC Press, 1990, 1–215.
6. Busconi L, Michel T: Endothelial nitric oxide synthase. *J Biol Chem* 1993; **268:** 8410–13.
7. Palmer RMJ, Ferrige AG, Moncada S. Nitric oxide release accounts for the biological activity of endothelium-derived relaxing factor: *Nature* 1987; **327:** 524–6.
8. Palmer RMJ, Ashtor DS, Moncada S. Vascular endothelial cells synthesize nitric oxide from L-arginine. *Nature* 1988; **333:** 664–6.
9. Radomski MW, Palmer RMJ, Moncada S. The anti-aggregating properties of vascular endothelium: interactions between prostacyclin and nitric oxide. *Br J Pharmac* 1987; **92:** 639–46.
10. Rapoport RM, Murad F. Agonist-induced endothelium-dependent relaxation in rat thoracic aorta may be mediated through cGMP. *Circulation Res* 1983; **52:** 352–7.
11. Yang Z, von Segesser L, Bauer E, Stulz P, Turina M, Lüscher TF. Different activation of endothelial L-arginine and cyclo-oxygenase pathway in human internal mammary artery and saphenous vein. *Circulation Res* 1991; **68:** 52–60.
12. Yang Z, Diederich D, Schneider K, *et al.* Endothelium-derived relaxing factor and protection against contractions induced by histamine and serotonin in the human internal mammary artery and in the saphenous vein. *Circulation* 1989; **80:** 1041–8.
13. Lüscher TF, Diederich D, Siebenmann R *et al.* Difference between endothelium-dependent relaxations in arterial and in venous coronary bypass grafts. *New Engl J Med* 1988; **319:** 462–7.

14. Yang Z, Siebenmann R, Studer M, Egloff L, Lüscher TF. Similar endothelium-dependent relaxation, but enhanced contractility of the right gastroepiploic artery as compared to the internal mammary artery. *J Thorac Cardiovasc Surg* 1992; **104:** 459–64.
15. O'Neil GS, Chester AH, Allen SP *et al.* Endothelial function of human gastroepiploic artery: Implications for its use as a bypass graft. *J Cardiovasc Surg* 1991; **102:** 561–5.
16. Ochiai M, Ohno M, Taguchi J *et al.* Responses of human gastroepiploic arteries to vasoactive substances – differences to internal mammary arteries and saphenous veins. *J Thorac Cardiovasc Surg* 1992; **104:** 453–8.
17. Hanet C, Schroeder E, Michel X *et al.* Flow-induced vasomotor response to tachycardia of the human internal mammary artery and saphenous vein grafts late following bypass surgery. *Circulation* 1991; **84 (Suppl.III):** III268–74.
18. Moncada S, Vane JR. Prostacyclin in the cardiovascular systems. *Adv Prostaglandin Thromboxane Leukotriene Res* 1980; **6:** 43–60.
19. Subramanian VA, Hernandez Y, Rtack-Goldman K, Grabowski EF, Weksler BB. Prostacyclin production by internal mammary artery as a factor in coronary artery bypass grafts. *Surgery* 1986; **100:** 376–83.
20. Oku T, Yamane S, Suma H *et al.* Comparison of prostacyclin production of human gastroepiploic artery and saphenous vein. *Ann Thorac Surg* 1990; **49:** 767–70.
21. Chaikhouni A, Crawford FA, Kochel PJ, Olanoff LS, Halushka PV. Human internal mammary artery produces more prostacyclin than saphenous vein. *J Thorac Cardiovasc Surg* 1986; **92:** 88–91.
22. Werner GS, Wiegand V, Kreuzer H. Effects of acetylcholine on arterial and venous grafts and coronary arteries in patients with coronary artery disease. *Eur Heart J* 1990; **11:** 127–37.
23. Yanagisawa M, Kurihara H, Kimura S *et al.* A novel potent vasoconstrictor peptide produced by vascular endothelial cells. *Nature* 1988; **332:** 411–15.
24. Xu D, Emoto N, Giaid A *et al.* ECE-1: a membrane-bound metalloprotease that catalyzes the proteolytic activation of big endothelin-1. *Cell* 1994; **78:** 473–85.
25. Lüscher TF, Yang Z, Tschudi M *et al.* Interaction between endothelin-1 and endothelium-derived relaxing factor in human arteries and veins. *Circulation Res* 1990; **66:** 1088–4.
26. Seo BG, Oemar BS, Siebenmann R, Von Segesser L, Lüscher TF. Both ET_A and ET_B receptors mediate contraction to endothelin-1 in human blood vessels. *Circulation* 1994; **89:** 1203–8.
27. Dohi Y, Lüscher TF. Endothelin in hypertensive resistance arteries: intraluminal and extraluminal dysfunction. *Hypertension* 1991; **18:** 543–9.
28. Clozel M, Gray GA, Breu V, Loffler BM, Osterwalder R. The endothelin ETB receptor mediates both vasodilation and vasoconstriction in vivo. *Biochem Biophys Res Commun* 1992; **186:** 867–73.
29. Yang Z, Bauer E, von Segesser L, Stulz P, Turina M, Lüscher TF. Different mobilization of calcium in endothelin-1-induced contractions in human arteries and veins: Effects of calcium antagonists. *J Cardiovasc Pharmac* 1990; **16:** 654–60.
30. Boulanger C, Lüscher TF. Release of endothelin from the porcine aorta: Inhibition by endothelium-derived nitric oxide. *J Clin Invest* 1990; **85:** 587–90.
31. Yang Z, Richard V, von Segesser L *et al.* Threshold concentrations of endothelin-1 potentiate contractions to norepinephrine and serotonin in human arteries: A new mechanism of vasospasm? *Circulation* 1990; **82:** 188–95.
32. Yang Z, Bauer E, von Segesser L, Turina M, Lüscher TF. Different effects of angiotension converting enzyme inhibition in human arteries and veins. *J Cardiovasc Pharmac* 1993; **22** (Suppl. 5): S17–22.
33. Powell JS, Clozel J-P, Müller RKM *et al.* Inhibitors of angiotensin-converting enzyme prevent myointimal proliferation after vascular injury. *Science* 1989; **245:** 186–8.
34. Roux SP, Clozel J-P, Kuhn H. Cilazapril inhibits wall thickening of vein bypass graft in the rat. *Hypertension* 1991; **18** (Suppl. II): II43–6.
35. Coller BS. Platelets and thrombolytic therapy. *New Engl J Med* 1990; **322:** 33–41.
36. Yang Z, Arnet U, Stulz P *et al.* Different interactions of platelets with arterial and venous coronary bypass vessels. *Lancet* 1991; **337:** 939–43.
37. Yang Z, Arnet U, Bauer E *et al.* Thrombin-induced endothelium-dependent inhibition and direct activation of platelet-vessel wall interaction: Role of prostacyclin, nitric oxide, and thromboxane A_2. *Circulation* 1994; **89:** 2266–72.
38. Li X-N, Stulz P, Siebenmann PR, Yang Z, Lüscher TF. Different effects of aggregating platelets in the right gastroepiploic artery and internal mammary artery. *J Thorac Cardiovasc Surg* 1992; **104:** 1294–302.
39. Predel HG, Yang Z, von Segesser L, Turina M, Bühler FR, Lüscher TF. Implications of pulsatile stretch on growth of saphenous vein and mammary artery smooth muscle. *Lancet* 1992; **340:** 878–9.
40. Angelini GD, Soyombo AA, Newby AC. Smooth muscle cell proliferation in response to injury in an organ culture of human saphenous vein. *Eur J Vasc Surg* 1991; **5:** 5–12.
41. Yang Z, Noll G, Lüscher TF. Calcium antagonists differently inhibit proliferation of human coronary smooth muscle cells in response to pulsatile stretch and platelet-derived growth factor. *Circulation* 1993; **88:** 832–6.
42. Yang Z, von Segesser L, Stulz P, Bauer E, Turina M, Lüscher TF. Cellular and molecular mechan-

isms of growth of human coronary bypass graft smooth muscle cells in response to PDGF and pulsatile stretch. *Eur Heart J (Abstract)* 1993; **14;** 713.

43. Loop FD, Lytle BW, Cosgrove DM *et al.* Influence of the internal mammary-artery graft on 10-year survival and other cardiac events. *New Engl J Med* 1986; **314:** 1–6.

44. Lytle BW, Loop FD, Cosgrove DM, Ratliff NB, Easley K, Taylor PC. Long-term (5 to 12 years) serial studies of internal mammary artery and saphenous vein coronary bypass grafts. *J Thorac Cardiovasc Surg* 1985; **89:** 248–58.

4 Biological and vasomotor properties of the gastroepiploic and inferior epigastric arteries

Adrian H. Chester and Magdi H. Yacoub

The success of the internal thoracic artery (ITA) is believed to be due in part to specific properties of the vascular smooth muscle and endothelial cells.[1–5] Although arteries share many characteristics recent work has shown that different arteries appear to have specific properties with regard to vascular reactivity and smooth muscle cell proliferation.

The credential for a successful arterial conduit is that it should be able to deliver an adequate supply of blood to sustain myocardial function. Since there are great variations in myocardial oxygen demand under different physiological conditions, arterial conduits should be able to respond to such requirements via constriction or relaxation of the vessel wall in response to receptor activation by hormones and drugs as well as physical stimuli such as shear stress and pulsatility. It is believed that specific differences in the vascular biology of arterial and venous grafts may explain the superior performance of arterial conduits.[6–10] The aims of this chapter are to compare and contrast endothelial and smooth muscle mechanisms in these two vessels, and attempt to equate how this may affect their performance as coronary artery bypass grafts.

Endothelial function

Arterial endothelial cells have a high capacity to secrete endothelial dilators, such as nitric oxide (NO) and prostacylin which guard against the vasoconstrictors produced in the endothelium, or released locally from aggregating platelets and other circulating blood cells.[4,5] This may be an important cellular mechanism that contributes to the superior patency rates of arterial grafts. NO may be released either basally or via a number of different stimuli such as shear stress and viscous drag caused by blood flow as well as pharmacological stimuli.[11] Subsequent relaxation of vascular smooth muscle is mediated by activation of guanylate cyclase, leading to an increase in cyclic guanosine monophosphate (cGMP).

It has been shown that the stimulated and basal activity of the L-arginine–nitric oxide pathway is much greater in the ITA and the gastroepiploic artery (GEA) compared to that of the saphenous vein (SV).[6,7,12] On the other hand, the formation of NO in both the ITA and GEA is similar with respect to receptor agonist responses, although the GEA appears to be able to generate significantly greater amounts of the second messenger cyclic GMP.[6,13,14] In a similar fashion the endothelial function of the inferior epigastric artery (IEA) has been assessed with substance P, acetylcholine, bradykinin and histamine. Values for the maximum effect of these agents appear greater in the IEA than in the ITA (Fig. 4.1).[15,16]

Recently the reactivity of the GEA has been compared to that of the radial artery (RA).[17] In terms of endothelial function, the RA had a comparable response to endothelium-dependent vasodilators. Both the RA and the GEA had a significantly higher contractile response to noradrenaline and 5-HT than segments of ITA when the endothelium was intact. The authors concluded that the ITA may have a greater basal release of endothelium-derived NO than either the RA or the GEA, which could be considered comparable.

The endothelium also generates the vasoconstrictor peptide endothelin; its contractile effects on

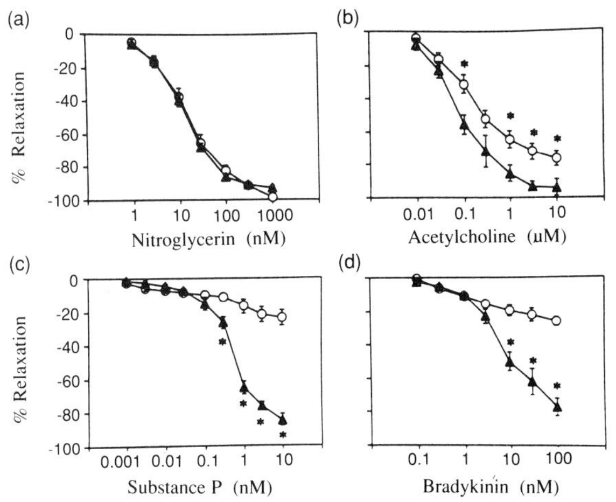

Fig. 4.1 Vasodilator effects of (a) nitroglycerin, (b) acetylcholine, (c) substance P and (d) bradykinin in isolated segments of human ITA (○) and IEA (▲). ⋆ =P<0.05. Reproduced with permission from Mugge *et al.*[16]

vascular smooth muscle exceed those of norepinephrine (NA), angiotensin II and 5-hydroxytryptamine (5-HT).[18] The amounts of endothelin formed in coronary bypass grafts remains to be established; however, thrombin, angiotensin II and transforming growth factor-β (TGF-β) (which is released from platelets) may stimulate its production.[18,19] However, neither the contractile or mitogenic responses of this peptide have been determined in the GEA or IEA and the physiological role of endothelin remains unclear, but it has been shown that endothelin can potentiate the effect of other vasoconstrictors in human arteries.[20,21]

Smooth muscle function

The contractile properties of coronary bypass vessels are determined by the size of the blood vessels, the thickness of the media, its histological composition and the receptor profile on the smooth muscle cells. Vascular smooth muscle cells are the most important component of the media. They are primary regulators of vascular tone and, therefore, of local blood flow. In addition, they can change their phenotype (phenotypic modulation), secrete substances, migrate and proliferate all of which have important implications for graft function.[22]

Several studies have reported a variation in the response of the ITA, GEA and IEA to a range of constrictor agents that may be encountered in the circulation, either as endogenous mediators of vessel tone or as a result of drug therapy associated with cardiac surgical procedures (Fig. 4.2).[16,23–26] Thus, the muscular arteries, such as the GEA, exhibit marked contractile responses to agonists such as NA, 5-HT and potassium chloride, while in elastic arteries such as the ITA, the absolute increase in tension is less pronounced. A study comparing the RA, ITA and GEA demonstrated that the RA had a much stronger contractile smooth muscle function than both of the other arteries.[17] This difference in response to agonists is partly a result of the variations in the subtypes of receptors, as well as their density and location in the vessel wall. The effects mediated by a range of receptor systems have been characterized in various arterial conduits: adrenergic, serotonin, muscarinic, histamine, dopamine and peptide receptors have all been examined. In many of these studies the maximum response to potassium chloride by the smooth muscle has been employed as an index for comparing receptor-mediated contractility. Various studies have demonstrated that the maximum force generated by the GEA and IEA is significantly greater than seen in the ITA.[23,25,26] This is probably due to histological differences in the muscle and elastin content of the vessel wall.[27]

Adrenergic receptors

The sympathetic (neurogenic) control of vessel tone is probably important in the regulation of blood flow when arteries are employed as pedicled grafts. However, free grafts will also be exposed to endogenous or exogenous catecholamines to which the full range of adrenoceptors may respond. Catecholamines may exert both contraction (α-adrenoceptor response) and relaxation (β-adrenoceptor response) of human arteries.

In the ITA, these receptors have been characterised and found to be primarily of α_1-adrenoceptor type.[28] These studies also indicate that the potent vasoconstrictor effect of these hormones in the vessels may have important implications for their perioperative administration. In a more recent study, the IEA has been shown to have a contractile response to NA and dopamine which is similar to that seen in the ITA.[23]

Dopamine receptors

Apart from the adrenergic receptors, dopamine can also exert its effects by acting at its own specific receptor subtypes, termed dopamine-1 (D_1) and dopamine-2 (D_2) receptors. These receptors have been reported to mediate a relaxing effect on a large number of blood vessels, including the coronary arteries.[29] However, these receptors have not yet been comprehensively studied in the arteries used as bypass conduits. The only observations that have been made have shown that dopamine can induce moderate vasoconstrictions at higher doses in both the ITA, GEA and IEA.[23,24] It is not clear whether

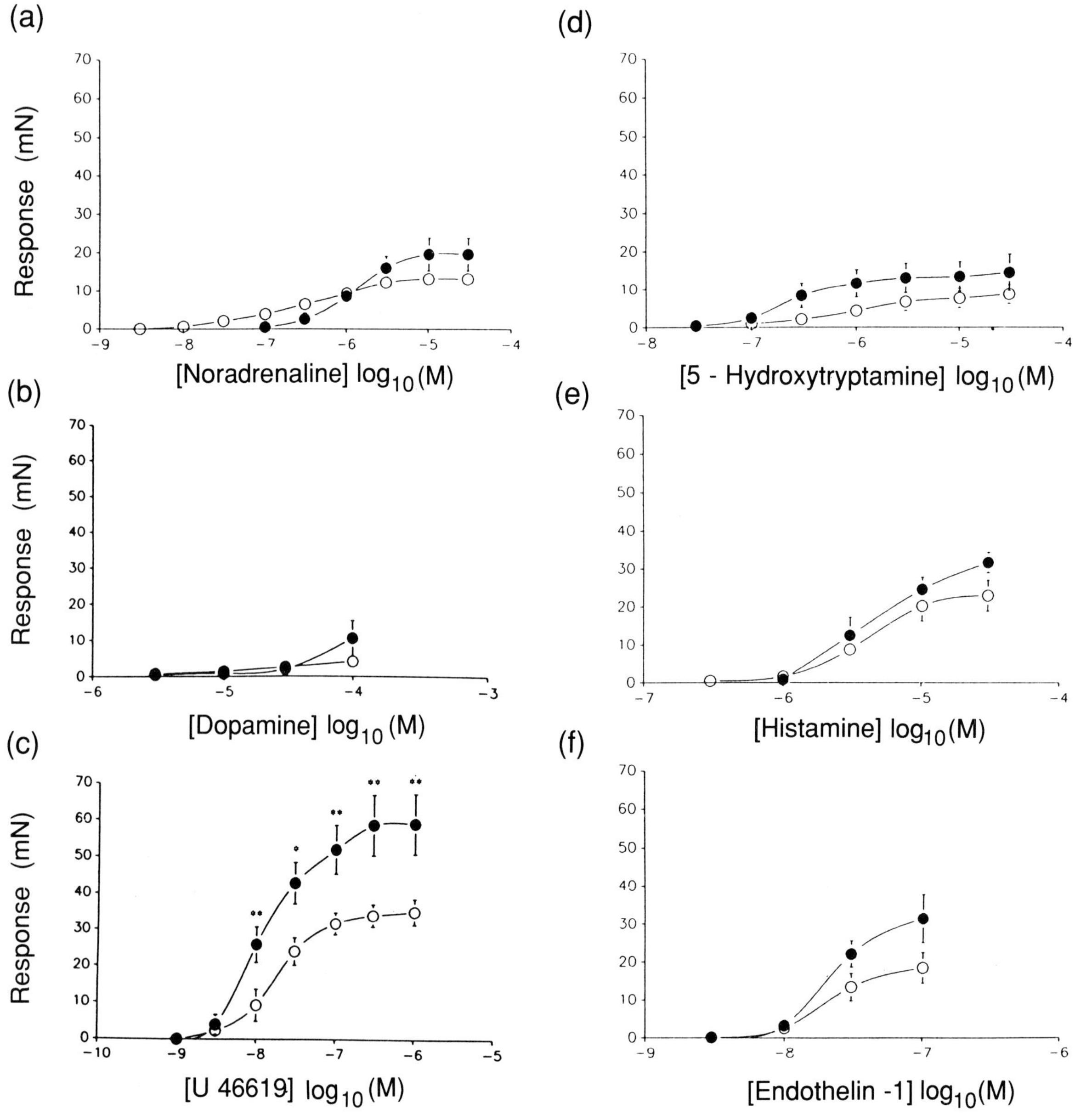

Fig. 4.2 Vasoconstrictor profile of (a) noradrenaline, (b) dopamine, (c) thromboxane mimetic U46619, (d) 5-hydroxytryptamine, (e) histamine and (f) endothelin-1 on isolated segments of human ITA (○) and IEA (●). ⋆ =$P<0.05$, ⋆⋆ =$P<0.01$. Reproduced with permission from Tadjkarimi *et al.*[23]

these responses are mediated specifically by a subtype of dopamine receptors or by a non-specific effect on adrenoceptors.

Muscarinic (cholinergic) receptors

Acetylcholine may induce relaxation in some isolated human arteries via stimulation of endothelial muscarinic receptors and contraction via activation of muscarinic receptors directly on smooth muscle cells. In those arteries that are used as arterial conduits, the ITA has the best documented response to acetylcholine, yielding a maximal endothelium-dependent relaxation.[6] However, the response seen in the IEA in one study does not appear to be as great.[15] This may reflect a difference in the muscarinic receptor profile, since the IEA retains maximum endothelium-dependent responses to other agonists.[15,16] At a higher concentration of acetylcholine ($<10^{-6}$ M) a contractile response can generally be seen via an action on smooth muscle receptors.

Histamine receptors

Histamine has a divergent response in most human arteries studied. It can produce both contraction via H_1-receptors and relaxation via either H_2-receptors on smooth muscle or a H_2-receptor acting through an endothelium-dependent mechanism.[30] This divergent response is seen in both the ITA and the IEA, each artery having a constrictor and dilator component.[15,23,31] However, although the GEA has a potent endothelium-dependent and independent dilator response to histamine, this artery is devoid of any constrictor response to this amine (Fig. 4.3).[24]

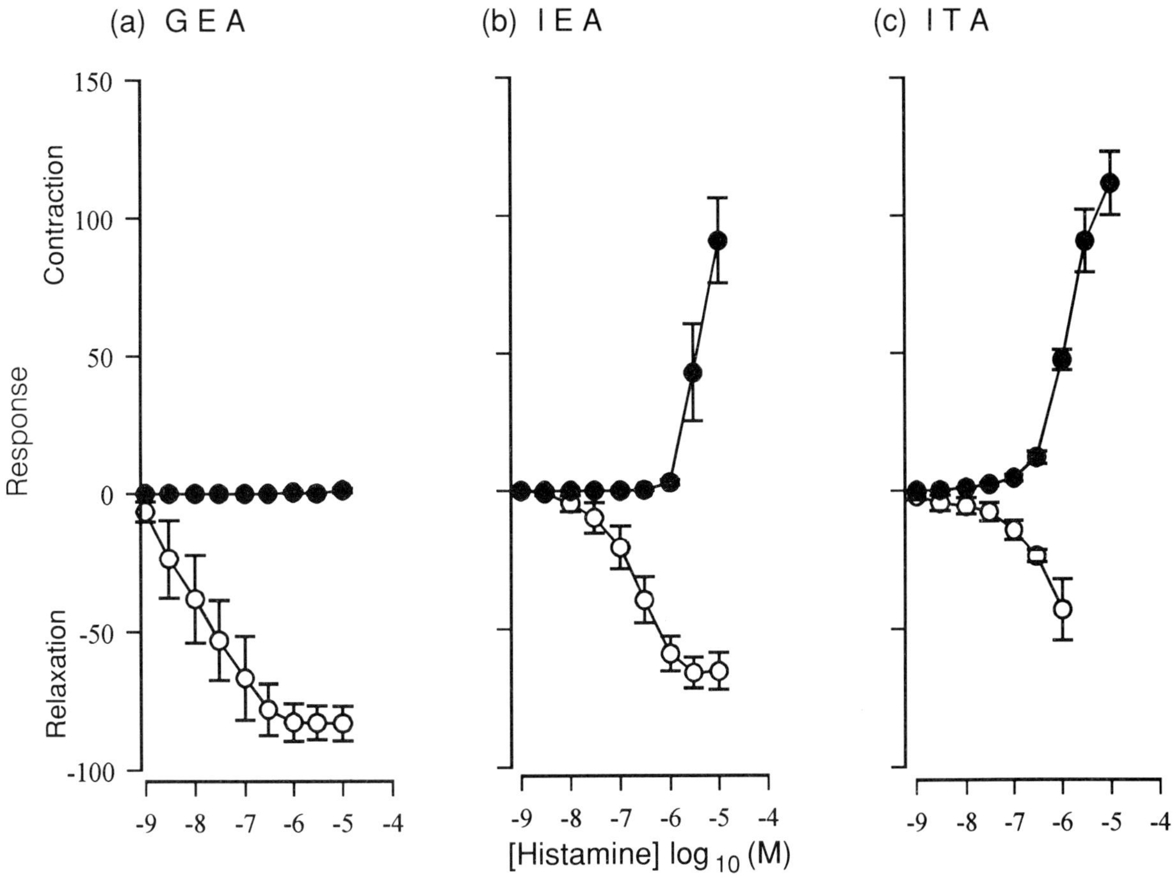

Fig. 4.3 Comparison of the divergent vasoactive effects of histamine on isolated segments of human (a) GEA, (b) IEA and (c) ITA. Contraction was measured on quiescent vessels (●) while relaxation was assessed in segments given an active tone with U46619 (○). (Unpubl. obs.)

One may speculate that there is a heterogeneity in the histamine receptor profile between the arteries used as bypass conduits. Since it has been shown that levels of histamine are raised in patients with ischaemic heart disease and following cardiopulmonary bypass, the response of each artery to histamine may be important in governing its short- and long-term performance.

5-Hydroxytryptamine receptors

Although the profile of the 5-HT receptors has not yet been defined in arterial conduits, it has been shown that the maximum effect of 5-HT on the ITA is approximately 50 per cent of that in the SV.[8] Comparison of GEA and ITA showed that the 5-HT receptor-mediated response was greater in the ITA, while a separate study demonstrated that the 5-HT response was comparable in the ITA and the IEA.[24,26] The precise 5-HT receptor profile in the ITA, GEA or IEA has not been determined. However it is known that both the human saphenous vein and coronary artery have 5-HT_1-like and 5-HT_2 receptors, both of which can mediate contraction. 5-HT is of particular interest since it is released in large concentrations locally by aggregating platelets at the site of thrombus formation. The potential role of 5-HT in inducing coronary and arterial vasospasm is increased since the effect mediated by 5-HT_1-like receptors has been shown to be enhanced by thromboxane A_2 in human coronary arteries.[32] Whether this mechanism is important in the initiation of bypass graft spasm requires further study.

Peptide receptors

Recent studies have shown that vasoactive peptides can play an important role in the control of vascular tone and homeostasis of blood flow and electrolyte balance. These compounds can act directly on vessels through their own receptors or modulate neuronal control as they are co-localized and/or co-released with acetylcholine and noradrenaline and capable of neuromodulation of these and other neurotransmitters. Peptides that have drawn much interest include the neuropeptide Y (NPY) and calcitonin gene-related peptide (CGRP), which have both been reported to have potent vasoactive effects in human arteries.[33,34] The effect of these two peptides has recently been compared on the ITA and GEA (Luu T.N. *et al.* unpublished data). The GEA was shown to exhibit a greater relaxant response to CGRP, but a less pronounced contraction to NPY compared to the ITA. The constriction induced by NPY could be significantly enhanced by removal of the endothelium in ITA segments but not GEA segments.

The comparative role of neuropeptides on the ITA and GEA has also recently been investigated. Those peptides such as vasoactive intestinal peptide (VIP), bombesin and gastrin, which have been associated with the gastrointestinal tract, were shown to have preferential vasodilator function on the GEA compared to the ITA.[35] Indeed, reports have been able to show an increase in flow in GEA grafts but not ITA grafts following the patients eating a meal.[36,37] The role of these peptides on the IEA remains to be determined.

Conclusion

Arterial grafts share some biological characteristics which render them potentially superior to vein grafts. However, recent studies have also shown heterogeneity of the biological, structural and functional properties of different arterial conduits, some of which have been outlined in this chapter. An extensive knowledge of these characteristics in the different grafts will aid in the choice and optimization of the performance of each particular conduit.

References

1. Loop FD, Lytle BW, Cosgrove DM *et al.* Influence of the internal mammary artery graft on 10 year survival and other cardiac events. *New Engl J Med* 1986; **314:** 1–6.
2. Foster ED, Kranc MAT. Alternative conduits for aortocoronary bypass grafting circulation 1989; **79** (Suppl I): I34–9.
3. Chester AH, Yacoub M. Vascular reactivity and endothelial function of bypass grafts. *Curr Opin Cardiol* 1990; **5:** 733–6.
4. Lüscher TF. Vascular biology of coronary bypass grafts. *Curr Opin Cardiol* 1991; **6:** 868–76.
5. Lüscher TF, Boulanger CM, Yang Z, Noll G, Dohi Y. Interactions between endothelium-derived relaxing and contracting factors in health and cardiovascular disease. *Circulation* 1993; **87** (Suppl V): V36–44.
6. Lüscher TF, Diedrich D, Siebenman R *et al.* Difference between endothelium-dependent relaxation in arterial and in venous coronary bypass grafts. *New Engl J Med* 1988; **319:** 462–7.

7. Yang Z, von Segesser L, Bauer E, Shulz P, Turina M, Lüscher TF. Different activation of the endothelial L-arginine and cyclo-oxygenase pathway in the human internal mammary artery and saphenous vein. *Circulation Res* 1991; **68:** 52–60.
8. Yang Z, Diederich D, Schneider K *et al.* Endothelium-derived relaxing factor and protection against contractions induced by histamine and serotonin in the human internal mammary artery and in the saphenous vein. *Circulation* 1989; **80:** 1041–8.
9. Allen SP, Chester AH, Dashwood MR, Tadjkarimi S, Piper PJ, Yacoub MH. Preferential vasoconstriction to cysteinyl leukotrienes in the human saphenous vein compared with the internal mammary artery: Implications for graft performance. *Circulation* 1994; **90:** 515–24.
10. Tadjkarimi S, O'Neil GS, Luu TN *et al.* Comparison of cyclic GMP in internal mammary artery and saphenous vein: implications for coronary artery bypass patency. *Cardiovasc Res* 1992; **26:** 297–300.
11. Bassenge E, Busse R. Endothelial modulation of coronary tone. *Prog Cardiovasc Dis* 1988; **30:** 349–80.
12. Akar F, Uydes BS, Ayrancioglu K *et al.* Endothelial function of human gastroepiploic artery in comparison with saphenous vein. *Cardiovasc Res* 1994; **28:** 500–4.
13. Rapoport RM, Murad F. Agonist-induced endothelium-dependent relaxation in rat thoracic aorta may be mediated through cGMP. *Circulation Res* 1983; **52:** 352–7.
14. O'Neil GS, Chester AH, Allen SP *et al.* Endothelial function of human gastroepiploic artery. Implications for its use as a bypass graft. *J Thorac Cardiovasc Surg* 1991; **102:** 561–5.
15. Tadjkarimi S, Chester AH, Borland JAA, Schyns CJ, O'Neil GS, Yacoub MH. Endothelial function and vasodilator profile of the inferior epigastric artery. *Ann Thorac Surg* 1994 (in press).
16. Mugge A, Barton MR, Cremer J, Frombach R, Lichtlen PR. Different vascular reactivity of human internal mammary and inferior epigastric arteries in vitro. *Ann Thorac Surg* 1993; **56:** 1085–9.
17. Chardigny C, Jebara VA, Acar C *et al.* Vasoreactivity of the radial artery. Comparison with the internal mammary and gastroepiploic arteries with implications for coronary artery surgery. *Circulation* 1993; **88** (part 2): 115–27.
18. Yanagisawa M, Kurihara H, Kimura S *et al.* A novel potent vasocontrictor peptide produced by vascular endothelial cells. *Nature* 1988; **332:** 411–15.
19. Boulanger C, Lüscher TF. Release of endothelin from the porcine aorta: inhibition by endothelium-derived nitric oxide. *J Clin Invest* 1990; **85:** 587–90.
20. Yang Z, Richard V, von Segesser L *et al.* Threshold concentrations of endothelin-1 potentiate contractions to norepinephrine and serotonin in human arteries: a new mechanism of vasospasm? *Circulation* 1990; **82:** 188–95.
21. Chester AH, O'Neil GS, Allen SP, Luu TN, Tadjkarimi S, Yacoub MH. Effect of endothelin on normal and diseased human coronary arteries. *Eur J Clin Invest* 1992; **22:** 210–13.
22. Klagsbrun M, Dluz S. Smooth muscle cell and endothelial cell growth factors. *Trends Cardiovasc Med* 1993; **3:** 213–17.
23. Tadjkarimi S, O'Neil GS, Schyns CJ, Borland JAA, Chester AH, Yacoub MH. Vasoconstrictor profile of the inferior epigastric artery. *Ann Thorac Surg* 1993; **56:** 1090–5.
24. O'Neil GS, Chester AH, Schyns CJ, Tadjkarimi S, Pepper JR, Yacoub MH. Vascular reactivity of human internal mammary and gastroepiploic arteries. *Ann Thorac Surg* 1991; **52:** 1310–14.
25. Yang Z, Siebenmann R, Studer M, Egloff L, Lüscher TF. Similar endothelium-dependent relaxation, but enhanced contractility of the right gastroepiploic artery as compared with the internal mammary artery. *J Thorac Cardiovasc Surg* 1992; **104:** 459–64.
26. Dignan RJ, Yeh T Jr, Dyke CM *et al.* Reactivity of gastroepiploic and internal mammary arteries: Relevance to coronary artery bypass grafting. *J Thorac Cardiovasc Surg* 1992; **103:** 116–23.
27. van Son JAM, Smedts F, Vincent JG, van Lier HJJ, Kubat K. Comparative anatomic studies of various arterial conduits for myocardial revascularization. *J Thorac Cardiovasc Surg* 1990; **99:** 703–7.
28. Weinstein JS, Grossman W, Weintraub RM, Thurer RL, Johnson RG, Morgan KG. Differences in α-adrenergic responsiveness between human internal mammary arteries and saphenous veins. *Circulation* 1989; **79:** 1264–70.
29. Hughes AD, Sever PS. Action of fenoldopam, a selective dopamine (DA_1) receptor agonist on isolated human arteries. *Blood Vessels* 1989; **26:** 119–27.
30. Toda N. Mechanism of histamine actions in human coronary arteries. *Circulation Res* 1987; **61:** 280–6.
31. Ochiai M, Ohno M, Taguchi J *et al.* Responses of human gastroepiploic arteries to vasoactive substances: Comparison with responses of internal mammary arteries and saphenous veins. *J Thorac Cardiovas Surg* 1992; **104:** 453–8.
32. Chester AH, Allen SP, Tadjkarimi S, Yacoub MH. Interaction between thromboxane A_2 and 5-hydroxytryptamine receptor subtypes in human coronary arteries. *Circulation* 1993; **87:** 874–80.
33. Franco-Cereceda A, Lundberg JM. Potent effects of neuropeptide Y and calcitonin gene-related peptide on human coronary vascular tone in vitro. *Acta Physiol Scand* 1987; **131:** 159–60.
34. Luu TN, Dashwood MR, Chester AH, Yacoub MH. Vasodilatory effect of calcitonin gene-related peptide and localization of its binding sites on

arteries used for coronary bypass surgery. *Eur Heart J* 1993; **14**: 388.

35. Luu TN, Chester AH, O'Neil GS, Tadjkarimi S, Pepper JR, Yacoub MH. Different responses of the human gastroepiploic and internal mammary arteries to vasoactive peptides. *Am J Physiol* 1993; **264:** H583–7.
36. Takayama T, Suma H, Wanibuchi Y. Postprandial flow physiology of the gastroepiploic artery graft. *J Thorac Cardiovas Surg* 1992; **104:** 848–9.
37. Takayama T, Suma H, Wanibuchi Y, Tohda E, Matsunaka T, Yamashita S. Physiological and pharmacological responses of arterial graft flow after coronary artery bypass grafting measured with an implantable ultrasonic doppler miniprobe. *Circulation* 1992; **86** (Suppl II): II-217–23.

5 Organ culture of arterial conduits

Cathy M. Holt, Sheila E. Francis and Gianni D. Angelini

The late failure of saphenous vein grafts and the established superiority of the left internal thoracic artery (LITA) graft has led to widespread use of arterial conduits.[1–4] The superior patency rate of the ITA has been attributed to its histological and biochemical properties.[5–12] Other mechanisms, however, have been proposed, including a difference in the susceptibility of venous and arterial conduits to the effect of surgical preparation. Understanding the basis of the biochemical differences between the saphenous vein and the internal thoracic artery may be helpful in developing strategies to reduce vein graft occlusion. In pursuit of this objective, the behaviour of segments of human saphenous vein and ITA in culture was evaluated. The influence of surgical preparation on intimal vascular smooth muscle cell proliferation was also investigated. Organ culture techniques were also used to obtain indirect evidence on the possible clinical behaviour of alternative arterial conduits such as the right gastroepiploic and inferior epigastric artery which have gained popularity despite incomplete detailed clinical assessments of their long-term performance.[13–15]

This experimental organ culture model offers advantages over histological studies since the progression of intimal thickening can be observed in human tissue over a convenient, short period under controlled and reproducible conditions. Furthermore, the use of organ culture rather than isolated cell culture studies, alows for the interaction of the different cell types within the vessel wall and the influence of the extracellular matrix to be considered.

Organ culture model

The organ culture model used in our laboratory is a modification of the method described by Pederson and Bowyer[16] for organ culture of rabbit aorta. Segments of arteries or vein were obtained from patients undergoing coronary artery bypass surgery. The distal (unused) portion of the ITA, gastroepiploic or inferior epigastric artery was collected after completion of mobilization and preparation for grafting. Saphenous vein segments were obtained either immediately after surgical exposure, 'freshly isolated',[17] or on completion of the last proximal anastomosis, 'surgically prepared'. Surgically prepared vein consisted of excess vein that had undergone adventitial removal, side branch ligation, gentle manual uncontrolled distention and storage in patient's heparinized blood at room temperature (23°C). Segments of vessel were subsequently transferred to the laboratory in HEPES buffered RPMI 1640 containing antibiotics and heparin, where organ cultures were subsequently performed. Vessels were kept moist and prepared for culture by carefully removing any loose adventitial tissue using microvascular scissors, care being taken not to damage the vessel wall.

Small segments of vessel were then opened longitudinally and pinned, intimal surface uppermost, into the base of a petri dish containing set sylgard resin. They were then pinned on top of a piece of polyester gauze in order to facilitate diffusion of nutrients to the adventitial surface. Organ cultures were maintained in RPMI 1640 culture medium containing sodium bicarbonate (2.0 g/litre) in place of HEPES and supplemented with glutamine (2 mmol/litre) and antibiotics as well as 30% fetal calf serum. Cultures were maintained at 37°C in a regulated atmosphere with 5% (vol/vol) CO_2 in air. Culture medium was replaced every 2–3 days and cultures were maintained for periods of up to 2 weeks. Cultures were pulse labelled with [^{3}H] thymidine for the last 24 hours of the culture period.

Tissue viability

Adenosine triphosphate (ATP), and adenosine diphosphate (ADP) were chosen as markers of viability of the predominant cell type, the vascular smooth muscle cell.[18–20] Indeed, we have previously shown that removal of the endothelium did not detectably affect these parameters.[21] We observed that the ATP/ADP ratio of freshly isolated vein and artery segments was maintained after 2 weeks in organ culture (Table 5.1). DNA concentration was also measured to give an indication of cell density and whether cell death had taken place during the culture period. DNA concentration of ITA segments remained constant during culture, whereas that of freshly isolated and surgically prepared veins declined probably due to necrosis of cells, tissue oedema, formation of extracellular matrix or a combination of these factors (*see* Table 5.1).

Scanning and transmission electron microscopy were performed to assess endothelial coverage of the segments of artery and vein both before and after 14 days in culture. Freshly isolated arteries and saphenous vein had a virtually undamaged endothelial layer except for occasional gaps between cells and minor areas of denudation at the cut edges. After 14 days in culture, the endothelial monolayer was still intact with the endothelial cells slightly enlarged but maintaining a typical cobblestone appearance. These findings were confirmed by transmission electron microscopy and immunostaining of transverse paraffin embedded sections with a monoclonal antibody, QB-END/10. Thus, the culture method provided adequate vascular smooth muscle cell and endothelial viability.

Cell proliferation

The primary aim was to investigate the rate of vascular smooth muscle cell proliferation and the development of intimal thickening in culture. In order to do this, cell proliferation was determined following the addition of [^{3}H]thymidine to the culture medium for the last 24 hours of the culture period. Total incorporation of [^{3}H]thymidine by the vein and artery segments and subsequent autoradiography of transverse paraffin sections of the vessel enabled us to accurately quantify global [^{3}H]thymidine incorporation as well as localize proliferating cells within the vessel wall.

The intimal thickening which developed in segments of vessel after 2 weeks in culture was quantified using digital image analysis of transverse histological sections stained with Alcian blue/Millers elastic/Van Gieson. The morphology of the vessel segments after culture was similar to that of uncultured vessel. However, a clearly defined neointimal layer was now visible (*see* Fig. 5.1). This new intima was easily distinguished as an elastin poor, mucopolysaccharide rich layer consisting of loosely packed cells as opposed to pre-existing intima, which where present was elastin rich and densely compacted.

Electron microscopy showed that this layer consisted of extracellular matrix and smooth muscle-like cells containing an abundance of rough endoplasmic reticulum and few actin filaments. This was indicative of a synthetic rather than a contractile smooth muscle cell phenotype. Autoradiography revealed that proliferating cells were present predominantly in the intima with fewer proliferating cells in the media (*see* Table 5.2). Thus, vascular

Table 5.1 ATP/ADP ratio and DNA concentration of saphenous vein and internal thoracic artery segments before and after 14 days in culture

	ATP/ADP		*DNA (μg/mg wet weight)*	
Days in culture	*0*	*14*	*0*	*14*
Freshly-isolated vein	2.05 ± 0.14(16)	1.88 ± 0.16(12)	0.51 ± 0.05(15)	0.38 ± 0.03(11)[a]
Surgically-prepared vein	0.99 ± 0.11(14)[b]	2.99 ± 0.34(11)[c]	0.35 ± 0.03(16)	0.25 ± 0.03(13)[a]
Internal thoracic artery	1.54 ± 0.16(12)	2.12 ± 0.23(10)[a]	0.24 ± 0.03(13)	0.21 ± 0.04(12)

[a] $P<0.025$ vs day 0.
[b] $P<0.0005$ vs freshly-isolated vein day 0.
[c] $P<0.0005$ vs day 0.
Values are means ± SEM for the number of experiments shown in parenthesis.

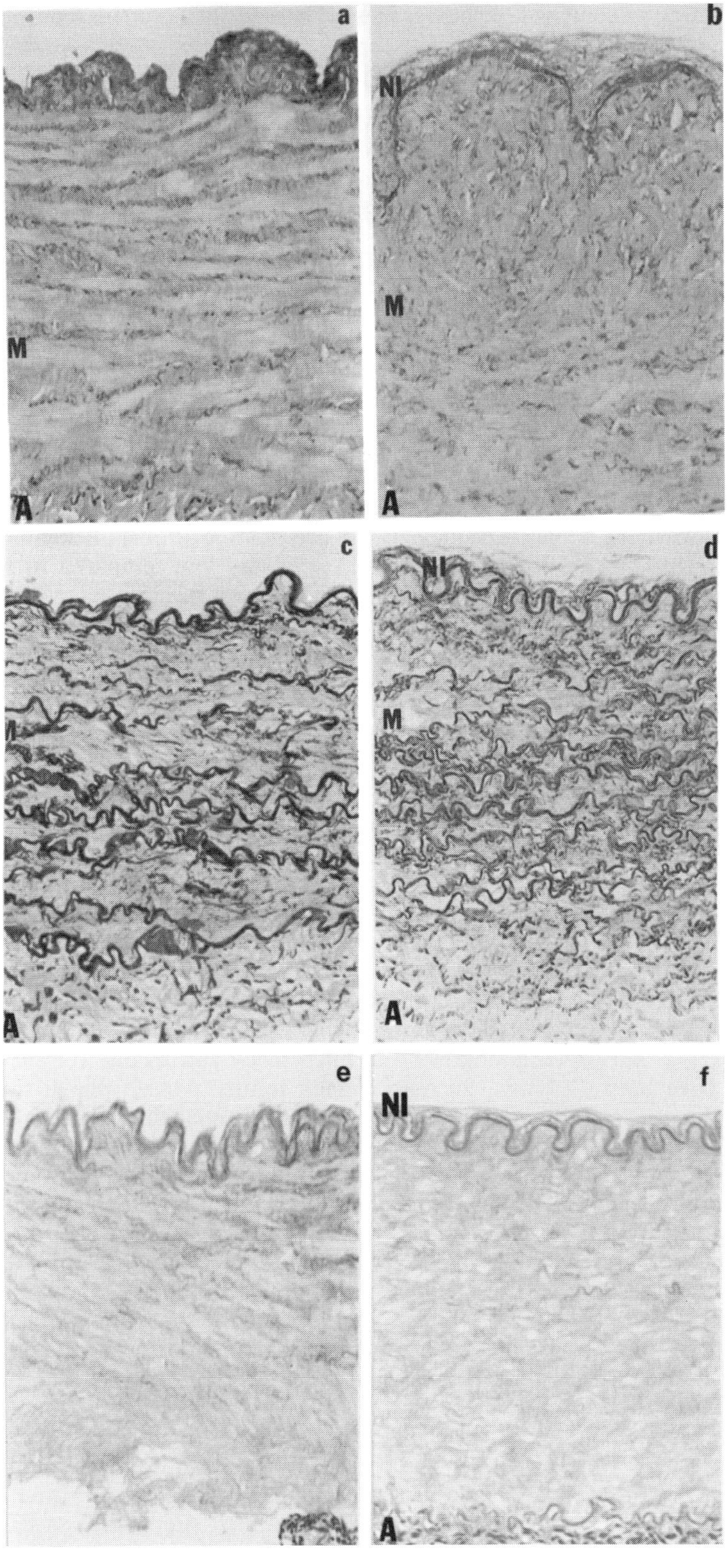

Fig. 5.1 Representative photomicrographs of surgically prepared saphenous vein, (a,b) internal thoracic artery (c,d) and inferior epigastric artery (e,f) before (a,c,e) and after 14 days in culture (b,d,f). Above the adventitia (A) the muscle layers in the media (M) of the saphenous vein and inferior epigastric artery both before and after culture can be seen. Note the predominance of elastic fibres in the media of the internal thoracic artery. A new intimal layer (NI) is visible after culture in the saphenous vein and internal thoracic and inferior epigastric arteries. Reproduced with permission from Holt *et al.*[20]

Table 5.2 Neointimal thickness and cell proliferation occuring in saphenous vein and internal thoracic artery segments after 14 days in culture

	Freshly isolated vein	*Surgically prepared vein*	*Internal thoracic artery*
Neointimal thickness (μm)	44 ± 8(10)[a]	72 ± 13(11)	34 ± 4(13)[a]
[^{3}H] Thymidine labelled nuclei/mm neointimal length	4.6 ± 2.0(9)	7.1 ± 1.2(11)	5.2 ± 1.0(10)
[^{3}H] Thymidine labelled nuclei/mm medial length	0.8 ± 0.3(9)[a]	2.8 ± 1.0(11)	0.6 ± 0.3(10)[a]
Total [^{3}H] Thymidine incorporation (dpm/μg DNA)	868 ± 90(11)[bc]	1682 ± 207(13)	1130 ± 100(13)[b]

[a]$P<0.05$ vs surgically prepared vein.
[b]$P<0.025$ vs surgically prepared vein.
[c]$P<0.05$ vs internal thoracic artery.
Values are means ± SEM for the number of experiments shown in parenthesis.

smooth muscle cell proliferation was directed to the subendothelial layers of the vessel despite exposure of all vessel surfaces, including the adventitia, to the culture medium.

Immunocytochemistry was used to identify specific cell types within the vessel wall before and after culture. QB-END 10[22] recognises the CD34 antigen on the endothelial cells and staining was seen on the intimal surface both before and after 14 days in culture. Alpha smooth muscle cell actin antibodies were used to identify vascular smooth muscle cells and these cells were seen throughout the media and neointima of both cultured artery and vein segments. Antibodies to the proliferating cell nuclear antigen (PCNA) which identifies cells traversing the cell cycle[23] were also used to quantify proliferation.

Surgical intervention

Different responses to surgical injury have been proposed to explain the dissimilarity in long-term behaviour of saphenous vein and ITA grafts. Measurements of tissue viability showed a fall in ATP concentrations in surgically prepared vein compared with freshly isolated vein obtained from the same patient. ATP/ADP ratios for ITA were intermediate between those for surgically prepared and freshly isolated saphenous vein (*see* Table 5.1). After culture, freshly isolated and surgically prepared vein and ITA segments all exhibited a neointima consisting of several layers of cells embedded in an extensive extracellular matrix (*see* Fig. 5.1). There was no apparent morphological difference in the neointima of freshly isolated and surgically prepared veins. The neointima differed morphologically from that in arteries in that it was composed of more densely packed material and was more cellular. The incidence of pre-existing intimal thickening in segments of ITA was very low compared with saphenous vein, in which it was invariably present. A significant correlation was found between this pre-existing intima and the degree of neointimal thickening that developed during culture in freshly isolated vein ($r=0.9$) surgically prepared vein ($r=0.9$) and ITA ($r=0.8$).

The degree of intimal thickening and vascular smooth muscle cell proliferation observed in culture was greater in surgically prepared when compared with freshly isolated saphenous vein and ITA (*see* Table 5.2). Medial cell proliferation as determined by autoradiography, was also much greater in surgically prepared than in either freshly isolated saphenous vein or ITA (*see* Table 5.2). Freshly isolated saphenous vein and ITA segments had a similar high degree of endothelial preservation judged by scanning electron microscopy and medial cell viability. Such minimally injured vessels showed a similar reduced degree of intimal thickening and intimal and medial smooth muscle cell proliferation. Thus, the response of uninjured saphenous vein and ITA in culture appeared similar, despite the intrinsic differences in histological and biochemical properties.

These findings therefore emphasize the importance of injury in promoting smooth muscle cell proliferation and imply that its different prevalence in saphenous vein and ITA grafts may be due to different susceptibilities to injury. Furthermore, one can speculate that reducing the amount of injury to the saphenous vein may reduce intimal proliferation and increase long-term graft patency. Injury probably occurs during surgical preparation of the conduits as well as after grafting, because of the altered haemodynamics of blood flow and the interruption of adventitial structures such as the *vasa vasorum*. The ITA is usually dissected on a pedicle to minimize adventitial disruption and due to its fragility and small calibre great care is taken in its mobilisation. In contrast to this, the saphenous vein is usually subjected to adventitial stripping and is often distended at high pressure. This is known to be a principal cause of medial and endothelial injury.[24,25]

Techniques to minimize surgical preparative injury have been described,[17,26,27] and can easily be applied without radical change in surgical practice. The clear evidence that this reduces early graft thrombosis,[28] and the wealth of circumstantial evidence, including that presented here for a reduction in smooth muscle cell proliferation, justify the widespread application of these techniques.

Other applications of organ culture models

Comparison with other arterial conduits

Alternative arterial conduits such as the inferior epigastric and the gastroepiploic arteries are being used more frequently in coronary artery surgery. Whereas the ITA is an elastic artery with clearly defined internal and external elastic laminae and numerous elastic lamellae in the media, the inferior epigastric and gastroepiploic arteries are muscular arteries with the medial layer composed primarily of smooth muscle cells. However, these arterial conduits are similar with respect to their absence of pre-existing intima. Studies of vascular reactivity have reported inconsistent findings with respect to the properties of these conduits.[10–12]

In general, some degree of intimal proliferation was observed in gastroepiploic and inferior epigastric artery segments maintained in culture for 14 days. This consisted of several loose layers of extracellular matrix with embedded smooth muscle cells, very similar in appearance and extent to that which was seen in cultured ITA. This observation taken together with the histological and biochemical properties suggest speculation of an intermediate tendency for the gastroepiploic and inferior epigastric grafts to develop intimal thickening.

Modulation of organ culture conditions

Manipulation of the culture conditions, e.g. the oxygen tension in the culture medium using specialized incubators, may affect the nature and amount of the intimal thickening which occurs in organ cultures of arterial and venous conduits. Arteries and veins in their normal habitats have defined levels of oxygenation and this may change when the conduit is used for myocardial revascularization. Indeed, recent work shows that hypoxia can markedly alter gene expression in human endothelial cells exposed to an oxygen tension of 14–18 Torr for 16 hours and this may be a significant factor in the development of intimal hyperplasia.[29]

Short-term (24 hours) and long-term (up to 14 days) co-culture of arterial conduit segments with human monocytes as previously performed with saphenous vein[30,31] may help to clarify further the mechanisms of acute interactions (e.g. cell adhesion) and longer term (e.g. growth regulation) controls.

The precise mechanisms involved in intimal proliferation remain poorly understood. However there is increasing evidence that growth factors and cytokines released by the cells that make up the vessel wall may be involved. Serum-free organ culture allows the identification of growth factors released from artery segments and correlation with any pre-existing intimal thickening.[32]

Effects of pressure and flow

A limitation of the organ culture methodology described is that it is a static system. The arterial conduit under study is pinned out in a glass petri dish in the absence of flow. A perfused organ culture system is currently under development, where viable, intact vessels can be maintained under varying conditions of pressure and flow. With the use of such techniques it is hoped that the effect of pressure and flow simulation on vascular smooth muscle cell proliferation and the development of intimal thickening can be investigated. Furthermore, acute studies can be performed to investigate the effect of high pressure on the expression of early response genes, e.g. *c-fos* and *c-jun* and growth factor genes using methods of gene expression analysis.

The organ culture model may prove useful as a tool to mathematically model flow along non-uniform conduits. Blood flow through a conduit may modulate the development of intimal thickening at various sites and in arterial conduits with pre-existing intima this may significantly alter shear stress within the vessel itself. This may be particularly important *in vivo* at branch points within the vessel or at the site of anastomosis.

Inhibitors of smooth muscle cell proliferation

The organ culture system described is fully quantitative and so allows the statistical evaluation of data obtained with inhibitors of smooth muscle cell proliferation. Given the underlying variability, approximately eight paired samples are needed to test for a 50 per cent reduction with 95 per cent confidence to achieve $P < 0.05$. Potential inhibitors of smooth muscle cell proliferation that have been studied using the organ culture model include analogues of cAMP and cGMP as well as the phosphodiesterase inhibitor isobutylmethylxanthine. These have all been shown to inhibit intimal thickening[33] although heparin[34] and a prostacyclin analogue (T. Taylor and G.D. Angelini; unpublished observations) were ineffective. Other novel inhibitors that are currently being investigated include antisense oligonucleotides as well as antagonists of specific growth factors.

Conclusions

These organ culture studies demonstrate that cell viability is maintained during culture and intimally directed vascular smooth muscle cell proliferation occurs consistently. A positive correlation was found between the degree of existing intima and neointimal thickening. This suggests that a neointima may be more likely to develop where previous migration of smooth muscle cells from the medial layer has already taken place.

Intimal thickening and medial smooth muscle cell proliferation were similar in undamaged freshly isolated saphenous vein and ITA segements, but were significantly greater in damaged surgically prepared vein. This raises the possibility that the greater intimal proliferation seen clinically in saphenous vein graft may arise not from extrinsic differences in arterial and venous smooth muscle cells, but from a greater susceptibility to injury. The similar behaviour in culture of the gastroepiploic and inferior epigastric arteries provides encouraging indirect evidence allowing prediction of their long-term patency rates.

The organ culture model represents a relatively new tool in the armoury of the cardiovascular researcher. It has unique advantages for studying a progressive process such as intimal thickening in human vessels. Furthermore, since intimal vascular smooth muscle cell proliferation is the initial common denominator to other vascular pathologies, including restenosis following angioplasty and coronary artery atheroscelerosis, the organ culture model can shed light on the underlying mechanisms of these processes and suggest targets for rational therapeutic intervention.

Acknowledgements

This work was supported by grants from the British Heart Foundation and the National Heart Research Fund.

References

1. Loop FD, Lytle BW, Cosgrove DM *et al.* Influence of the internal mammary artery graft on 10 year survival and other cardiac events. *New Engl J Med* 1986; **314:** 1–6.
2. Angelini GD, Bryan AJ. Extending the use of autologous arterial conduits in myocardial revascularisation. *Br Heart J* 1992; **68:** 161–2.
3. Okies JE, Page US, Bigelow JC, Krause AH, Salomon NW. The left internal mammary artery: the graft of choice. *Circulation* 1984; **70** (Suppl.I): 213–21.
4. Cameron A, Davis KB, Green GE, Myers WO, Pettinger M. Clinical implications of internal mammary artery bypass grafts: the Coronary Artery Surgery Study experience. *Circulation* 1988; **77:** 815–19.
5. Sims FH. The internal mammary artery as a bypass graft? *Ann Thorac Surg* 1987; **44:** 2–3.
6. van Son JAM, Smedts F, Vincent JG, van Lier HJJ, Kubat K. Comparative anatomic studies of various arterial conduits for myocardial revascularization. *J Thoracic Cardiovasc Surg* 1990; **99:** 703–7.
7. van Son JAM, Smedts F. Histology of arterial conduits as a predictor of their long-term patency as coronary bypass conduits. *Eur J Cardiothorac Surg* 1993; **7:** 277–8.
8. Lüscher TF, Diederich D, Siebenmann R *et al.* Difference between endothelium-dependent relaxation in arterial and in venous coronary bypass grafts. *New Engl J Med* 1988; **319:** 462–7.
9. Mugge A, Barton MR, Cremer J, Frombach R, Lichtlen PR. Different vascular reactivity of human internal mammary and inferior epigastric arteries in vitro. *Ann Thorac Surg* 1993; **56:** 1085–9.
10. Tadjkarimi S, O'Neil GS, Schyns CJ, Borland JAA, Chester AH, Yacoub MH. Vasoconstrictor profile of

the inferior epigastric artery. *Ann Thorac Surg* 1993; **56:** 1090–5.
11. Dignan RJ, Yeh T, Dyke CM *et al.* Reactivity of gastroepiploic and internal mammary arteries. *J Thorac Cardiovasc Surg* 1992; **103:** 116–23.
12. O'Neil GS, Chester AH, Schyns CJ, Tadjkarimi S, Pepper JR, Yacoub MH. Vascular reactivity of human internal mammary artery and gastroepiploic arteries. *Ann Thorac Surg* 1991; **52:** 1310–14.
13. Vincent JG, van Son JAM, Skotnicki SH. Inferior epigastric artery as a conduit in myocardial revascularization: The alternative free arterial graft. *Ann Thorac Surg* 1990; **49:** 323–5.
14. Perrault LP, Carrier M, Hebert Y *et al.* Clinical experience with the right gastroepiploic artery in coronary artery bypass grafting. *Ann Thorac Surg* 1993; **56:** 1082–4.
15. Suma H, Fukumoto H, Takeuchi A. Coronary artery bypass grafting by utilizing in situ right gastroepiploic artery: Basic study and clinical application. *Ann Thorac Surg* 1987; **44:** 394–7.
16. Pederson DC, Bowyer DE. Endothelial injury and healing in vitro. *Am J Pathol* 1985; **119:** 264–72.
17. Gottlob R. The preservation of venous endothelium by dissection without touching and by an atraumatic technique of vascular anastomosis. *Minerva Chir* 1977; **32:** 693–700.
18. Soyombo AA, Angelini GD, Bryan AJ, Newby AC. Intimal proliferation in an organ culture of human saphenous vein. *Am J Pathol* 1990; **137:** 1401–10.
19. Angelini GD, Soyombo AA, Newby AC. Smooth muscle cell proliferation in response to injury in an organ culture of human saphenous vein. *Eur J Vasc Surg* 1991; **5:** 5–12.
20. Holt CM, Francis SE, Newby AC *et al.* Comparison of response to injury in organ culture of human saphenous vein and internal mammary artery. *Ann Thorac Surg* 1993; **55:** 1522–8.
21. Holt CM, Francis SE, Rogers S *et al.* Intimal proliferation in an organ culture of human internal mammary artery. *Cardiovasc Res* 1992; **26:** 1189–94.
22. Anthony PP, Ramani P. Endothelial markers in malignant vascular tumours of the liver: Superiority of QB-END/10 over Von Willebrand factor and Ulex europaeus agglutinin 1. *J Clin Path* 1991; **44:** 29–32.
23. Hall PA, Levison DA, Woods AL *et al.* Proliferating cell nuclear antigen (PCNA) immunolocalization in paraffin sections: An index of cell proliferation with evidence of deregulated expression in some neoplasms. *J Pathol* 1990; **162:** 285–94.
24. Angelini GD, Breckenridge IM, Butchart EG *et al.* Metabolic damage to human saphenous vein during preparation for coronary artery bypass grafting. *Cardiovasc Res* 1985; **19:** 326–34.
25. Ramos JR, Berger K, Mansfield PB, Sauvage LR. Histological fate and endothelial changes of distended and nondistended vein grafts. *Ann Surg* 1976; **183:** 205–28.
26. Haudenschild CC, Gould KE, Quist WC, LoGerfo FW. Protection of endothelium in vessel segments excised for grafting. *Circulation* 1981; **64** (Suppl. II): 101–107.
27. Angelini GD, Breckenridge IM, Williams HM, Newby AC. A surgical preparative technique for coronary bypass grafts of human saphenous vein which preserves medial and endothelial functional integrity. *J Thorac Cardiovasc Surg* 1987; **94:** 393–8.
28. Angelini GD, Bryan AJ, Williams HM, Morgan R, Newby AC. Distention promotes platelet and leukocyte adhesion and reduces short-term patency in pig arteriovenous bypass grafts. *J Thorac Cardiovasc Surg* 1990; **99:** 433–9.
29. Karakurum M, Shreeniwas R, Chen J *et al.* Hypoxic induction of interleukin-8 gene expression in human endothelial cells.. *J Clin Invest* 1994; **93:** 1564–70.
30. Cooper JP, Newby AC. Monocyte adhesion to human saphenous vein in vitro. *Atherosclerosis* 1991; **91:** 85–95.
31. Cooper JP, Soyombo A, Williams A, Newby AC. Monocytes inhibit intimal smooth muscle proliferation: in vitro studies with human saphenous vein. *Br Heart J* 1992; **68:** 93.
32. Holt CM, Francis SM, Gadsdon PA, Violaris A, Izzat MB, Angelini GD. Release of platelet derived growth factor in serum-free organ culture of human coronary artery. *Cardiovasc Res* 1994; **28:** 1–6.
33. Soyombo A, Newby AC. Inhibition of smooth muscle cell proliferation by cyclic nucleotides in an organ culture of human saphenous vein. *J Mol Cell Cardiol* 1991; **23:** S114.
34. Francis SE, Holt CM, Taylor T, Gadsdon PA, Angelini GD. Heparin and neointimal thickening in an organ culture of human saphenous vein. *Atheroscelerosis* 1992: **93:** 155–6.

6 Flow through arterial conduits

Graham J. Cooper and Gianni D. Angelini

The unique flow properties of the internal thoracic artery (ITA) have been recognized since the earliest days of its use; Effler noted that a number of arteries implanted as a Vineberg procedure were in spasm but that these 'dry' arteries were patent when studied postoperatively.[1] It is now established that the pattern of flow through ITA grafts is substantially different from that through saphenous vein grafts. However, the relationship of flow to the clinical results obtained with use of the ITA remains largely speculative. Although flow early postoperatively may be inadequate, in the longer term ITA grafts retain the ability to adapt to changes in myocardial blood flow demand.[2] Most flow data concern ITA grafts but there is enough information to make some observations on right gastroepiploic artery (GEA) and inferior epigastric artery (IEA) grafts.

Flow pattern and volume through ITA grafts

Theoretically blood flow through a tube with the dimensions of the ITA is laminar, at rates up to 1000 ml/min.[3] In practice ITA grafts show the regular, parabolic, cross-sectional velocity profile characteristic of laminar flow.[4] Flow through ungrafted ITAs is principally systolic[5–8] whereas that through grafted arteries is modulated from predominantly systolic proximally to predominantly diastolic distally[9] (Figs 6.1 and 6.2). Saphenous vein grafts show diastolic flow predominance throughout their length.[9] The rise in diastolic flow velocity in ITA grafts is greater and more sustained than in saphenous vein grafts.[10] Flow velocity through ITA grafts is higher than that through saphenous vein grafts and, given their smaller diameter produces greater wall shear stress.[9] This beneficially modulates endothelial responses,[11–13] resists neutrophil adhesion[14] and inhibits smooth muscle cell proliferation.[15] Reduction of wall shear stress leads to a decrease in arterial diameter.[16] The development of intimal hyperplasia and atherosclerosis may represent an attempt to increase wall shear stress by vascular remodelling.[17]

The volume of flow through ITA grafts is influenced by coronary artery diameter[18] and the graft/coronary artery diameter ratio.[19] It also correlates

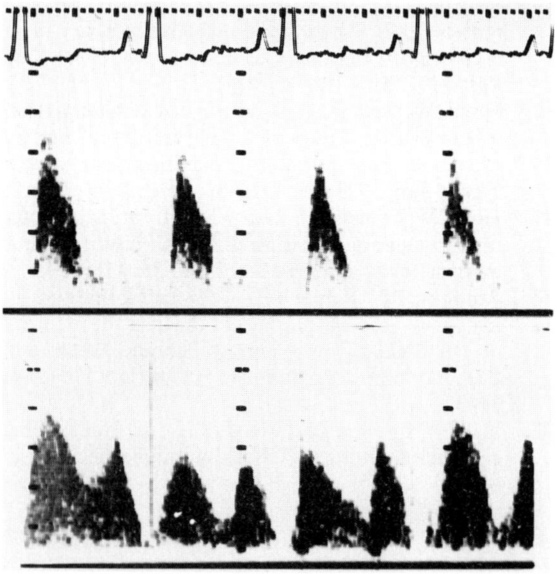

Fig. 6.1 Flow through an ungrafted right ITA (top) is principally systolic whilst that through the left ITA to LAD graft (bottom) has a large diastolic component. Reproduced courtesy of Dr John Chambers, Department of Cardiology, Guy's Hospital, London.

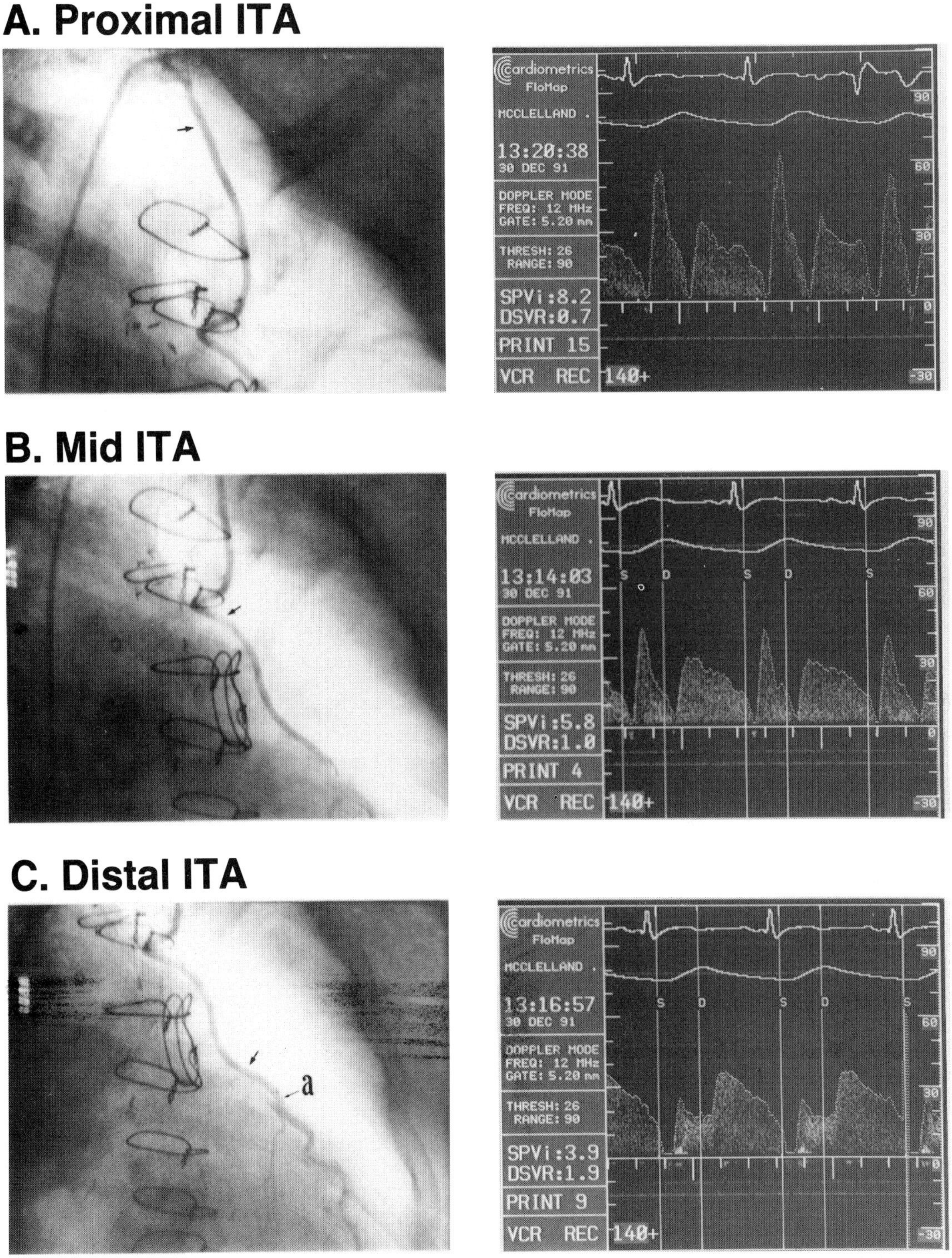

Fig. 6.2 Intravascular ultrasound recording showing the modulation of flow through a grafted ITA from predominantly systolic to predominantly diastolic in the (a) proximal, (b) mid and (c) distal portions of the graft. Reproduced with permission from Bach *et al.*[9]

with a flow-independent measurement of coronary artery resistance[5] and the regional ejection fraction of the left ventricular apex when the left anterior descending (LAD) coronary artery is grafted.[20] The relative importance of these factors is not established and comparisons of flow through ITA and vein grafts suggest that the resistance to flow imposed by the ITA itself is also important (see below).

After anastomosis, flow through left ITA grafts to the LAD is around 50 ml/min (range 36–70).[19–30] Although this may increase in the first few hours after cardiopulmonary bypass,[26,27] weeks later resting flow remains around 50 ml/min.[4,31] Flow through left ITA and right ITA grafts to circumflex branches is also about 50 ml/min.[24,25,29] Flow through right ITA grafts to the LAD or right coronary artery is around 33 ml/min.[19,24,25] Free right ITA grafts to the LAD have a similar flow to *in-situ* left grafts.[28] The significance of these differences is unclear although there may be a relationship between graft flow and patency.

Postanastomotic flow is significantly higher through ITA grafts patent at 1 year[32] and up to 10 years[33] than that through occluded grafts but this is not a universal finding.[19] Flow velocity, rather than flow volume, may be a more important determinant of graft closure.[34] However, reports of ITAs that are apparently occluded subsequently reopening[35–38] argue against either flow volume or flow velocity being an important determinant of anatomical patency. This ability of ITA grafts to remain anatomically patent when apparently occluded at angiography possibly explains the conflicting data on patency and intraoperative flow. The diameter of ITA grafts is reduced with high native coronary artery flow[39] and may progress to angiographic occlusion.[38] Low intraoperative graft flow may, therefore, only reflect competitive flow from a native vessel with a relatively minor stenosis.[40,41] Although low graft flow may be related to loss of angiographic patency, loss of angiographic patency does not necessarily imply loss of anatomical patency and the relationship of graft flow to anatomical patency is not established.

Problem of inadequate flow through ITA grafts

Spasm of ITA grafts may occur early postoperatively,[42,43] or years later[44] even producing myocardial infarction.[45] The incidence of haemodynamic collapse due to inadequate ITA graft flow immediately postoperatively is variable but low; 0.3–1.8 per cent.[46–49] Although inadequate flow may be due solely to spasm in the graft[42] more often a non-spastic ITA graft fails to meet myocardial demand. This is more likely when the recipient artery is the LAD[47–49] with at least an 80 per cent proximal stenosis,[47,48] and a diameter greater than the ITA.[46,47] The risk of inadequate flow is especially pronounced in reoperative surgery.[46,47,50] Replacement of a patent vein graft to a blocked LAD graft is an independent predictor of operative mortality and this has been attributed to myocardial hypoperfusion.[50]

Although the incidence of clinically manifest inadequate flow is low, there is increasing evidence that, compared to saphenous vein grafts, ITA grafts to the LAD are associated with subtle reductions in left ventricular function for up to 1 month postoperatively. Patients with ITA grafts have similar postoperative coronary flow reserve,[51,52] regional myocardial perfusion,[53] exercise capacity[51,54,55] and increases in global ejection fraction[55] to those with saphenous vein grafts. However, immediately after cardiopulmonary bypass, 17 per cent of patients revascularized with an ITA show a deterioration in regional left ventricular function which is seen in only 4 per cent of patients revascularized with saphenous vein.[56] Inability to deliver antegrade cardioplegia through *in situ* ITA grafts may have impaired myocardial protection in these patients.[57] However, similar reductions of regional ventricular function in areas supplied by ITA grafts have been observed in a series in which over half the patients received both antegrade and retrograde cardioplegia.[58] Anterior wall motion in areas supplied by left ITA grafts had recovered by 4 hours postoperatively but posterior wall motion in areas supplied by right ITA grafts remained depressed at 4 hours.[58] One month postoperatively, 22 per cent of patients with ITA grafts have exercise-induced wall motion abnormalities in areas perfused by these grafts which are not found in patients with saphenous vein grafts.[55] Furthermore, a fall in ejection fraction with maximal exercise, indicative of myocardial ischaemia, is found in 21 per cent of patients with a single ITA graft, in 38 per cent with multiple arterial grafts but in none with saphenous vein grafts.[59] In this study, however, the work rate achieved at maximal exercise was greater in patients with arterial grafts than those with vein grafts alone.[59] Although, flow through arterial grafts may only be inadequate at work rates higher than those achieved by patients with vein grafts alone and the clinical consequence is only the avoidance of strenuous exercise in the first postoperative month,[57] the experimental finding that progressive reduction of ITA graft flow produces regional and then global left ventricular dysfunction[60] leaves some cause for concern.

In the absence of a clinical method for quantifying the amount of myocardium supplied by an artery and the oxygen demand of that myocardium, it is not possible to define the minimum acceptable flow through a coronary artery bypass graft. In considering the adequacy of ITA flow there are good reasons for using vein graft flow as the reference. Firstly, the occurrence of haemodynamic collapse associated with inadequate ITA flow is generally reversed by prompt placement of a supporting vein graft.[48,50] Secondly, progressive impairment of left ventricular function results from progressive reductions in ITA graft flow.[60]

Comparisons of early postoperative flow through saphenous vein and ITA grafts reveal some important differences. In a controlled clinical study, mean flow through vein grafts to the LAD was 117 ml/min and that in ITA grafts to the same vessel, 43 ml/min.[21] This difference had a significant effect on the adequacy of myocardial blood supply assessed by the diastolic pressure time index/tension time index ratio.[61] The mean ratio for vein grafts was 0.81 and that for ITA grafts 0.47.[21] Other clinical studies have been less well controlled. Overall, flow through ITA grafts is less than that through saphenous vein grafts to the LAD coronary artery[20,22,62] and circumflex coronary artery[63] but is similar if free flow through the artery is at least 100 ml/min,[23,25] if free flow is at least 40 ml/min and the diameter of the coronary artery is 1.0 mm or less[18] and if the diameter of ITA and coronary artery are similar.[19] However, although flows through both ITAs and vein grafts increase with increasing coronary artery diameter, that through vein grafts remains significantly greater at coronary artery diameters of up to 2.5 mm[18] and when the diameter of the ITA is less than that of the coronary artery.[19] Two weeks after surgery, ITA grafts with a free flow of greater than 50 ml/min have a significantly lower flow than saphenous vein grafts[31] and this difference persists for up to 19.5 months.[64]

The lower flow through the ITA is explained by its smaller diameter compared to saphenous vein. The pressure drop across the ITA, an index of its resistance to flow, increases exponentially at diameters below 3 mm;[3,20] at operation the diameter of

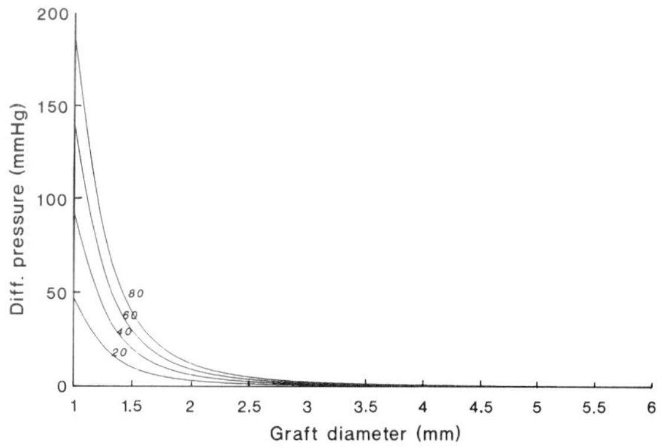

Fig. 6.3 The relationship between the pressure drop across a cylindrical tube and its internal diameter at flows of 20, 40, 60 and 80 ml/min. Viscosity = 0.035 Poise; graft length = 10 cm. Reproduced with permission from Louagie *et al.*[20]

the vessel is within this critical range[2,65,66] (Fig. 6.3).

Attention has been directed to improving free flow through the artery. Although this may not correlate with postanastomotic flow,[20] the previously reviewed evidence suggests that if free flow is at least 100 ml/min postanastomotic flow is equivalent to that through a vein graft regardless of recipient coronary artery diameter. Whether this level is applicable to the elderly[67] and those with a small body surface area[68] requires clarification. Accepting a free flow of at least 50 ml/min does not protect against hypoperfusion.[48] Although it has been reported that postoperative complications are not associated with low free flow rates,[20] this study lacks the statistical power to make this negative assertion with any confidence. After mobilization, but before division, ITA flow is low.[20,30] After division, free flow is around 20 ml/min[65,69] with little spontaneous improvement.[69] Free flow rates in excess of 100 ml/min may be obtained using topical sodium nitroprusside.[69] intraluminal injection of papaverine[70] or hydrostatic dilatation with papaverine[65] or isosorbide dinitrate.[71]

Adaptability of ITA and competitive flow

ITA grafts retain the ability to dilatate in response to increased myocardial blood flow demand[2] and vasoactive drugs.[72] Five years postoperatively 12 per cent of *in situ* ITA grafts have increased in diameter as a result of vein graft occlusion, progression of native vessel atherosclerosis or myocardial hypertrophy.[73] By 11 years, with the increased attrition of vein grafts, 31 per cent of ITA grafts have increased in diameter.[74] In children, *in situ* right ITA and left ITA grafts increase in length and diameter in proportion to the growth of the child.[75,76]

This adaptability of the ITA may also result in a reduction in diameter of the vessel. Although in a canine model competitive flow through the native coronary artery does not reduce ITA graft flow acutely[77] or chronically[78] there is evidence that the phenomenon of competitive flow occurs in man. Two situations are described. An ITA grafted to a vessel with a minor stenosis may close initially but subsequently regain patency if the stenosis increases;[35–37] or, a graft that is initially patent apparently occludes with regression of the native coronary artery stenosis,[38] anatomical patency of the graft can be demonstrated by temporary occlusion of the native coronary artery.[38] At 5 years, 5 per cent of ITA grafts have decreased in diameter, half as a result of competitive flow.[73] There is no increase in this number by 11 years.[74] The degree of coronary artery stenosis determines ITA graft diameter[39] and flow volume through the graft.[40,41]

Right GEA and IEA grafts

Less data is available for right GEA and IEA grafts. As these conduits are not usually used to graft the LAD, concern about inadequate flow may be less marked. Limited clinical experience with the right GEA as a LAD graft is good.[79]

The diameter of the distal left ITA[3,65,66] is similar to that of the GEA[80,81] and IEA.[66,82] The length of the left ITA as an *in situ* graft to the LAD is 15 to 16 cm,[83,84] an *in situ* right GEA graft is longer at 24 cm,[81] but similar at 18 cm[81] when used as a free graft. The length of the IEA is around 11 cm.[66,82] From these data the greater length of an *in-situ* right GEA graft may impose a greater resistance to flow than an ITA, free GEA or IEA graft. In addition, grafts originating from the descending aorta show less diastolic flow than those originating from the ascending aorta[85,86] (Fig. 6.4). Flow through *in situ* right GEA grafts may therefore be further compromised by their origin from the coeliac axis.

Despite these observations, in patent, *in situ* GEA grafts around two thirds of flow occurs in diastole[87] as it does in left ITA grafts.[5] After intraluminal injection of papaverine, free flow through GEAs is similar to that through left ITAs.[88,89] However, postanastomotic flow through GEA grafts is slightly less than that through ITA grafts with a lower flow velocity.[27,90] Flow rates through IEA[66,91] grafts are similar to those through ITA grafts.

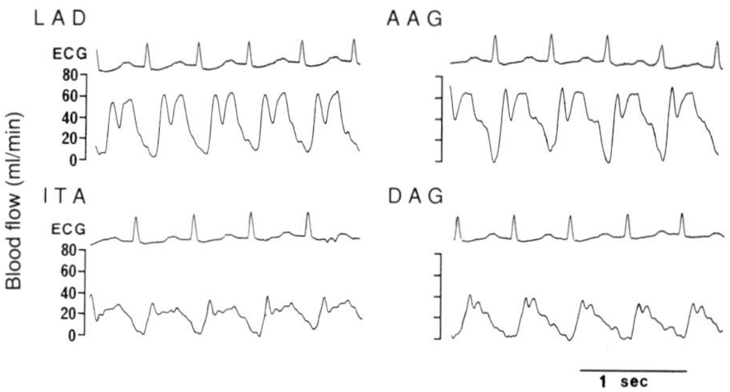

Fig. 6.4 Blood flow in the LAD coronary artery and grafts arising from the ascending aorta (AAG), subclavian artery, ITA and descending aorta (DAG). Reproduced with permission from Tedoriya *et al.*[86]

The capacity of right GEA grafts to increase their flow velocity in response to exercise is similar to that of ITA grafts[90,92] and they have the unique property of showing a marked postprandial increase in flow.[90,93] Areas of the myocardium revascularized by GEAs show an increase in myocardial blood flow[94] although changes in regional ejection fraction in response to exercise have not been reported as they have for ITA grafts. Preliminary evidence suggests that *in situ* GEA grafts show a similar growth potential to ITA grafts.[95] Right GEA grafts are susceptible to angiographically demonstrated rather than clinically apparent postoperative spasm[96,97] which is more common in free grafts.[81]

Conclusion

The majority of the data on flow through arterial conduits concerns ITA grafts. Although there is no direct evidence linking the excellent flow characteristics of ITA grafts with the long-term benefits associated with their use, it seems reasonable to assume that they play an important part. Long-term reduction in the diameter of ITA grafts, often an adaptation to competitive flow through native coronary arteries, does not necessarily represent a loss of anatomical patency and is a manifestation of the preserved vasoreactivity of the graft. In the immediate postoperative period, low flow through ITA grafts to the LAD may have serious consequences. This risk is especially pronounced when an ITA is used to graft a LAD with a greater diameter and an 80 per cent proximal stenosis or to replace a patent vein graft to this vessel. Under these circumstances it is prudent to use an ITA only if it has a free flow of at least 100 ml/min and to be prepared to place a supporting vein graft if there is any evidence of hypoperfusion. The significance of early exercise-induced reductions in left ventricular function in patients with arterial grafts remains to be clarified. The data available on the flow properties of GEA grafts suggests that these may be inferior to those of the ITA; lower flow velocity and, when used *in situ*, possibly a smaller diastolic flow component. Until further data are available GEA and IEA should not be used to graft the LAD when the left ITA is available.

References

1. Effler DB, Sones FM, Groves LK, Shorez E. Myocardial revascularisation by Vineberg's internal mammary artery implant. Evaluation of postoperative results. *J Thorac Cardiovasc Surg* 1965; **50:** 527–33.
2. Singh RN, Beg RA, Kay EB. Physiological adaptability: the secret of success of the internal mammary artery grafts. *Ann Thorac Surg* 1986; **41:** 247–50.
3. Dobrin P, Canfield T, Moran J, Sullivan H, Pifarré R. Coronary artery bypass. The physiological basis for differences in flow with internal mammary artery and saphenous vein grafts. *J Thorac Cardiovasc Surg* 1977; **74:** 445–54.
4. Fujiwara T, Kajiya F, Kanazawa S *et al.* Comparison of blood flow velocity waveforms in different coronary artery bypass grafts. Sequential saphenous vein grafts and internal mammary artery grafts. *Circulation* 1988; **78:** 1210–17.
5. de Bono DP, Samani NJ, Spyt TJ, Hartshorne T, Thrush AJ, Evans DH. Transcutaneous ultrasound measurement of blood flow in internal mammary artery to coronary artery grafts. *Lancet* 1992; **339:** 379–81.
6. Krijne R, Lyttwin RM, Höltgen R, Heinrich KW, Marx R, Sons H. Combined two dimensional and Doppler echocardiographic examination of internal mammary artery grafts from the supraclavicular fossa. *Int J Cardiol* 1992; **37:** 61–64.
7. Van Son JA, Van Asten WN, Peters MB, Skotnicki SH. Noninvasive preoperative and postoperative serial hemodynamic assessment of the internal mammary artery in myocardial revascularisation. *J Thorac Cradiovasc Surg* 1993; **106:** 750–2.
8. Van Son JA, Skotnicki SH, Peters MB, Pijls NH, Noyez L, Van Asten WN. Noninvasive hemodynamic assessment of the internal mammary artery in myocardial revascularization. *Ann Thorac Surg* 1993; **55:** 404–9.
9. Bach RG, Kern MJ, Donohue TJ, Aguirre FV, Caracciolo EA. Comparison of phasic blood flow velocity characteristics of arterial and venous coronary artery bypass conduits. *Circulation* 1993; **88** (Suppl. II): II133–40.
10. Fusejima K, Takahara Y, Sudo Y, Murayama H, Masuda Y, Inagaki Y. Comparison of coronary hemodynamics in patients with internal mammary artery and saphenous vein coronary artery bypass grafts: A noninvasive approach using combined two-dimensional and Doppler echocardiography. *J Am Coll Cardiol* 1990; **15:** 131–9.
11. Rubanyi GM, Romero JC, Vanhoutte PM. Flow induced release of endothelium derived relaxant factor. *Am J Physiol* 1986; **250:** H1145–9.
12. Diamond SL, Eskin SG, McIntire LV. Fluid flow stimulates tissue plasminogen activator secretion by cultured human endothelial cells. *Science* 1989; **243:** 1483–5.
13. Sharefkin JB, Diamond SL, Eskin SG, McIntire LV, Dieffenbach CW. Fluid flow decreases preproendothelin mRNA levels and suppresses endothelin-1 peptide release in cultured human endothelial cells. *J Vasc Surg* 1991; **14:** 1–9.
14. Lawrence MB, Smith CW, Eskin SG, McIntire LV. Effect of venous shear stress on CD-18 mediated neutrophil adhesion to cultured endothelium. *Blood* 1990; **75:** 227–37.
15. Sterpetti AV, Cucina A, D'Angelo LS, Cardillo B, Cavallaro A. Shear stress modulates the proliferation rate, protein synthesis and mitogenic activity of arterial smooth muscle cells. *Surgery* 1993; **113:** 691–9.
16. Langille L, O'Donnell F. Reductions in arterial diameter produced by chronic decreases in blood flow are endothelium dependent. *Science* 1986; **231:** 405–7.
17. Glagov S, Zarius C, Giddens DP, Ku DN. Hemodynamics and atherosclerosis. Insights and perspectives gained from studies of human arteries. *Arch Pathol Lab Med* 1988; **112:** 1018–31.
18. Tyras DH, Barner HB, Kaiser GC, Codd JE, Pennington DG, Willman VL. Bypass grafts to the left anterior descending coronary artery: Saphenous vein versus internal mammary artery. *J Thorac Cardiovasc Surg* 1980; **80:** 327–33.
19. Grondin CM, Lespérance J, Bourassa MG, Campeau L. Coronary artery grafting with the saphenous vein or internal mammary artery. Comparison of late results in two consecutive series of patients. *Ann Thorac Surg* 1975; **20:** 605–18.

20. Louagie YAG, Haxhe JP, Buche M, Schoevaerdts JC. Intraoperative electromagnetic flowmeter measurements in coronary artery bypass grafts. *Ann Thorac Surg* 1994; **57**: 357–64.
21. Flemma RJ, Singh HM, Tector AJ. Lepley D, Frazier BL. Comparative hemodynamic properties of vein and mammary artery in coronary bypass operations. *Ann Thorac Surg* 1975; **20**: 619–27.
22. Green GE, Spencer FC, Tice DA, Stertzer SH. Arterial and venous microsurgical bypass grafts for coronary artery disease. *J Thorac Cardiovasc Surg* 1970; **60**: 491–503.
23. Geha AS, Baue AE. Early and late results of coronary revascularization with saphenous vein and internal mammary artery grafts. *Am J Surg* 1979; **137**: 456–63.
24. Geha AS, Krone RJ, McCormick JR, Baue AE. Selection of coronary bypass. Anatomic, physiological and angiographic considerations of vein and mammary artery grafts. *J Thorac Cardiovasc Surg* 1975; **70**: 414–31.
25. McCormick JR, Kaneko M, Baue AE, Geha AS. Blood flow and vasoactive drug effects in internal mammary and venous bypass grafts. *Circulation* 1975; **52** (Suppl. I): I72–8.
26. Takayama T, Suma H, Wanibuchi Y *et al.* Doppler miniprobe to measure arterial graft flow in coronary artery bypass grafting. *Ann Thorac Surg* 1991; **52**: 322–4.
27. Barner HB. The internal mammary artery as a free graft. *J Thorac Cardiovasc Surg* 1973; **66**: 219–21.
28. Geha AS. Crossed double internal mammary artery to coronary artery grafts: Indications, techniques and results. *Arch Surg* 1976; **111**: 289–92.
29. Barner HB. Blood flow in the internal mammary artery. *Am Heart J* 1973; **86**: 570–1.
30. Canver CC, Dame NA. Ultrasonic assessment of internal thoracic artery graft flow in the revascularized heart. Ann Thorac Surg 1994; **58**: 135–8.
31. Hamby RI, Aintablian A, Wisoff BG, Hartstein ML. Comparative study of post-operative flow in the saphenous vein and internal mammary artery bypass grafts. *Am Heart J* 1977; **93**: 306–15.
32. Barner HB, Mudd JG, Mark AL, Ahmad N, Dickens JF. Patency of internal mammary-coronary grafts. Circulation 1975; **54 (Suppl. III)**: III70–3.
33. Huddleston CB, Stoney WS, Alford WC *et al.* Internal mammary artery grafts: Technical factors influencing patency. *Ann Thorac Surg* 1986; **42**: 543–9.
34. Wilson RF, Marcus ML, White CW. Effects of coronary bypass surgery and angioplasty on coronary blood flow and flow reserve. *Prog Cardiovasc Dis* 1988; **31**: 95–114.
35. Dincer B, Barner HB. The 'occluded' internal mammary artery graft. Restoration of patency after apparent occlusion associated with the progression of coronary disease. *J Thorac Cardiovasc Surg* 1983; **85**: 318–20.
36. Aris A, Borrás X, Ramió J. Patency of internal mammary artery grafts in no flow situations. *J Thorac Cardiovasc Surg* 1987; **93**: 62–4.
37. Suma H. Internal thoracic artery and competitive flow. *J Thorac Cardiovasc Surg* 1991; **102**: 639–40.
38. Kitamura S, Kawachi K, Seki T, Sawabata N, Morita R, Kawata T. Angiographic demonstration of no flow anatomical patency of internal thoracic–coronary artery bypass graft. *Ann Thorac Surg* 1992; **53**: 156–9.
39. Seki T, Kitamura S, Kawachi K *et al.* A quantitative study of post-operative luminal narrowing of the internal thoracic artery graft in coronary artery bypass surgery. *J Thorac Cardiovasc Surg* 1992; **104**: 1532–8.
40. Jones EL, Lutz JF, King SB, Powelson S, Knopf W. Extended use of the internal mammary artery graft: Important anatomic and physiologic considerations. *Circulation* 1986; **74** (Suppl III): III42–7.
41. Jones EL, Lattouf O, Lutz JF, King SB. Important anatomical and physiological considerations in performance of complex mammary–coronary artery operations. *Ann Thorac Surg* 1987; **43**: 469–77.
42. Sarabu MR, McClung JA, Fass A, Reed GE. Early postoperative spasm in left internal mammary artery bypass grafts. *Ann Thorac Surg* 1987; **44**: 199–200.
43. Frierson JH, Bigelow JC, Duke DJ, Mahoney TM, Dimas AP. Treatment of perioperative mammary artery spasm with nifedepine. *Am Heart J* 1993; **125**: 884–6.
44. Kong B, Kopelman H, Segal BL, Iskandrian AS. Angiographic demonstration of spasm in a left internal mammary artery used as a bypass to the left anterior descending coronary artery. *Am J Cardiol* 1988; **61**: 1363.
45. Stone GW, Hartzler GO. Spontaneous reversible spasm in an internal mammary artery graft causing acute myocardial infarction. *Am J Cardiol* 1989; **64**:822–3.
46. Von Segesser L, Simonet F, Meier B, Finci L, Faidutti B. Inadequate flow after internal mammary–coronary artery anastomoses. *Thorac Cardiovasc Surg* 1987; **35**: 352–4.
47. Jones EL, Lattouf OM, Weintraub WS. Catastrophic consequences of internal mammary artery hypoperfusion. *J Thorac Cardiovasc Surg* 1989; **98**: 902–7.
48. Vajtai P, Ravichandran PS, Fessler CL *et al.* Inadequate internal mammary artery graft as a cause of postoperative ischaemia: diagnosis and management. *Eur J Cardiothorac Surg* 1992; **6**: 603–8.
49. Tector AJ, Amundsen S, Schmal TM, Kress DC, Peter M. Total revascularization with T grafts. *Ann Thorac Surg* 1994; **57**: 33–9.
50. Navia D, Cosgrove DM, Lytle BW *et al.* Is the

internal thoracic artery the conduit of choice to replace a stenotic vein graft? *Ann Thorac Surg* 1994; **57**: 40–4.

51. Johnson AM, Kron IL, Watson DD, Gibson RS, Nolan SP. Evaluation of post-operative flow reserve in internal mammary artery bypass grafts. *J Thorac Cardiovasc Surg* 1986; **92**: 822–6.
52. Hodgson JM, Singh AK, Drew TM, Riley RS, Williams DO. Coronary flow reserve provided by sequential internal mammary artery grafts. *J Am Coll Cardiol* 1986; **7**: 32–7.
53. Schmidt DH, Blau F, Hellman C, Grzelak L, Johnson WD. Isoproterenol induced flow responses in mammary and vein bypass grafts: *J Thorac Cardiovasc Surg* 1980; **80**: 319–26.
54. Siegel W, Loop FD. Comparison of internal mammary artery and saphenous vein bypass grafts for myocardial revascularisation. Exercise test and angiographic correlations. *Circulation* 1976; **54** (Suppl. III): III1–3.
55. Kawasuji M, Tsujiguchi H, Tedoriya T, Taki J, Iwa T. Evaluation of post-operative flow capacity of internal mammary artery. *J Thorac Cardiovasc Surg* 1990; **99**: 696–702.
56. Simon P, Owen A, Neumann F *et al.* Immediate effects of mammary artery revascularisation versus saphenous vein on global and regional myocardial function. An intra-operative echocardiographic assessment. *Thorac Cardiovasc Surg* 1991; **39** (Suppl. 3): 228–32.
57. Loop FD, Thomas JD. Hypoperfusion after arterial bypass grafting. *Ann Thorac Surg* 1993; **56**: 812–13.
58. Friesewinkel O, Sorg S, Eckel L, Beyersdorf F. Immediate postoperative recovery of regional wall motion after unilateral and bilateral internal mammary artery revascularization. *Eur J Cardiothorac Surg* 1994; **8**: 395–9.
59. Kawasuji M, Tedoriya T, Takemura H, Sakakibara N, Taki J, Watanabe Y. Flow capacities of arterial grafts for coronary artery bypass grafting. *Ann Thorac Surg* 1993; **56**: 957–2.
60. Harris LJ, Crooke GA, LaMendola CL, Grossi EA, Baumann G, Esposito RA. Effects of graded reductions in internal mammary artery bypass flow on left ventricular function. *Ann Thorac Surg* 1993; **56**: 1348–50.
61. Hoffman JI, Buckberg GD. Pathophysiology of subendocardial ischaemia. *Br Med J* 1975; **1**: 76–9.
62. Orszulak TA, Schaff HV, Chesebro JH, Holmes DR. Initial experience with sequential IMA bypass grafts to the LAD and LAD-diagonal coronary arteries. *Mayo Clin Proc* 1986; **61**: 3–8.
63. Barner HB. Double internal mammary coronary artery bypass. *Arch Surg* 1974; **109**: 627–30.
64. Kay EB, Naraghipour H, Beg RA *et al.* Internal mammary artery bypass graft. Long term patency rate and follow up. *Ann Thorac Surg* 1974; **18**: 269–79.
65. Mills NL, Bringaze WL. Preparation of the internal mammary artery graft. Which is the best method? *J Thorac Cardiovasc Surg* 1989; **98**: 73–7.
66. Barner HB, Naunheim KS, Fiore AC, Fischer VW, Hariss HH. Use of the inferior epigastric artery as a free graft for myocardial revascularization. *Ann Thorac Surg* 1991; **52**: 429–36.
67. Dignan RJ, Yeh T, Dyke CM, Lutz HA, Wechsler AS. The influence of age and sex on human internal mammary artery size and reactivity. *Ann Thorac Surg* 1992; **53**: 792–7.
68. Suma H, Takeuchi A, Kondo K *et al.* Internal mammary artery grafting in patients with smaller body structure. *J. Thorac Cardiovasc Surg* 1988; **96**: 393–9.
69. Cooper GJ, Wilkinson GAL, Angelini GD. Overcoming perioperative spasm of the internal mammary artery: Which is the best vasodilator? *J Thorac Cardiovasc Surg* 1992; **104**: 465–8.
70. Green GE. Rate of blood flow from the internal mammary artery. *Surgery* 1971; **70**: 809–13.
71. Eckel L, Skupin M, Schräder R *et al.* Adequate flow through the internal mammary artery graft achieved with a dilatation technique. *Thorac Cardiovasc Surg* 1990; **38**: 157–60.
72. Singh RN, Sosa JA. Internal mammary artery. A 'live' conduit for coronary bypass. *J Thorac Cardiovasc Surg* 1984; **87**: 936–8.
73. Björk VO, Ivert T, Landou C. Angiographic changes in internal mammary artery and saphenous vein grafts 2 weeks, 1 year and 5 years after coronary artery bypass grafting. *Scand J Thorac Cardiovasc Surg* 1981; **15**: 23–30.
74. Ivert T, Huttunen K, Landou C, Bjork VO. Angiographic studies of internal mammary artery grafts 11 years after coronary artery bypass. *J Thorac Cardiovasc Surg* 1988; **96**: 1–12.
75. Kitamura S, Seki T, Kawachi K *et al.* Excellent patency and growth potential of internal mammary artery grafts in pediatric coronary artery bypass surgery. New evidence for a 'live' conduit. *Circulation* 1988; **78** (Suppl. I): I129–39.
76. Kitamura S, Kawachi K, Seki T *et al.* Bilateral internal mammary artery grafts for coronary artery bypass operations in children. *J Thorac Cardiovasc Surg* 1990; **99**: 708–15.
77. Spence PA, Lust RM, Zeri RS *et al.* Competitive flow from a fully patent coronary artery does not limit acute mammary graft flow. *Ann Thorac Surg* 1992; **54**: 21–5.
78. Lust RM, Zeri RS, Spence PA *et al.* Effect of chronic native flow competition on internal thoracic artery grafts. *Ann Thorac Surg* 1994; **57**: 45–50.
79. Suma H, Amano A, Fukuda S *et al.* Gastroepiploic artery graft for anterior descending coronary artery bypass. *Ann Thorac Surg* 1994; **57**: 925–7.
80. Suma H, Fukimoto H, Takeuchi A. Coronary artery bypass grafting by utilizing in-situ right gastroepiploic artery: Basic study and clinical application.

Ann Thorac Surg 1987; **44:** 394–7.
81. Mills NL, Everson CT. Right gastroepiploic artery: A third arterial conduit for coronary artery bypass. *Ann Thorac Surg* 1989; **47:** 706–11.
82. Milgalter E, Pearl JM, Laks H *et al.* The inferior epigastric arteries as coronary bypass conduits. Size preoperative duplex scan assessment of suitability and early clinical experience. *J Thorac Cardiovasc Surg* 1992; **103:** 463–5.
83. Dregelid E, Heldal K, Andersen KS, Stangeland L, Svendsen E. Dilatation of the internal mammary artery by external papaverine application to the pedicle. An improved method. *Eur J Cardiothorac Surg* 1993; **7:** 158–62.
84. Vander Salm TJ, Chowdhary S, Okike ON, Pezella AT, Pasque MK. Internal mammary artery grafts: The shortest route to the coronary artery. *Ann Thorac Surg* 1989; **47:** 421–7.
85. Wakabayashi A, Beron E, Lou MA *et al.* Physiological basis for systemic to coronary artery bypass graft: Inadequacy of the internal mammary artery for this purpose and appraisal of the ascending aorta as its proximal site. *Arch Surg* 1970; **100:** 17–19.
86. Tedoriya T, Kawasuji M, Ueyama K, Sakakibara N, Takemura H, Watanabe Y. Physiologic characteristics of coronary artery bypass grafts. *Ann Thorac Surg* 1993; **56:** 951–6.
87. Nishida H, Endo M, Koyanagi H, Nakamura K. Coronary artery bypass grafting with the right gastroepiploic artery and evaluation of flow with transcutaneous Doppler echocardiography. *J Thorac Cardiovasc Surg* 1994; **108:** 532–9.
88. Verkkala K, Järvinen A, Keto P, Virtanen K, Lehtola H, Pellinen T, Right gastroepiploic artery as a coronary bypass graft. *Ann Thorac Surg* 1989; **47:** 716–19.
89. Suma H, Takeuchi A, Hirota Y. Myocardial revascularisation with combined arterial grafts utilising the internal mammary and gastroepiploic arteries. *Ann Thorac Surg* 1989; **47:** 712–15.
90. Takayama T, Suma H, Wanibuchi Y, Tohda E, Matsunaka T, Yamashita S. Physiological and pharmacological responses of arterial graft flow after coronary artery bypass grafting measured with an implantable Doppler miniprobe. *Circulation* 1992; **86** (Suppl. II): II217–23.
91. Puig LB, Ciongolli W, Cividanes GV *et al.* Inferior epigastric artery as a free graft for myocardial revascularization. *J Thorac Cardiovasc Surg* 1990; **99:** 251–5.
92. Kusukawa J, Hirota Y, Kawamura K *et al.* Efficacy of coronary artery bypass surgery with gastroepiploic artery. Assessment with Thallium 201 myocardial scintigraphy. *Circulation* 1989; **80** (Suppl. I): I135–40.
93. Takayama T, Suma H, Wanibuchi Y. Postprandial flow physiology of the gastroepiploic artery graft. *J Thorac Cardiovasc Surg* 1992; **104:** 848–9.
94. Suma H, Wanibuchi Y, Terada Y, Fukuda S, Takayama T, Furata S. The right gastroepiploic graft. Clinical and angiographis midterm results in 200 patients. *J Thorac Cardiovasc Surg* 1993; **105:** 615–22.
95. Isomura T, Hisatomi K, Hirano A, Ohishi K, Inoue O, Kato H. The right gastroepiploic artery and its growth potential. *J Thorac Cardiovasc Surg* 1994; **108:** 592–3.
96. Suma H. Spasm of the gastroepiploic artery graft. *Ann Thorac Surg* 1990; **49:** 168–9.
97. Mills NL, Hockmuth DR, Everson CT. Robart CC. Right gastroepiploic artery used for coronary artery bypass grafting. Evaluation of flow characteristics and size. *J Thorac Cardiovasc Surg* 1993; **106:** 579–85.

7 Patient selection and contraindications

Alan J. Bryan and Nicholas T. Kouchoukos

Coronary artery bypass surgery has evolved over the last 25 years and can now be performed expeditiously with low operative risk. There is a general perception that the increased application of arterial conduits in myocardial revascularization may lead to improvements in early and late patient outcome.[1,2] This has been based on the established favourable impact of the pedicled left internal thoracic artery (ITA) graft anastomosed to the left anterior descending coronary artery (LAD) on graft patency, need for reoperation and late survival.[3] While the use of a single ITA graft to the LAD may be regarded as standard practice,[4] the indications and selection of patients for additional arterial conduits can only be based on the outcome of well organized clinical research.[2] In particular, modifications in operative technique which might potentially increase early morbidity and mortality or increase operative time inordinately, may not be justified as routine procedures[1] despite the promise of late improvements in clinical outcome. Currently, technical skills and knowledge of long-term outcome are evolving but are still incomplete for some of the more recently introduced arterial conduits.

Factors influencing the use of arterial conduits

A multitude of factors interact to provide a rational basis for surgeons to use the arterial conduits currently available for myocardial revascularization. Principal among these is the overall benefit to the patient, which is largely dependent upon early and late graft patency. While a significant body of knowledge now exists about the late performance of ITA grafts, the long-term patency of the right gastroepiploic artery (GEA) and inferior epigastric artery (IEA) and other potential arterial grafts is not known. It is important to recognize that both early and late patency may be subject to variables which reflect more than just different biological characteristics of particular conduits. A conduit which is technically difficult to harvest and prepare or implant may occlude early, despite excellent biological characteristics which would predict optimal late patency.[5] An example of this is the reduced early patency of free ITA grafts, which has been attributed to difficulties with the proximal aortic anastomosis;[6] this appears still to reduce overall patency.[7] Similarly, early experience routing right ITA grafts through the transverse sinus produced unsatisfactory results,[8] although increasing experience suggests that these problems have been largely resolved.[7]

The interest and experience of individual surgeons may be an important consideration, and only procedures that can be completed without large increases in operating time and are within the range of technical competence of the majority of surgeons are ever likely to become widely applicable.[9] More complex arterial reconstructions inevitably require relatively long myocardial ischaemic times.[7] A further confounding influence is that if certain arterial conduits are used only in situations where other conduits are scarce or in other specific but rare situations, then lack of experience and familiarity with their use may result in less satisfactory outcomes.

Many patient-related variables will also influence patterns of usage of arterial grafts. Clearly, the age of the patient should be considered, since in the very elderly, in particular, the simplest procedure which gives the best early outcome should be used in most instances. One of the more common factors which determines the use of arterial conduits is the lack of suitable venous conduit (i.e. greater and lesser saphenous vein), since reoperations account for up to 20 per cent of all myocardial revascularization procedures in some North American centres.[1] Diabetes mellitus and obesity may also dissuade surgeons from use of additional arterial conduits, since use of bilateral internal thoracic artery grafts is associated with increased wound infection.[10–12] A number of other factors may need to be considered, and these will be discussed further in relation to each conduit.

Vascular disease within arterial conduits themselves or in the vessels from which they originate should also be considered as a potential contraindication to their use. This would include atherosclerosis, dissection or arteritis. Finally, the precise coronary anatomy and the biological significance of certain aspects of the atherosclerotic disease may influence the use of arterial conduits. It is clear that the favourable impact of the left ITA graft to the LAD coronary artery is based not only on the excellent characteristics of the graft, but also on the biological importance of the LAD. This has been cited as the dominant influence on outcome after coronary artery bypass grafting.[1,13] This may explain in part the apparent lack of positive survival benefits from the addition of further arterial grafts. Lack of sufficient length of certain arterial grafts may also limit their usefulness.

It is clear that factors that may influence an individual surgeon's choice of material for grafting, either arterial or venous, are many. These are related not only to the surgeon's skill or familiarity with a particular conduit, but also to the characteristics of the conduit and the particular patient, as well as anatomical aspects of the coronary arterial system.

Left ITA graft

A large body of information now exists regarding the use of the left ITA graft. The experience from the Cleveland Clinic provided the first data which demonstrated the superiority of the left ITA over the saphenous vein graft when anastomosed to the LAD coronary artery.[3] Since the mid 1980s, this graft has been widely used[4] and it is employed in a large percentage of revascularization procedures in the UK[14] and North America.[4] There are now few contraindications to its use.[15]

Atherosclerosis of the ITA is relatively rare, occurring in 2–6 per cent of individuals evaluated by angiography.[16–18] Thus the suitability of the left ITA for use as a bypass graft is judged primarily by the free flow observed after harvesting. Duplex ultrasound imaging of the artery before operation can provide information about patency and flow.[19] However, the low incidence of abnormalities mitigates against its routine use in preoperative evaluation. Duplex ultrasound may be of more value in reoperative surgery when there is uncertainty about the integrity and size of the ITA. Acute dissection of the ITA, either in localized areas[20] or in its entirety, may occur, and significant haematomas in the ITA pedicle should be viewed with suspicion. Dissection of the ITA can be largely avoided by careful mobilization but can result in sudden death if it occurs early postoperatively.[21] If there is any suspicion of dissection, the left ITA should be discarded. Anatomical anomalies of the left ITA are relatively common[22] but few of these lead to any significant modification of the surgical procedure, or preclude its use. While some investigators have encouraged the use of routine angiography of the ITA,[22] few centres actually practise this, because it is expensive and probably unnecessary. More careful assessment of the ITA is required in patients with widespread vasculopathy. Clinical assessment should always include auscultation for bruits at the base of the neck and measurement of the blood pressure in both arms as crude indicators of potentially reduced ITA flow (Fig. 7.1). It has been demonstrated in a small number of patients that percutaneous transluminal angioplasty (PTA) of significant subclavian stenoses to increase ITA flow can be undertaken before or after myocardial revascularization, with good results.[23] However, the long-term function of pedicled left ITA grafts after PTA of the subclavian artery is unknown. A significant incidence of restenosis might be anticipated.[24] The occurrence of catastrophic lower limb ischaemia after left ITA harvesting, when this vessel forms an important collateral in the presence of an obstructed aorta–iliac system, has been reported, and this possibility should be borne in mind when use of the ITA is contemplated in patients with severe vascular disease.[25,26] Similarly, the ITA should not be used as a pedicled graft in patients with dissection involving the aortic arch.

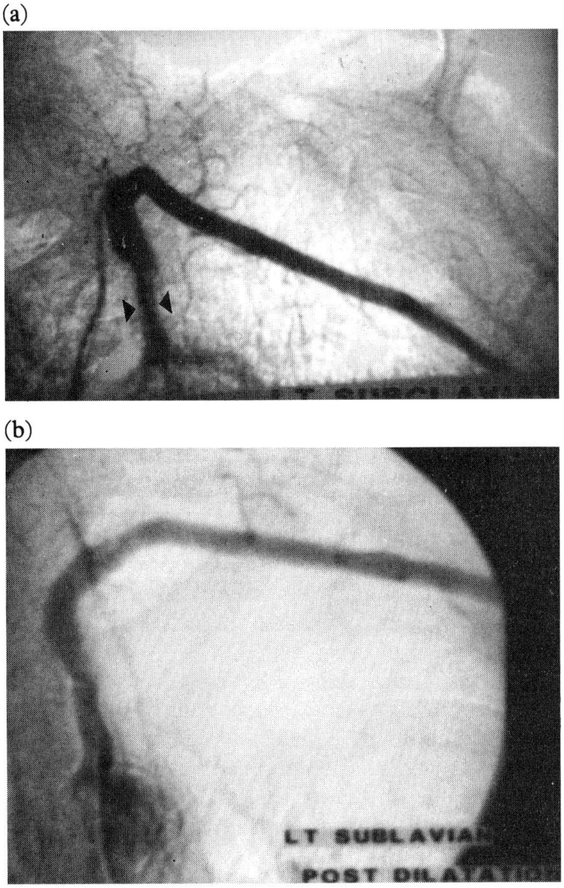

Fig. 7.1 (a) Digital subtraction angiogram showing haemodynamically significant proximal left subclavian stenosis; and (b) satisfactory immediate post-angioplasty appearances.

Deformities of the chest wall or previous thoracic operations may contraindicate use of the ITA. Severe pectus excavatum may make harvesting of the ITA technically difficult. Previous anterior or lateral thoracotomy for trauma or other indications may have damaged the left ITA. Irradiation of the chest wall for mediastinal or breast malignancies may injure the ITA. Arteritis can develop both in the ITA and in the coronary circulation, and although the ITA has been used successfully in this situation,[27] others have advocated caution.[15] Extensive pleural or pericardial involvement with asbestosis can make mobilization of the ITA difficult or impossible.

Age is not a contraindication to the use of the ITA,[28–30] and the observation that short-term as well as long-term outcome after operation is improved with its use[31,32] obviates the argument that improvements in long-term survival is the only major benefit of the ITA graft. In our view, the poor quality of the available vein, and the increased prevalence of substantial atherosclerosis in the ascending aorta in elderly patients provides additional justification for the use of at least one ITA graft in the elderly.

The clinical status of the patient is important and in emergency situations, prompt revascularization is essential.[15] In haemodynamically unstable patients cardiopulmonary bypass should be instituted first and then ITA mobilization may follow;[33] although this can be considered as a contraindication to arterial grafting[1,15] it is still often possible. The most common situation in which this arises is failed angioplasty. Reports suggest that even in this group, a significant proportion of patients (40–85 per cent) may undergo left ITA grafting with excellent survival.[33–36] It is unclear at present whether the use of reperfusion catheters results in improved myocardial salvage.[35,36] Recently published data demonstrates that patients who receive an ITA graft during emergency surgery or following a failed percutaneous transluminal coronary angioplasty (PTCA) have a reduced mortality.[31,32] In two recent studies, operative mortality was reduced in all subgroups who received an ITA graft when compared to those patients who received vein grafts only. This included patients with poor left ventricular function, recent infarction and left main coronary artery disease.[31,32] There now appears to be fewer recognized contraindications to the use of ITA grafts than in the past.[37,38] A note of caution is required since, while such analyses are useful, they may still be subject to the effects of factors beyond the limits of the analysis – they are not prospective randomized trials. However, in any clinical situation the ultimate decision regarding operative strategy rests with the operating surgeon to judge what is likely to result in the best early outcome for an individual patient.

Although the surgical group of the Cleveland Clinic has advocated the use of ITA grafts in reoperations,[39] they have shown that replacing a stenotic vein graft to an occluded LAD coronary artery with an ITA graft results in a significant increase in morbidity and mortality. This presumably is the result of inadequate blood flow through the ITA graft and hypoperfusion of the myocardium.[39] When this situation exists three options are available: to leave the stenotic vein graft in continuity, to add a graft to the LAD or to add a vein graft to a diagonal branch of the LAD.

A further relative contraindication to the use of the left ITA graft is to territories other than the LAD coronary artery, when the LAD is not significantly diseased. Some investigators have argued that the native left ITA should be preserved, since progression of native coronary disease might necessitate reoperation for LAD disease. We believe that the use of left ITA graft to the circumflex system represents an optimal primary operation and that reoperation will be necessary in only a small proportion of patients. Anatomically the left ITA has sufficient length to revascularize any of the branches of the left coronary system[40] and further advantage may be gained by careful routing or lengthening procedures.[40–42] If reoperation on the LAD is required, the right ITA could still be used providing it was not used in the initial operation.

Bilateral, sequential and complex ITA grafting

The indications for more complex ITA grafting are less clear. This is partly because of variability in the ways in which arterial conduits are used and the fact that in general, the series reported represent highly selected groups of patients operated on by individuals or in centres with high levels of expertise.[7,8,43–45] Barner has alluded to some of the problems associated with multiple arterial grafts, and cautions against over-zealous application.[9] Several authors have suggested that if one arterial graft is good, then two or three may be better.[1,2] However, arriving at a definitive answer may be more difficult.

Bilateral ITA grafting is not associated with increased operative risk[44] though similarly in the medium term it has shown little benefit.[13] In the long term there is the suggestion that overall symptom relief and risk of reoperation may be improved[43,46,47] but late survival benefits remain unclear.[48] Overall, this leads us to conclude that these procedures are predominantly indicated in young patients with well preserved left ventricular function though what this constitutes in exact chronological terms is open to debate. Bilateral ITA grafting has been widely used in reoperations particularly in situations where conduit is scarce, since it does not apparently increase operative risk and can yield excellent results.[49,50]

If the ascending aorta is severely atherosclerotic (Fig. 7.2), calcified (Fig. 7.3) or aneurysmal, it may not be possible or advisable to anastomose vein grafts to it, and manipulation and clamping should be minimized. In this setting, bilateral pedicled ITA grafts or complex arterial grafting techniques based on pedicled grafts may be of particular value.[51] In the setting of acute dissection of the ascending aorta,

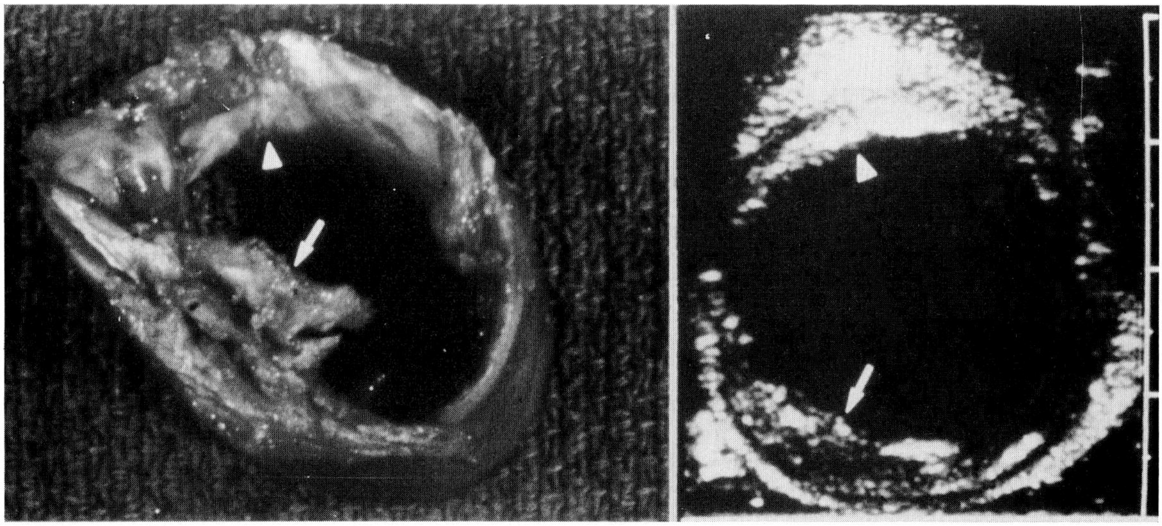

Fig. 7.2 Severely atherosclerotic ascending aorta resected at operation (left); atherosclerotic plaques, arrowed, presented with accompanying intraoperative epivascular ultrasound image (right). Reproduced with permission from Wareing *et al.*[79]

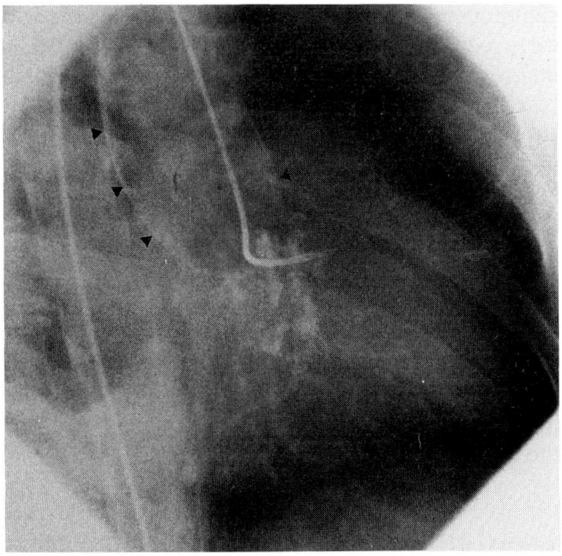

Fig. 7.3 Severe calcification of the ascending aorta ('Porcelain aorta') in an elderly female requiring concomitant aortic valve replacement and myocardial revascularization; arterial grafts may be particularly indicated in this situation to avoid proximal aortic anastomoses.

particularly when all of the dissection is not excised, there is a risk of subclavian dissection and flow through pedicled grafts may be compromised.

A further indication for extensive use of ITA grafts is in patients with Kawasaki syndrome, where accelerated atherosclerosis in saphenous vein grafts is particularly problematic, given the young age of the patients.[52] A clear survival benefit with the use of the left ITA graft has been demonstrated and arterial conduits should be used whenever possible.[52]

The use of sequential ITA grafting has been advocated by several groups using both internal thoracic arteries in a variety of complex configurations, including T-grafts and Y-grafts with excellent results.[53,54] The most widely used sequential configurations are those involving two marginal branches of the circumflex artery or the LAD and its diagonal branch.[45,55] A successful outcome requires appropriate judgement, attention to the detail of surgical technique and suitable anatomy.[56]

This use of bilateral ITA grafting may be somewhat limited by excluding obese or diabetic patients and the very elderly where the risk of significant wound infection appears to be elevated.[10–12,43] The weight of evidence suggests that bilateral ITA grafting does increase wound problems, at least in certain subgroups, and that this in itself may result in morbidity and indeed mortality.[32]

Based upon the foregoing observations, bilateral ITA grafting should be applied liberally in young patients, in patients in whom other conduit is scarce or unavailable, in reoperations or where lower extremity vein may be required for peripheral vascular reconstructions. While more complex ITA grafting procedures involving multiple distal anastomoses are appealing, they should be used selectively and by those with the technical expertise to achieve consistently excellent results.[45,55,56].

Right GEA graft

This graft has been in clinical use for more than 5 years and there have been many short-term reports of satisfactory early results.[57–60] The long-term results are unknown and further observational studies with careful follow-up involving angiography are necessary. The precise role of the GEA in myocardial revascularization is unclear but its greatest application so far has been as a pedicled graft to branches of the right coronary system. It can be used in other coronary territories[61] but experience has shown that its use as a free graft may be associated with lower patency,[57] presumably due to technical difficulties with the proximal anastomosis to the aorta.[57,60] Some have favoured free grafts and argue for their potential advantages which, it is suggested, might include greater ease of axial orientation and haemostasis.[62] In addition, late reoperation with elevation of the heart may necessitate division of the conduit with a pedicled graft, and subsequent upper abdominal surgery does not entail any risk of graft injury if a free graft is used.

While it inevitably adds to the operative time, harvesting the GEA is not difficult and does not increase operative risk.[63] Early and medium term patency rates of pedicled GEA grafts are excellent.[57] Whether preoperative superior mesenteric angiography is necessary prior to use of the GEA, particulary in patients with abdominal aortic atherosclerosis, is unclear.[64] It is probably not necessary on a routine basis since atherosclerosis in the artery itself is very uncommon[65] and in only about 5 per cent of patients will use of the GEA be impossible due to its small anatomical size.[57] A flow of less than 50 ml/min after intraluminal papaverine is regarded as the lowest recommended flow for use of the graft.[57]

Previous abdominal surgery and obesity are only

relative contraindications to its use and there are now several reports of successful upper abdominal and gastric surgery in patients who have undergone previous GEA grafting.[66,67]

The GEA is established as a useful arterial graft predominantly in young patients where total arterial revascularization is the aim.[7] It also has a major role in reoperations if conduit is scarce and in procedures where proximal aortic anastomoses need to be avoided, e.g. severe atherosclerosis or calcification of the ascending aorta.[68,69]

IEA graft

This conduit has been evaluated for a relatively short period,[70] and as a consequence reported experience is much less than with other arterial grafts.[70–72] However, there is sufficient information to define broadly its likely application. Two IEA grafts may be used, again most commonly in young patients where total revascularization is the aim or when conduit is scarce in reoperations.[70–72] Ultrasound and histological assessment has shown it to be largely free of atheroma and when this occurs it is limited to the proximal portion, adjacent to the external iliac artery.[70–74] It can only be used as a free graft and early patency is clearly inferior to pedicled ITA or GEA grafts.[72,73] Despite encouraging early results from some centres, poor results reported from at least one excellent unit (early patency rate 60 per cent) dictates caution in its use.[5] Since a proximal anastomosis is required it might be anticipated that the reduced early patency is related to the proximal anastomosis as it may be with free ITA grafts.[6] The IEA has limited length, the mean being around 10–12 cm, and for this reason its use is largely limited to revascularization of the proximal right, diagonal and high circumflex branches[71] though it has also been used as a T-graft or a Y-graft.[71] For the present, when other arterial conduits are available such as the ITA, these should be preferred, particularly for revascularization of the LAD system.

Radial artery and other arterial conduits

Early experience with the radial artery graft reported failure rates of 35–60 per cent with short-term follow-up.[75–77] However, a recent re-evaluation of this conduit by Acar *et al.* applying contemporary preparation techniques, resulted in early patency in 29 of 31 grafts at 6–13 months with no incidence of upper extremity ischaemia.[78] These results suggest that the radial artery may represent another alternative conduit and further reports of its use are awaited.

A number of other arterial conduits, including the splenic artery, the subscapular artery and the lateral costal and intercostal arteries have been used successfully for myocardial revascularisation, either reported as single cases or in small numbers of patients. In all of the above, the overall level of knowledge makes it impossible to define specific indications for their use, except to say that they are bound to be limited, given the number and scope of the other arterial conduits now available.

Conduit selection for total arterial revascularization

As we have already indicated, there are two main groups of patients where extensive use of arterial conduits may be justified: young patients and patients in whom other suitable conduits are absent or scarce. In most young patients bilateral ITA grafts to the LAD and circumflex systems and a GEA graft to the right coronary system could be considered an optimal combination.[7] In diabetics and in the obese, the left ITA only should be used to reduce the risk of sternal complications, and can be supplemented by the right GEA[57] or an IEA graft if appropriate. Use of both ITA grafts and both IEAs may not be advisable since superficial necrosis of the abdominal wall has been reported.[70] In general, strategies entailing several arterial inflows are to be recommended[9] rather than multiple sequential anastomoses[45] or reliance on single ITA inflow.[53]

In reoperative situations and where conduit is scarce, bilateral ITA grafting still represents the simplest and most effective option, if both arteries are available. Use of alternative arterial conduits depends on their availability, the coronary anatomical requirements, and the skill and experience of the operator.

References

1. Orszulak TA. Are arterial grafts better or worse than applied physiology teaches? *Ann Thorac Surg* 1993; **56:** 809–11.

2. Angelini GD, Bryan AJ. Extending the use of arterial conduits in myocardial revascularisation. *Br Heart J* 1992; **68:** 161–2.
3. Loop FD, Lytle BW, Cosgrove DM *et al.* Influence of the internal mammary artery graft on 10 year survival and other cardiac events. *New Engl J Med* 1986; **314:** 1–6.
4. Kirklin JW and Subcommittee on Coronary Artery Bypass Graft Surgery. Guidelines and indications for coronary artery bypass graft surgery [ACC/AMA Task Force]. *J Am Coll Cardiol* 1991; **17:** 543–89.
5. Perrault LP, Carrier M, Hebert Y, Cartier R, Leclerc Y, Pelletier LC. Early experience with the inferior epigastric artery in coronary artery bypass grafting. *J Thorac Cardiovasc Surg* 1993; **106:** 928–30.
6. Loop FD, Lytle BW, Cosgrove DM *et al.* Free (aorta-coronary) internal mammary artery graft. Late results. *J Thorac Cardiovasc Surg* 1986; **92:** 827–31.
7. Dion R, Etienne PY, Verhelst R *et al.* Bilateral mammary grafting – clinical, functional and angiographic assessment in 400 consecutive patients. *Eur J Cardiothorac Surg* 1993; **7:** 287–94.
8. Rankin JS, Newman GE, Bashore TM *et al.* Clinical and angiographic assessment of complex mammary artery bypass grafting. *J Thorac Cardiovasc Surg* 1986; **92:** 832–46.
9. Barner HB. Use of the internal thoracic artery: simple, complex, or with a backup? *Ann Thorac Surg* 1994; **57:** 8–9.
10. Loop FD, Lytle BW, Cosgrove DM *et al.* Sternal wound complications after isolated coronary artery bypass grafting: early and late mortality, morbidity and cost of care. *Ann Thorac Surg* 1990; **49:** 179–87.
11. Kouchoukos NT, Wareing TH, Murphy SF, Pelate C, Marshall WG. Risks of bilateral internal mammary artery bypass grafting. *Ann Thorac Surg* 1990; **49:** 210–19.
12. He G-W, Ryan WH, Acuff TE *et al.* Risk factors for operative mortality and sternal wound infection in bilateral internal mammary artery grafting. *J Thorac Cardiovasc Surg* 1994; **107:** 196–202.
13. Morris JJ, Smith R, Glower DD *et al.* Clinical evaluation of single versus multiple mammary artery bypass. *Circulation* 1990; **82** (Suppl. IV): IV214–23.
14. Izzat MB, West RR, Bryan AJ, Angelini GD. Coronary artery bypass surgery: current practice in the United Kingdom. *Br Heart J* 1994; **71:** 382–5.
15. Loop FD, Lytle BW, Cosgrove DM. New arteries for old. *Circulation* 1989; **79** (Suppl I): I40–5.
16. Singh RN. Atherosclerosis and the internal mammary arteries. *Cardiovasc Intervent Radiol* 1983; **6:** 72–7.
17. Kryne R, Deng MCHK, Heinrich KW, Sons H, Krian A. Semiselective angiography of the internal mammary artery as a preparation for coronary bypass surgery. *Am J Cardiol* 1990; **66:** 377–8.
18. Sons HJ, Godehardt E, Kunert J, Losse B, Bircks W. Internal thoracic artery: prevalence of atherosclerotic changes. *J Thorac Cardiovasc Surg* 1993; **106:** 1192–5.
19. Canver CC, Ricotta JJ, Bhayana JN, Fiedler RC, Mentzer Jr RM. Use of duplex imaging to assess suitability of the internal mammary artery for coronary artery surgery. *J Vasc Surg* 1991; **13:** 294–301.
20. Treasure T. Damage to an internal mammary graft at dissection. *Br Heart J* 1993; **70:** 390.
21. Dougenis D, Robinson MC, Brown AH. Acute dissection of the internal mammary artery; a fatal complication of coronary artery bypass grafting. *J Cardiovasc Surg* (Torino)1990; **31:** 589–591.
22. Bauer EP, Bino MC, von Segesser LK, Laske A, Turina M. Internal mammary artery anomalies. *Thorac Cardiovasc Surg* 1990; **38:** 312–15.
23. Perrault LP, Carrier M, Hudon G, Lenarbre L, Hebert Y, Pelletier LC. Transluminal angioplasty of the subclavian artery in patients with internal mammary grafts. *Ann Thorac Surg* 1993; **56:** 927–30.
24. McGrath LB (Invited commentary of Perrault LP *et al*). *Ann Thorac Surg* 1993; **56:** 930.
25. Kitamura S, Inoue K, Kawachi K *et al.* Lower extremity ischaemia secondary to internal thoracic coronary artery bypass grafting. *Ann Thorac Surg* 1993; **56:** 157–9.
26. Dietzek AM, Goldsmith J, Veith FJ. Interruption of critical aortoiliac collateral circulation during nonvascular operations: A case of acute limb threatening ischemia. *J Vasc Surg* 1990; **12:** 645–53.
27. van Son JAM, Noyez L, van Asten WNJC. Use of internal mammary artery in myocardial revascularisation after mediastinal irradiation. *J Thorac Cardiovasc Surg* 1992; **104:** 1539–44.
28. Wareing TH, Saffitz JE, Kouchoukos NT. Use of single internal mammary artery grafts in older patients. *Circulation* 1990; **82** (Suppl. IV): 224–8.
29. Azariades M, Fessler CL, Floten HS, Starr A. Five-year results of coronary bypass grafting for patients older than 70 years: role of internal mammary artery. *Ann Thorac Surg* 1990; **50:** 940–5.
30. Mullany CJ, Darling GE, Pluth JR *et al.* Early and late results after isolated coronary artery bypass surgery in 159 patients aged 80 years and older. *Circulation* 1990; **82** (Suppl. IV): 229–36.
31. Edwards FH, Clark RE, Schwartz M. Impact of internal mammary artery conduits on operative mortality in coronary revascularisation. *Ann Thorac Surg* 1994; **57:** 27–32.
32. Grover FL, Johnson RR, Marshall G, Hammermeister KE, Department of Veterans Affairs Cardiac Surgeons. Impact of mammary grafts on coronary bypass operative mortality and morbidity. *Ann Thorac Surg* 1994; **57:** 559–69.
33. Caes FL, van Nooten GJ. Use of internal mammary artery for emergency grafting after failed coronary angioplasty. *Ann Thorac Surg* 1994; **57:** 1295–9.

34. Zapolinski A, Rosenblum J, Myler RK *et al.* Emergency coronary artery bypass surgery following failed balloon angioplasty: role of the internal mammary artery graft. *J Cardiac Surg* 1991; **6:** 439–48.
35. Ferguson TB, Hinohara T, Simpson J, Stack RS, Wechsler AS Catheter reperfusion to allow optimal coronary bypass grafting following failed transluminal coronary angioplasty *Ann Thorac Surg* 1986; **42:** 399–405.
36. Kereiakis DJ, Abbottsmith CW, Callard GM, Flege JB Emergent internal mammary artery grafting following failed percutaneous transluminal angioplasty: Use of transluminal catheter reperfusion *Am Heart J* 1987; **113:** 1018–20.
37. Lefrak EA The internal mammary artery bypass graft: praise versus practice *Tex Heart Inst J* 1987; **14:** 139–43.
38. Angelini GD, Bryan AJ, West RR, Newby AC, Breckenridge IM Coronary artery bypass surgery: Current practice in the United Kingdom *Thorax* 1989; **44:** 721–4.
39. Navia D, Cosgrove DM, Lytle BW *et al* Is the internal thoracic artery the conduit of choice to replace a stenotic vein graft? *Ann Thorac Surg* 1994; **57:** 40–4.
40. Vander Salm TJ, Chowdhary S, Okike ON, Pezzella AT, Pasque MK Internal mammary artery grafts: The shortest route to the coronary arteries *Ann Thorac Surg* 1989; **47:** 421–7.
41. Cosgrove DM, Loop FD Techniques to maximise mammary artery length *Ann Thorac Surg* 1985; **40:** 78–9.
42. Pacifico AD, Sears NJ, Burgos C Harvesting, routing and anastomosing the left internal mammary artery graft *Ann Thorac Surg* 1986; **42:** 708–10.
43. Galbut DL, Traad EA, Dorman HJ *et al* Seventeen year experience with bilateral internal mammary artery graft *Ann Thorac Surg* 1990; **49:** 195–201.
44. Lytle BW, Cosgrove DM, Loop FD, Borsh J, Goormastic M, Taylor PC Perioperative risk of bilateral internal mammary artery grafting analysis of 500 cases from 1971–1984 *Circulation* 1986; **74** (Suppl. III): III37–52.
45. van Sterkenberg SMM, Ernst SMPG, Brutel de la Riviere A *et al* Triple sequential grafts using the internal mammary artery: An angiographic and short-term follow-up study *J Thorac Cardiovasc Surg* 1992; **104:** 60–5.
46. Cameron A, Kemp Jr MG, Green GE Bypass surgery with the internal mammary artery graft: 15 year follow up *Circulation* 1986; **74** (Suppl. III): III30–I6.
47. Fiore AC, Naunheim KS, Dean P *et al* Results of internal thoracic artery grafting over 15 years: Single versus double grafts *Ann Thorac Surg* 1990; **49:** 202–9.
48. Naunheim KS, Barner HB, Fiore AC 1992 update: Results of internal thoracic artery grafting over 15 years: Single versus double grafts *Ann Thorac Surg* 1992; **53:** 716–18.
49. Loop FD, Lytle BW, Cosgrove DM Bilateral internal thoracic artery grafting in reoperations *Ann Thorac Surg* 1991; **52:** 3–4.
50. Galbut DL, Traad EA, Dorman HJ Bilateral internal mammary artery grafts in reoperative and primary coronary bypass surgery *Ann Thorac Surg* 1991; **52:** 20–8.
51. Peigh PS, DiSesa VJ, Collins Jr JJ, Cohn LM Coronary bypass grafting with totally calcified or acutely dissected ascending aorta *Ann Thorac Surg* 1991; **5:** 102–4.
52. Kitamura S, Kameda Y, Seki T *et al* Long term outcome of myocardial revascularisation in patients with Kawasaki coronary artery disease *J Thorac Cardiovasc Surg* 1994; **107:** 663–74.
53. Tector AJ, Amundsen S, Schmal TM, Kress DC, Peter M Total revascularisation with T grafts *Ann Thorac Surg* 1994; **57:** 33–9.
54. Slater AD, Gott JP, Gay Jr LA Extended use of bilateral internal mammary arteries for coronary artery disease *Ann Thorac Surg* 1990; **49:** 1014–15.
55. Palatianos GM, Bolooki H, Horowitz MD *et al* Sequential internal mammary artery grafts for coronary artery bypass *Ann Thorac surg* 1993; **56:** 1136–40.
56. Jones EL, Lattouf O, Lutz JF, King SB Important anatomical and physiological considerations in performance of complex mammary coronary artery operations *Ann Thorac Surg* 1987; **43:** 469–77.
57. Suma H, Wanibachi Y, Terada Y, Fukuda S, Takayama T, Furuta S The right gastoepiploic artery graft. Clinical and angiographic midterm results in 200 patients *J Thorac Cardiovasc Surg* 1993; **105:** 615–23.
58. Grandjean JG, Boonstra PW, den Heyer P, Ebels T. Arterial revascularisation with the right gastroepiploic artery and internal mammary arteries in 300 patients *J Thorac Cardiovasc Surg* 1994; **107:** 1309–16.
59. Perrault LP, Carrier M, Hebert Y *et al.* Clinical experience with the right gastrepiploic artery in coronary artery bypass grafting *Ann Thorac Surg* 1993; **56:** 1082–4.
60. Lytle BW, Cosgrove DM, Ratliff NB, Loop FD. Coronary artery bypass grafting with the right gastrepiploic artery *J Thorac Cardiovasc Surg* 1989; **97:** 826–31.
61. Suma H, Amano A, Fukuda S *et al.* Gastroepiploic artery graft for anterior descending coronary artery bypass *Ann Thorac Surg* 1994; **57:** 925–7.
62. Barner HB New arterial conduits for coronary bypass surgery *Thorac Cardiovasc Surg* 1994; **6:** 76–80.
63. Suma H, Wanibuchi Y, Furuta S, Takeuchi A. Does use of the gastroepiploic artery graft increase surgical risk? *J Thorac Cardiovasc Surg* 1991; **101:** 121–5.

64. Mills NL (Discussion of Suma H *et al*). *J Thorac Cardiovasc Surg* 1993; **105:** 615–23.
65. Suma H, Wanibuchi Y, Furuta S, Isshiki T, Yamaguchi T, Takanashi R. Comparative study between the gastroepiploic and the internal thoracic artery as a coronary bypass graft *Eur J Cardiothorac Surg* 1991; **5:** 244–7.
66. Perrault LP, Rheault MJ, Carrier M. Total gastrectomy in a patient with an *in situ* right gastroepiploic artery graft *Ann Thorac Surg* 1994; **57:** 751–2.
67. Terada Y, Suma H. Cholecystectomy after coronary artery bypass grafting using right gastroepiploic artery *Ann Thorac Surg* 1994; **57:** 1369–74.
68. Suma H. Coronary artery bypass grafting in patients with calcified ascending aorta: aortic no-touch technique *Ann Thorac Surg* 1989; 48: 728–30.
69. Mills N, Everson C. Atherosclerosis of the ascending aorta and coronary artery bypass pathology, clinical correlates and operative management *J Thorac Cardiovasc Surg* 1991; **102:** 546–53.
70. Puig LB, Ciongolli W, Cividanes GV *et al.* Inferior epigastric artery as a free graft for myocardial revascularisation *J Thorac Cardiovasc Surg* 1990; 99: 251–5.
71. Barner HB, Naunheim KS, Fiore AC, Fischer VW, Harris HH. Use of the inferior epigastric artery as a free graft for myocardial revascularisation *Ann Thorac Surg* 1991; **52:** 429–37.
72. Buche M, Schoevaerdts JC, Louagie Y *et al.* Use of the inferior epigastric artery for coronary bypass *J Thorac Cardiovasc Surg* 1992; **103:** 665–70.
73. Cremer J, Mugge A, Schulze M *et al.* The inferior epigastric artery for coronary bypass grafting. Functional assessment and clinical results *Eur J Cardiothorac Surg* 1993; **7:** 423–7.
74. Milgalter E, Laks H, Elami A, Louie H, Permut L, Baker JD. Preoperative Duplex scan assessment of the inferior epigastric artery as a coronary bypass conduit *Ann Thorac Surg* 1991; **52:** 567–8.
75. Carpentier A, Guermonprez JL, Deloche A *et al.* The aorta-to-coronary radial artery bypass graft *Ann Thorac Surg* 1973; **16:** 111–18.
76. Curtis JJ, Stoney WS, Alford WC. Jr Intimal hyperplasia: A cause of radial artery to aorto-coronary bypass graft failure *Ann Thorac Surg* 1975; **20:** 628–35.
77. Fisk RL, Brooks CH, Callaghan JC, Dvorkin J. Experience with the radial artery graft for coronary artery bypass *Ann Thorac Surg* 1976; 21: 513–18.
78. Acar C, Jebara VA, Portoghese M *et al.* Revival of the radial artery for coronary bypass grafting: Revival of an old conduit *Ann Thorac Surg* 1992; **54:** 652–60.
79. Wareing TH, Davila-Roman VG, Barzilai B *et al.* Management of the severely atherosclerotic ascending aorta during cardiac operations: a strategy for detection and treatment. *J Thorac Cardiovasc Surg* 1992; **103:** 453–62.

Part II
Internal thoracic artery

8 Surgical Techniques

Robert Dion and Gianni D. Angelini

In recent years the internal thoracic artery (ITA) has become the universally accepted conduit of choice for coronary artery bypass surgery.[1,2] Its superior long-term patency rate over saphenous vein has been attributed to the fact that the ITA is a 'living graft'. The functional viability of the ITA depends to a large extent on the way it is mobilized, prepared and anastomosed for grafting. Several important considerations should therefore be taken into account:

1. dissection of the ITA should be performed to eliminate or minimise any possible damage to its vascular walls;
2. the maximum length of ITA should be mobilized to be used for multiple distal anastomoses;
3. early ITA flow should be maximized to maintain adequate myocardial perfusion and function;
4. the ideal mediastinal and epicardial course should be chosen together with reliable anastomotic techniques to optimize the result of sequential ITA grafts.

Mobilization of the ITA pedicle

In most routine coronary surgery, mobilization is performed prior to exposure of the heart and institution of cardiopulmonary bypass. All the pericardial dissection is completed and the isthmus of the thymus is divided. A retractor is then used to lift the appropriate side of the divided sternum to expose the ITA. Several retractors have been designed specifically for this purpose and fall into two groups:

1. Table-mounted retractors like the Favaloro[3] and the Omnitract,[4] although providing excellent exposure, take time to set up, tend to intrude in the operating field and require complex manoeuvres to move them aseptically if both ITAs need to be mobilized. Injury to the lower trunk of the brachial plexus and the radial nerve in the spiral groove has also been reported in association with the use of table-mounted retractors.[5]
2. Other types, similar to sternal retractors, work on the principal of lifting and everting the sternal edge on the side of the ITA to be mobilized while depressing the opposite side[5,6,7]. They are much less cumbersome to use and can be readily transferred to the opposite side without the potential for wound contamination.

Sternal retraction can be improved by dividing the attachment of the diaphragm to its lower end and by mobilizing slightly the strap muscles from the back of the sternum until its top border can be visualized. Once the sternum has been lifted the reflection of the mediastinal pleura is dissected from the anterior chest wall, following which a pleurotomy extending from the apex near the subclavian vein to the diaphragm is performed. The outlines of the ITA can be seen through the endothoracic fascia. Some surgeons advocate leaving the pleura intact using extrapleural access to reduce the incidence of postoperative pleural effusion and hemidiaphragm impairment.[8] This technique, however, tends to displace the ITA pedicle anteriorly and may produce undesirable angulation by the inflated upper lobe of the lung. The medial aspect of the endothoracic fascia is then incised at the most accessible portion of the ITA, usually at the level of the middle and distal third.

Techniques of dissection vary and there may be almost as many methods as there are cardiac surgeons. Electrocautery (coagulation) is undoubtedly the most widely used method in the 'en bloc' technique where the entire vascular pedicle is taken down with about 1–2 cm of surrounding tissue on either side. Excessive heat, causing separation of the intima has been reported[9] and an optimal crest factor current of 10–11 has been recommended to prevent this from happening.[10] Caution is also needed to prevent the electrocautery blade touching the ITA wall, or coming into contact with a haemostat metal clip placed at the base of a major side branch of the ITA. A combination of electrocautery and ultrasonic aspiration has also been described to reduce bleeding and shorten the mobilization time.[11]

With smooth-tipped forceps the endothoracic fascia is then drawn away and peeled down from the chest wall using frequent, gentle pushes with the flat of the (non-operational) electrocautery blade. At this stage perforating intercostal branches can be identified, clipped and divided and downward traction applied gently to facilitate distal dissection. As the pedicle falls away from the chest wall the surgeon's finger or a tape can be passed around it and downward traction applied gently to facilitate distal dissection to beyond the ITA bifurcation. The larger of the two branches (usually the superior epigastric artery) may be used for anastomosis. If both branches are of good calibre the ITA may be used as a Y-graft to two adjacent coronary arteries. The dissection is then continued upward to the level of the first intercostal vessels which are divided in the same manner. The advantages of the 'en bloc' technique are its ease, the fact that mobilization can be carried out without handling the artery directly and the theoretical preservation of venous and lymphatic drainage.

Some surgeons prefer the isolated or 'skeleton' technique where the ITA is identified at a convenient point as it crosses a costal cartilage (where there are no branches) and directly dissected out. The artery is then followed proximally and distally by meticulous dissection, clipping and dividing every branch. Bipolar diathermy can be used to cauterize branches. The advantage of this technique is that it yields more graft length by freeing the artery of surrounding tissue. A combination of the 'en bloc' and 'skeleton' techniques can be used; the block of tissue surrounding the ITA is divided at 2–3 cm intervals down to the arterial wall. To gain additional mobility and length of the ITA pedicle, the large penetrating thymic branches of the internal thoracic vein can be divided. However, attention should be paid to spare the pericardiophrenic artery, the first branch of the ITA serving as the major blood supply to the phrenic nerve.[12] Dissection of the ITA can be extended up to its origin with the subclavian artery. In situations where there is hyperinflation of the lung obscuring visualization of the ITA–subclavian junction, cardiopulmonary bypass can be instituted allowing deflation of the lung and easy access to the most proximal portions of the ITA. However, the possibility of injury to the phrenic nerve that lies medially and posterior to the ITA pedicle must be appreciated. After systemic heparinization, the ITA pedicle distal to the bifurcation is divided and a soft vascular clamp placed across the bleeding end.

Flow considerations

The greater patency rate of ITA grafts compared to saphenous vein grafts has often been attributed to the ability of the ITA to adapt to changes in blood flow demand by the myocardium.[13–15] This vasoreactivity, however, also accounts for the vasospasm and flow reduction which follows mobilization of the ITA. Under normal haemodynamic conditions flow through the ITA is laminar and is governed by the systemic arterial blood pressure and the resistance imposed by the artery.[16] The scope to alter the blood pressure in order to improve the ITA's flow is limited by the need to maintain a balance between myocardial perfusion and work. The resistance to flow offered by the ITA is related to the viscosity of the blood, the length and radius of the artery and the coronary resistance. Given that the first two factors and the coronary resistance are outside the surgeon's control, the radius of the artery is the only parameter amenable to change. Since the resistance to flow is inversely proportional to the fourth power of the radius, dilating the ITA will produce a major increase in flow. Therefore various pharmacological and physical methods have been proposed to overcome perioperative spasm of the ITA.

Pharmacological approach to vasospasm

After mobilization, vasospasm often reduces flow through the ITA and little spontaneous improvement occurs in the time prior to granting.[17,18] A time-honoured method of relaxing the ITA and increasing flow is to wrap it in a papaverine-soaked swab. More recently, however, *in vitro* studies on

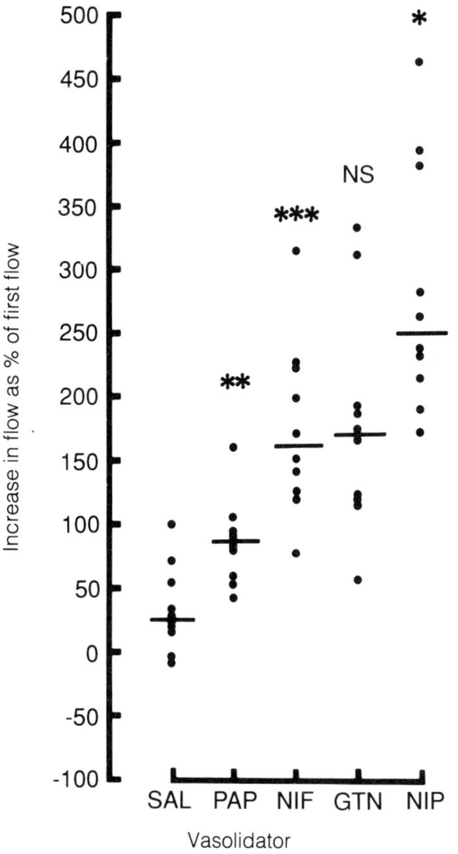

Fig. 8.1 ITA free flow expressed as percentage of control. SAL = normal saline; PAP = papaverine; NIF = nifedipine; GTN = glyceryl trinitrate; NIP = sodium nitroprusside. **P* <0.05; ***P* <0.01; ****P* <0.001 versus previous group. Reproduced with permission from Cooper *et al.*[17]

the reactivity of the ITA have suggested that glyceryl trinitrate and calcium antagonists may be superior to papaverine in relieving ITA spasm.[19,20] The isolated ITA contracts strongly in response to thromboxane and α-adrenoceptor agonists. Glyceryl trinitrate rapidly fully relaxes a precontracted ITA but it seems to be a very weak inhibitor if applied before the constrictor stimulus. Calcium entry blocking drugs and in particular nifedipine have a slow onset but fully relax precontracted ITA. These observations suggest that perioperative spasm is best prevented by pretreatment with calcium entry blocking drugs or specific receptor antagonists. If spasm occurs perioperatively glyceryl trinitrate will rapidly relax the tissue regardless of the nature of the constrictor stimulus. The poor response of the ITA to β-adrenoceptor[20] stimulation

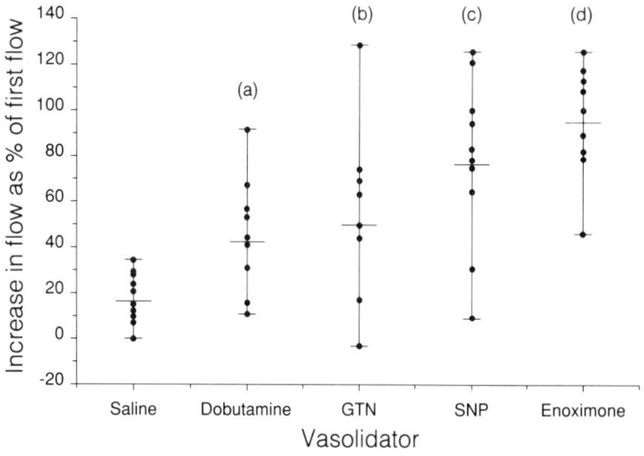

Fig. 8.2 ITA free flow expressed as a percentage of control. (a) = $P<0.1$ (vs normal saline); (b) = $P=0.02$ (vs normal saline); (c) = $P<0.05$ (vs dobutamine and normal saline); (d) = $P<0.01$ (vs dobutamine, GTN and normal saline). SAL = normal saline; GTN = glyceryl trinitrate; SNP = sodium nitroprusside. Reproduced with permission from Izzat *et al.*[18]

also implies that perioperative administration of catecholamine or sympathicomimetic amines are unlikely to dilate the ITA. These *in vitro* observations were recently tested in the clinical setting. A study on the effect of topical vasodilators on the ability to overcome ITA spasm showed that papaverine, with a modest 70 per cent increase in free flow, was the least effective of the agents investigated.[17] Nifedipine and glyceryl trinitrate raised flow by 160 per cent. Sodium nitroprusside, however, with an increase in free flow of 250 per cent over control proved to be the most effective vasodilator (Fig. 8.1). The beneficial effect of topical vasodilators is, however, only temporary and may not prevent postoperative spasm of the ITA. In a recent clinical study[18] glyceryl trinitrate and sodium nitroprusside relieved ITA spasm when administered systemically. Both these agents, however, were not as effective as enoximone, a phosphodiesterase-III inhibitor (with a half-life of 3 hours)[21] which, when administered as a single bolus dose, produced the greatest increase in ITA free flow (Fig. 8.2).

Physical approach to vasospasm

Several physical means have been used to improve flow through the ITA. Amongst these are gentle massage of the pedicle, wrapping of the artery in a warm swab, injection of saline into the tissue adjacent to the ITA and the use of an appropriate size probe or a balloon catheter to dilate the entire length of the artery[22–25] Hydrostatic pressure has also been employed by using an olive-tip cannula to inject heparinized saline or other solution intraluminally.[24,26] All these methods are usually rewarded with a dramatic improvement in flow. The main concern about their use is that they may cause injury to the vessel wall, thereby compromising the early and late patency of the ITA. Probing of the ITA in the dog causes endothelial cell loss and impaired release of prostacyclin and endothelium-derived relaxing factor.[27] The reduced production of both these factors, which are important modulators of vascular tone and inhibitors of platelet adhesion and aggregation, may predispose the ITA to postoperative spasm and early graft thrombosis.[28–30] More recently intraluminal dilatation with dilute papaverine has been shown to produce a dramatic increase in ITA free-flow to a mean value of 229 ml/min, greater than the flow achieved with any other method.[26] This, however, poses the question of whether the increase in flow is due to the vasodilator action of the papaverine or is the direct consequence of overstretching of the smooth muscle cells in the ITA medial layer. Hydrostatic dilatation of the porcine ITA is known to produce disruption and fenestration of the internal elastic lamina and functional damage to the media.[31,32] A direct consequence of this may be a decreased capacity to generate adenosine, a potent vasodilator and antiplatelet aggregating factor.[33–34] Injury to the media which is known to stimulate smooth muscle cell proliferation fundamental to the development of intimal hyperplasia in saphenous vein grafts may have implications for the long-term performance of the ITA graft.[35–37] This may be further enhanced by disruption of the internal elastic lamina which in undamaged ITA is considered to act as a barrier to proliferation and suppression of intimal thickening.[1,38]

Techniques of anastomosis

Care is taken to keep the opening into the ITA somewhat longer than that into the coronary vessel, which is usually 3–4 mm in length. The 'parachute' technique and a running stitch of 8/0 Prolene suture is used for all of the ITA anastomoses.

Classical longitudinal anastomoses

Coronary vessel coursing towards the surgeon (sagittal plane) (Fig. 8.3)

If the heel of the anastomosis is considered as the

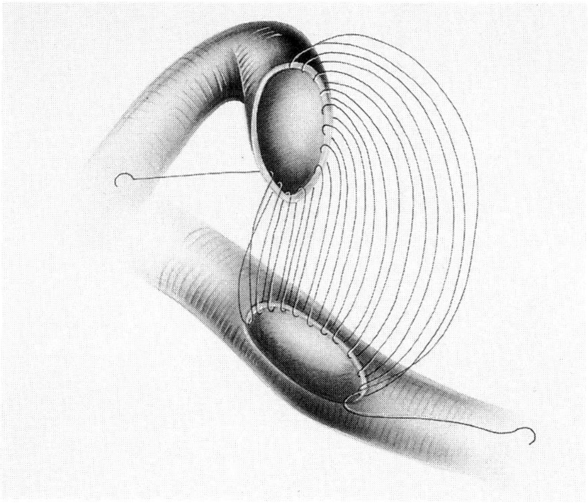

Fig. 8.3 Longitudinal end-to-side anastomosis in the length: the coronary vessel courses towards the surgeon (sagittal plane).

'six o'clock' spot, the first stitch is passed through the ITA wall from inside to outside at 'seven o'clock' and that part of the suture is clipped with rubber-shoed 'mosquito' forceps. The anastomosis is then continued counterclockwise, with the use of the other end of the suture, and care taken to pass the needle through the coronary artery wall from inside to outside. When the toe of the anastomosis is reached, the ITA is brought down to the coronary vessel by gently pulling both ends of the suture, and the second half of the anastomosis is performed *in situ*. The knot of the suture is therefore situated at 'seven o'clock'. Indeed, one should avoid placing a knot or a 'U'-shaped stitch at the heel and/or on the toe of an anastomosis. Also, the spacing of the stitches should be considerably reduced at these two sites (at least three or four stitches). By respecting these rules, we have never detected a so-called 'purse-string' effect in our angiographic restudies.[39,40]

Coronary vessel coursing in a frontal plane (Fig. 8.4)

Generally from the left to the right side of the surgeon, i.e. in the case of a wide angled diagonal artery. If the toe of the anastomosis is considered as the 'three o'clock' spot, the first stitch is passed through the ITA wall from inside to outside at 'two o'clock' and then clipped with rubber-shoed 'mosquito' forceps. The anastomosis is then continued clockwise, using the other end of the suture and care taken to pass the needle through the coronary artery wall from inside to outside. When the heel of the

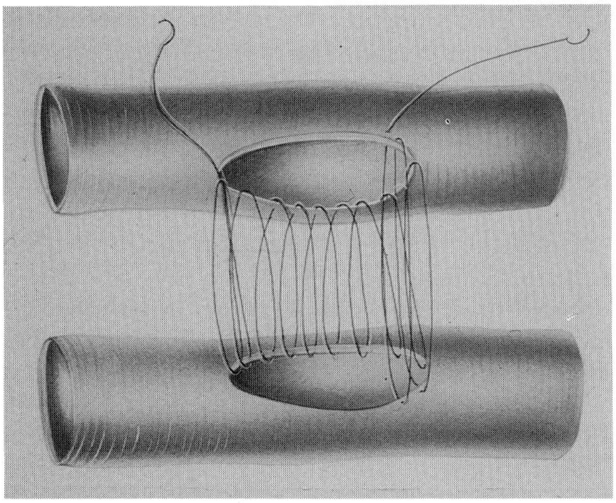

Fig. 8.4 Longitudinal side-to-side anastomosis: the coronary vessel courses in a frontal plane.

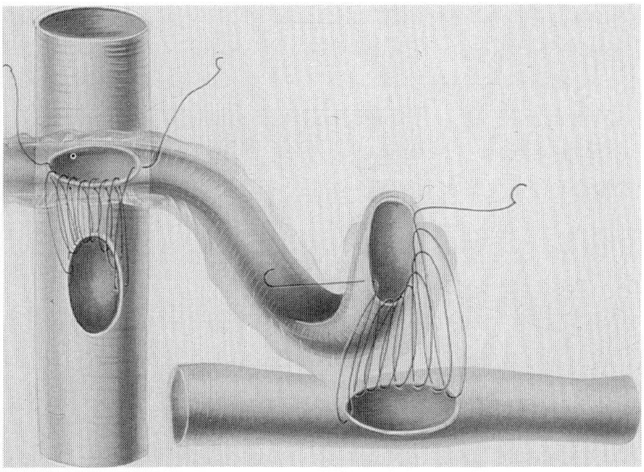

Fig. 8.5 Diamond-shaped anastomoses with the coronary vessels coursing in the sagittal plane (left) and in the frontal plane (right).

anastomosis is reached, the ITA is brought down to the coronary vessel by gently pulling both ends of the suture. The running stitch is then continued until the mid point between toe and heel. The other needle is then used again and passed from outside to inside the ITA wall (at 'two o'clock'), and the anastomosis is then completed, the tie being placed at the mid point of the lateral wall of the vessels.

Diamond shape anastomoses

Coronary vessel coursing towards the surgeon (Fig. 8.5)

The first stitch goes from outside to inside at the toe of the ITA arteriotomy, then from inside to outside at the mid point of the 'right' lateral wall of the coronary arteriotomy ('three o'clock'). The running suture continues clockwise towards the heel of the coronary vessel ('six o'clock') and further to the opposite 'left' lateral wall ('nine o'clock'). The ITA is then brought down to the coronary vessel by pulling on both ends of the suture. The last half of the anastomosis is then completed, counter-clockwise, starting with a 'U' shaped stitch (outside–inside the ITA) at 'three o'clock'. The knot is situated at 'nine o'clock', well away from the inflow and outflow sites of the coronary arteriotomy.

Coronary vessel coursing in a frontal plane (Fig. 8.5)

The first stitch goes from outside to inside near the mid point of the 'right' lateral wall of the ITA arteriotomy ('four o'clock'), then from inside to outside just over the toe of the coronary arteriotomy. The running suture continues clockwise until the heel of the coronary arteriotomy is reached. The ITA is then brought down by pulling on both ends of the suture. The suture is then continued clockwise only as far as the mid point between toe and heel of the coronary arteriotomy. The other needle is then passed through the ITA wall from outside to inside at 'four o'clock' ('U'-shaped stitch), and the anastomosis is completed by a couterclockwise running suture. The tie is placed at the mid point of the coronary arteriotomy, again well away from the inflow and the outflow sites of the coronary arteriotomy.

In our experience, the patency rates of those diamond-shaped anastomoses at 6 and at 13 months were 94.5 per cent and did not differ from those of the 'longitudinal' anastomoses.[39,40] The use of diamond-shaped anastomoses yields two major advantages: first, it helps to economize on the length of a pedicled ITA, and second it does not give rise to preferential flow towards the distal part of the coronary vessel. For instance, following sequential grafting of one or more diagonal arteries, the extremity of the left ITA pedicle may have to be anastomosed to a somewhat distal segment of the LAD coronary artery while the stenosis of this vessel may be quite proximal; in this configuration, a 'T' (diamond-shaped) anastomosis is to be preferred, because it should ensure equal perfusion of the LAD segments on each side of the anastomosis, while a 'longitudinal' anastomosis might preferentially perfuse the smaller distal territory (Fig. 8.6).

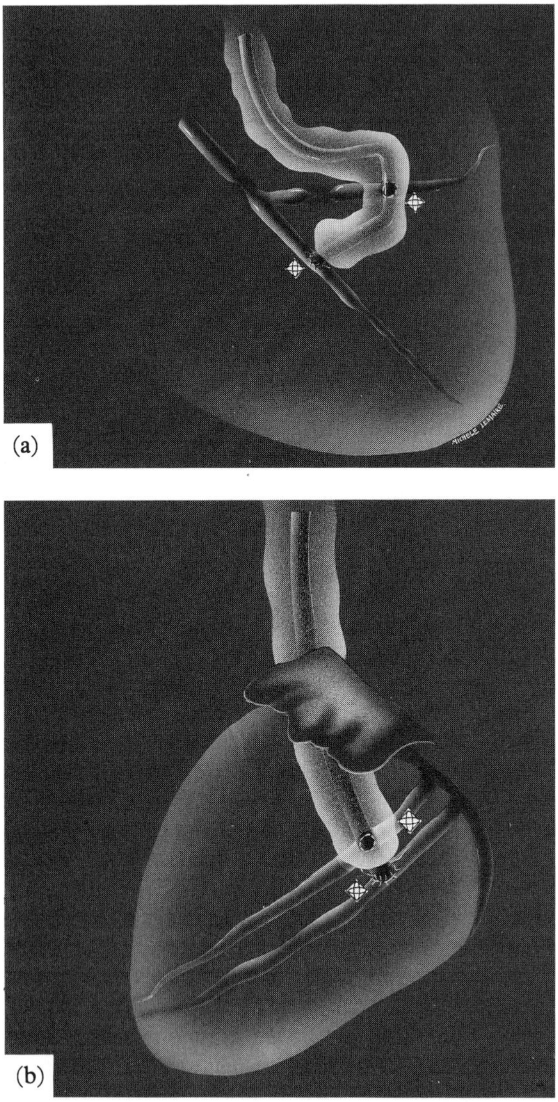

Fig. 8.6 Sequential diamond-shaped anastomoses (⊕): how they contribute to economy in ITA length and avoidance of placing an anastomosis on too distal a segment of LAD. (a) = left ITA to diagonal and LAD; (b) = right ITA to first and second circumflex arteries.

Sequential anastomoses

Sequential grafting is essential if a pedicled ITA graft is to be optimized.[41–43] In the LAD coronary artery area, we start with the most proximal side-to-side anastomosis: indeed the distance between the diagonal branches and the LAD will not increase with the filling of the heart, because the graft then parallels the solid interventricular septum. By contrast, in the circumflex area, we usually first graft the most dominant vessel to be revascularized, even if it is the most distal one; after completion of that important anastomosis, we decide about the other one(s) taking into account the remaining length of the ITA pedicle, the level of the arteriotomy(ies) on the other vessel(s), and last but not least, the potential increase of the heart diameter in the short axis after filling.

Side-to-side anastomoses may be constructed either longditudinally or in a diamond-shaped fashion; in the latter, the length of the coronary arteriotomy should not exceed the diameter of the ITA to avoid flattening of the anastomotic site. The ITA is approached through a generous 2 cm longitudinal incision in the ventral aspect of the pedicle, to prevent undesirable angulation due to the thickness of the pedicle. When sequential anastomoses are close to each other (≤2 cm), we prefer to incise the ventral aspect of the pedicle all along from the proximal anastomosis to the distal one. In a similar manner to sequential saphenous vein grafting, we prefer to place the distal anastomosis on the most dominant coronary vessel.

Coronary endarterectomy

In our experience, endarterectomy of the left coronary system is needed in approximately 5 per cent of cases. A venous hood is then used to close the long coronary arteriotomy and the ITA is then implanted into it as previously described (Fig. 8.7).[44] Where

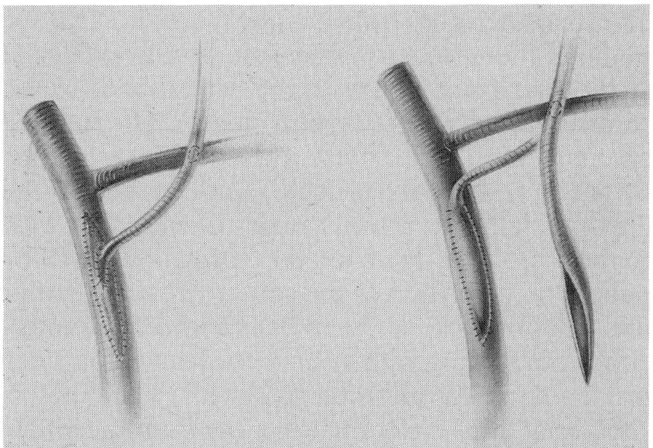

Fig. 8.7 Use of ITA after extensive coronary endarterectomy: (left) via a venous hood: easy anastomosis and economy of ITA length; (right) danger of flattening the narrow ITA over the extensive and broad coronary arteriotomy after endarterectomy; loss of ITA length.

extensive endarterectomy of the LAD area is required, we do not hesitate to supplement the ITA with a saphenous vein graft in order to provide immediately an optimal flow to the whole area of perfused myocardium.

Free ITA grafts

In a recent review of our first 127 free ITA grafts, we found a patency rate at 6 and at 13 months (84.6 per cent), significantly lower than that of pedicled ITA grafts (95 per cent): 67 had been anastomosed to the ascending aorta, either directly using a running suture of 7/0 Prolene, or via a venous hood when the aortic wall was judged unsuitable for direct suture (Fig. 8.8), with a patency rate of 80 per cent. In 60 cases, free grafts had been anastomosed to the proximal segment of a saphenous vein graft or to another ITA graft (8/0 Prolene) resulting in a patency rate of 88.8 per cent. However, we suspect that the proximal anastomosis is not the only factor responsible for this early attrition. Indeed, the segment of ascending aorta that is usually chosen for the proximal anastomosis of all free grafts (including saphenous vein grafts) is probably the least suitable part of the whole arterial system: the ascent of the systolic head of pressure (*dp/dt*) is there the highest, and, simultaneously, the coronary resistance is at its peak due to the contraction of the myocardium. This situation might favour disruption of the endothelium and the internal elastic lamina of free grafts and result in early intimal hyperplasia.

Loop *et al.*[45] reported similar patency rates within 18 months of operation. Hanet *et al.*[46,47] have suggested that the physiological adaptability of the free ITA graft is comparable to that of the pedicled graft. Van Son[48] has demonstrated that *vasa vasorum* of the ITA are confined to the adventitia, implying that using an ITA as a free graft should not induce any wall ischaemia. Furthermore, Aarnio *et al.*[49] have shown similar prostacyclin production in free and pedicled ITA grafts. These data tend to indicate that, beyond the early failures, free ITA graft patency rate should parallel that of the pedicled graft. Nevertheless, we tend to restrict their use, and, if we have no alternative, we anastomose them nowadays to the other pedicled ITA (8/0 Prolene), as reported by Calafiore *et al.* (Fig. 8.8 (right)).[50]

Strategy in ITA grafting

The longer the ITA pedicle, the smaller its calibre. Furthermore, the distal part of the ITA is known to be more muscular and less elastic, and therefore more prone to develop spasm and atherosclerosis. Therefore, it is important to minimize the length of ITA between its origin from the subclavian artery and the first distal anastomosis. In our experience, we achieve this by opening the ipsilateral pleura and by incising vertically the pleura and the pericardium down to the phrenic nerve. Other advantages of this manoeuvre are that the ITA pedicle then lies under the lung and away from the sternum, and that the pericardium, prolonged by the pleural fat, can easily be approximated at the end of the procedure. A variety of techniques to maximize the length of the pedicled ITA has been described.[51] We prefer a longitudinal incision of the ventral aspect of the pedicle onto the ITA itself from the distal end to the subclavian artery. (Fig. 8.9) The ITA vein can also

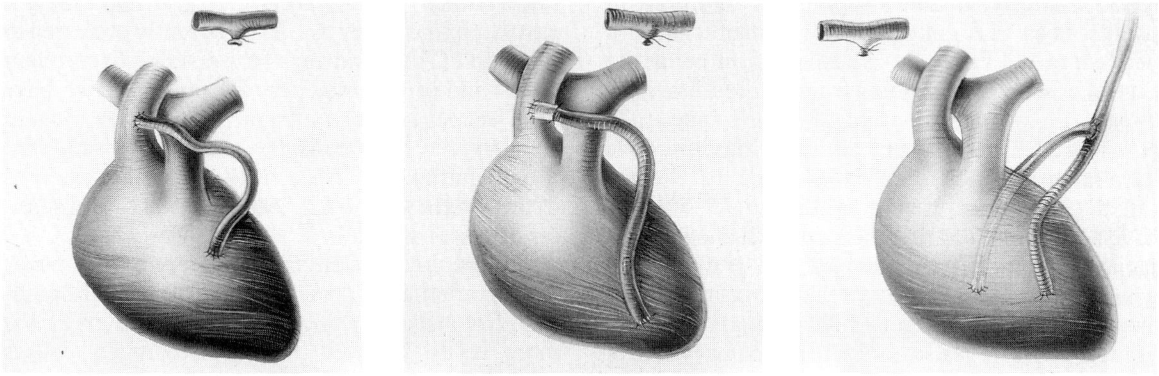

Fig. 8.8 Free ITA grafts; the three different types of proximal anastomosis: directly into the ascending aorta (left); via a venous hood (middle); into the other pedicled ITA artery (right).

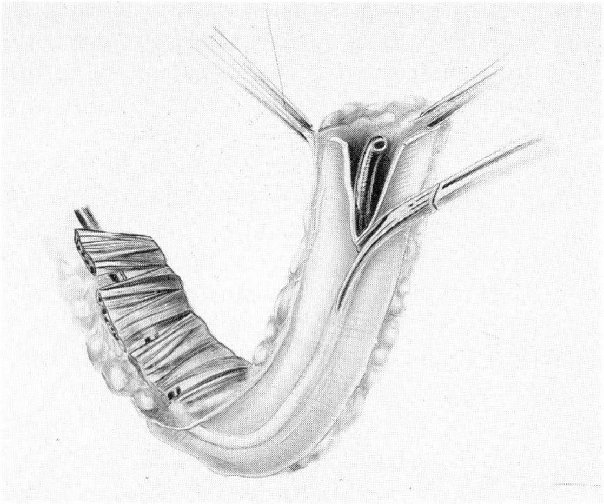

Fig. 8.9 Technique of maximizing the length of pedicled ITA.

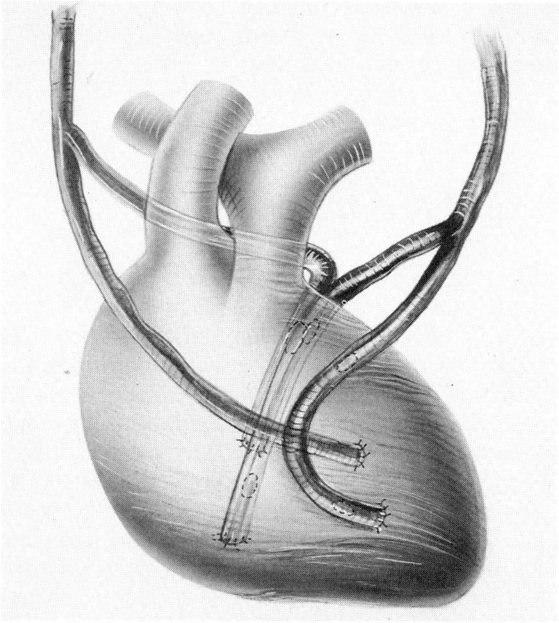

Fig. 8.10 Routing of left and right pedicled ITA arteries.

be divided as it drains into the innominate vein. These manoeuvres can provide additional length of up to 3 cm. Coronary artery disease may be progressive and so arterial grafts should be evenly distributed over the myocardium. Construction of sequential grafts should avoid grafting two adjacent coronary vessels with two different arterial grafts. Also, the anastomoses should be placed distal to any coronary lesion of significance, especially on the LAD and, here again, sequential grafting must be considered in doubtful cases.

Unlike many authors,[42,52–55] we have not taken into account the adequacy of ITA free cut-end flow, possible calibre discrepancy, the lack of a high-grade proximal coronary stenosis, or the amount of myocardium revascularized, even before sequential grafting.[39] However, we have not hesitated, intraoperatively, to add a saphenous vein graft in parallel to an ITA graft if ITA flow insufficiency (2 per cent of all ITA grafts) is suspected, either at the time of or soon after weaning from cardiopulmonary bypass. Following this strategy we have practically eliminated the occurrence of early postoperative haemodynamic deterioration ascribed to the so-called 'ITA insufficiency syndrome'.[53,55,56] We have been convinced that this approach allows more patients to benefit from complex ITA grafting than would do so if we respected the above-mentioned exclusion criteria. Angiographic restudy of these 'double grafts' reveals an 88 per cent patency rate of both the ITA and saphenous vein grafts to the same vessel. We, like others,[57–59] believe that the left ITA can maintain no-flow patency until saphenous vein graft failure occurs. Construction of diamond-shaped and sequential anastomoses and directing the right ITA through the transverse sinus[60] has enabled us to reperfuse an increasing number of coronary vessels with pedicled ITA grafts (*see* Fig. 8.10). Like Rankin,[54] we anastomose ITAs 'not so much to the best vessels, but to the best myocardium'. Our preferred grafting strategy consists of directing the left ITA to the LAD-diagonal area and the right ITA to the other most *dominant* diseased coronary vessel(s). In recent years, our initial strategy of complex ITA grafting has evolved into a strategy of complex arterial grafting: the right gastroepiploic artery (GEA) is currently preferred to the right ITA for grafting of the distal right coronary artery and/or its branches. By doing so, we have been encouraged to find that the patency rates of right ITA to right coronary – initially[39] somewhat disappointing (83.3 per cent) – returned to the level of those right ITA to LAD and right ITA to circumflex artery (Table 8.1).[40]

If more than one circumflex artery branch needs to be grafted and, provided that there is no significant diagonal artery to be reperfused, the left ITA is more easily directed to the circumflex vessels (diamond-shaped anastomoses), the right ITA then being anastomosed to the LAD area. We then protect the right ITA pedicle from the sternum using a

Table 8.1 Angiographic patency of ITA anastomoses. Correlation with grafted coronary vessel and with type of conduit. Patency rates were compared using the likehood ratio statistic G^2

	Pedicled left ITA			*Pedicled right ITA*		
	Restudied	*Patent*	*[%]*	*Restudied*	*Patent*	*[%]*
LAD	232	225	96.9	42	40	95.2
CX	45	43	95.6	90	86	95.2
RCA	–	–	–	31	29	93.5
Total	277	268	96.7	163	155	95.1
			NS (96.7 vs 95.1)			

LAD vs CX: NS

LAD vs CX, LAD vs RCA, CX vs RCA: NS

ITA = internal mammary artery; LAD = left anterior descending; CX = circumflex; RCA = right coronary artery.

pleuropericardial flap. More recently a sleeve made of Goretex (Preclude IMA Sleeve, W.L. Gore & Associates Inc., Flagstaff, AZ 86002–00500, USA) has been used for protection to allow easier identification of the right ITA pedicle at reoperation. If an ITA has to be used as a free graft, our current preference is for a proximal anastomosis into the other pedicled ITA.

Obviously, our confidence in applying ITAs to the whole spectrum of grafting situations has allowed us to maintain a flexible approach, and base our operative strategy on the intraoperative findings, thus enhancing the versatility of the conduit.

Our recent angiographic re-study[40] has been very encouraging with an average patency rate of ITA anastomoses after 13 months of 94.5 per cent. This was identical to that found after 6 months in a previous report[39] confirming our belief that the attrition rate of ITA anastomoses is minimal after the early months following surgery. Complex ITA grafting easily reaches the anterior and posterolateral walls of the left ventricle. In triple-vessel disease, the adjunct of right GEA grafting (complex arterial grafting) is often needed – currently in 18 per cent of our patients – to reach the inferior vessels. In an ideal operative situation i.e. in an elective case with no significant co-morbid disorder, every significant diseased coronary vessel should receive an arterial graft, (preferably pedicled). Saphenous vein grafts should be restricted to less dominant vessels when complete revascularization is needed.

References

1. Angelini GD, Bryan AJ. Extending the use of autologous arterial conduits in myocardial revascularisation. *Br Heart J* 1992; **68:** 161–2.
2. Lytle BW, Loop FD, Cosgrove DM, Ratliff NB, Easley K, Taylor PC. Long-term (5 to 12 years) serial studies of internal mammary artery and saphenous vein coronary grafts. *J Thorac Cardiovasc Surg* 1985; **89:** 248–58.
3. Favaloro RG. Unilateral self-rataining retractor for use in internal mammary artery dissection. *J Thorac Cardiovasc Surg* 1967; **53:** 864–5.
4. Pittman J, Fehrenbacher J, Pittman S, Beckman D. Improved visualisation of the internal mammary artery with a new retractor system. *Ann Thorac Surg* 1989; **48:** 869–70.
5. Brown EH, Dougenis D. Dissection of the two internal mammary arteries with minimal exposure and minimal adverse sequelae by means of an inexpensive, simple atraumatic retractor. *J Thorac Cardiovasc Surg* 1991; **102:** 753–6.
6. Angelini GD, Azzu AA. A retractor for harvesting the internal mammary artery, incorporating a fibreoptic transillumination system. *Ann Thorac Surg* 1990; **50:** 314–15.
7. Choux A, Blanche C. A new concept in sternal retraction: applications for internal mammary artery dissection and valve replacement surgery. *Ann Thorac Surg* 1986; **42:** 473–4.
8. Noera G, Pensa PM, Guelfi P, Biagi B, Lodi R, Carbone C. Extrapleural takedown of the internal mammary artery as a pedicle. *Ann Thorac Surg* 1991; **52:** 1292–4.

9. Lehtola A, Verkkola K, Järvinen A. Is electrocautery safe for internal mammary artery (IMA) mobilisation? A study using scanning electron microscopy (SEM). *Thorac Cardiovasc Surgeon* 1989; **37:** 55–7.
10. Mills NL. Physiological and technical aspects of internal mammary artery coronary artery bypass graft In: Cohn LH ed. *Modern techniques in surgery: cardiac – thoracic surgery*. Mount Kisco, New York: Futura Publishing Co Inc, 1982; 1–19.
11. Suma H, Fukumoto H, Takeuchi A. Application of ultrasonic aspirator for dissection of the internal mammary artery in coronary artery bypass grafting. *Ann Thorac Surg* 1987; **43:** 676–7.
12. O'Brien JW, Johnson SH, Van Steyn SJ *et al.* Effect of internal mammary artery dissection on phrenic nerve perfusion and function. *Ann Thorac Surg* 1991; **52:** 182–8.
13. Singh RN, Beg RA, Kay EB. Physiological adaptability: the secret of success of the internal mamary artery grafts *Ann Thorac Surg* 1986; **41:** 247–50.
14. Kitamura S, Kawachi K, Seki T *et al.* Bilateral internal mamary artery grafts for coronary artery bypass operations in children. *J Thorac Cardiovasc Surg* 1990; **99:** 708–15.
15. Ivert T, Huttunen K, London C, Bjork VO. Angiographic studies of internal mammary artery grafts 11 years after coronary artery bypass. *J Thorac Cardiovasc Surg* 1988; **96:** 1–12.
16. Dobrin P, Canfield T, Moran J, Sullivan J, Pifarré R. Coronary artery bypass. The physiological basis for differences in flow with internal mammary artery and saphenous vein grafts. *J Thorac Cardiovasc Surg* 1977; **74:** 445–54.
17. Cooper GJ, Wilkinson GAL, Angelini GD. Overcoming perioperative spasm of the internal mammary artery: which is the best vasodilator? *J Thorac Cardiovasc Surg* 1992; **104:** 465–8.
18. Izzat MB, West RR, Ragoonanan C, Angelini GD. Effect of systemic vasodilators on internal mammary artery. Implications for postoperative treatment after myocardial revascularisation. *J Thorac Cardiovasc Surg* 1994; **108:** 82–5.
19. He GW, Rosenfeldt FL, Buxton BF, Angus JA. Reactivity of human isolated internal mammary artery to constrictor and dilator agents Circulation 1989; **80** (Suppl. I): 141–50.
20. He GW, Buxton B, Rosenfeldt FL, Wilson AC, Angus JA. Weak beta-adrenoceptor-mediated relaxation in the human internal mammary artery. *J Thorac Cardiovasc Surg* 1989; **97:** 259–66.
21. Installe E, Gonzalez M, Jacquemart JL *et al.* Comparative effects on hemodynamics of enoximone, dobutamine and nitroprusside in severe congestive heart failure. *Am J Cardiol 1987;* **60:** 46C–52C.
22. Nashef SAH, Angelini GD. Preparation of the internal mammary artery. *Br J Hosp Med* 1990; **45:** 339–42.
23. John LCH, Edmondson SJ, Rees GM. Modified technique of internal mammary artery harvest. *Ann Thorac Surg* 1991; **52:** 157–8.
24. Jones EL. Preparation of the internal mammary artery for coronary bypass surgery. *J Card Surg* 1991; **6:** 326–9.
25. Fogarty TJ, Mollenauer KH. Preparation of the internal mammary artery for coronary artery bypass grafting. *J Card Surg* 1991; **6:** 322–5.
26. Mills NM, Bringaze WL. Preparation of the internal mammary artery graft: Which is the best method? *J Thorac Cardiovasc Surg* 1989; **98:** 73–9.
27. Johns RA, Peach MJ, Flanagan T, Kron IL. Probing of the canine mammary artery damages endothelium and impairs vasodilation resulting from prostacyclin and endothelium-derived relaxing factor. *J. Thorac Cardiovasc Surg* 1989; **97:** 252–8.
28. Vanhoutte PM. Platelets, endothelium and blood vessel wall. *Experimentia 1988*; **44:** 105–8.
29. Moncada S, Vane JR. Arachidonic acid metabolites and the interactions between platelets and blood vessel walls. *New Engl J Med* 1979; **300:** 1142–7.
30. Sneddon JM, Bearpark T, Vane JR. Endothelium derived relaxing factor (EDRF) inhibits platelet adhesion to bovine endothelial cells. *Br J. Pharmacol* 1988; **93:** 100P.
31. Cooper GJ, Gillot R, Francis SE, Angelini GD. Distension produces medial but not endothelial damage in porcine internal mammary artery. *Cardiovas Surg* 1995; **3:** 171–4.
32. van Son JAM, Tavilla G, Noyez L. Detrimental sequelae on the wall of the internal mammary artery caused by hydrostatic dilatation with diluted papaverine solution. *J Thorac Cardiovasc Surg* 1992; **104:** 972–6.
33. Berne RM. The role of adenosine in the regulation of coronary blood flow. *Circ Res* 1980; **47:** 807–13.
34. Haslam RJ, Davidson MML, Davies T, Lynham JA, McClenaghan MD. Regulation of blood platelet function by cyclic nucleotides. *Adv Cyclic Nucleotide Res* 1978; **9:** 533–52.
35. Fuster V, Chesebro JJ aortocoronary artery vein graft disease: experimental and clinical approach for the understanding of the role of platelets and plalelet inhibitors. *Circulation* 1985; **72** (Suppl. V): 65–70.
36. Angelini GD, Bryan AJ, Williams HMJ *et al.* Timecourse of media and intimal thickening in pig venous arterial grafts: relationship to endothelial injury and cholesterol accumulation *J Thorac Cardiovasc Surg* 1992; **103:** 1093–103.
37. Angelini GD, Newby AC. The future of saphenous vein as a coronary artery bypass conduit. *Eur Heart J* 1989; **10:** 273–80.
38. Sims FH. The internal mammary artery as a bypass graft. *Ann Thorac Surg* 1987; **44:** 2–3.
39. Dion RAE, Verhelst R, Rousseau M *et al.* Sequential mammary artery grafting: clinical, functional and angiographic assessment 6 months postopera-

tively in 231 consecutive patients. *J Thorac Cardiovasc Surg* 1989; **98:** 80–9.
40. Dion R, Etienne PY, Verhelst R *et al.* Bilateral mammary grafting. Clinical, functional and angiographic assessment in 400 consecutive patients. *Eur J Cardiothorac Surg* 1993; **7:** 287–94.
41. Tector AJ, Schmahl TM. Techniques for multiple internal mammary artery bypass grafts. *Ann Thorac Surg* 1984; **38:** 281–6.
42. Kamath ML, Matysik LS, Schmidt DH, Smith LL. Sequential internal mammary artery grafts. Expanded utilization of an ideal conduit. *J Thorac Cardiovasc Surg* 1985; **89:** 163–9.
43. van Sterkenburg SMM, Ernst SMPG, Brutel de la Rivière A *et al.* Triple sequential grafts using the internal mammary artery. An angiographic and short-term follow-up study. *J Thorac Cardiovasc Surg* 1992; **104:** 60–5.
44. Dion RAE, Noirhomme P, Wyns W, Van Dyck M, Goenen M, Ponlot R. Left-sided coronary thromboendarterectomy in complex internal mammary artery grafting. In: Ghosch PR, Unger F eds. *Cardiac Reconstructions.* Springer: Berlin, 1989: 319–26.
45. Loop FD, Lytle BW, Cosgrove DM, Golding LAR, Taylor PC, Stewart RW. Free (aorta-coronary) internal mammary artery graft: late results. *J Thorac Cardiovasc Surg* 1986; **92:** 827–31.
46. Hanet C, Wyns W, Decoster O, Pouleur H, Dion R, Rousseau M. Angiographic evaluation of vasomotor properties of internal mammary arteries before and after coronary artery bypass grafting in men. *Am J Cardiol* 1990; **65:** 918–21.
47. Hanet C, Michel X, Schroeder E *et al.* Vasomotor response of internal mammary artery and saphenous vein bypass grafts to increases in heart rate. *Circulation* (Suppl. Cardiovasc Surgery) Nov, 1991.
48. Van Son JAM, Smedts J, Vincent GJ, Van Lier HJJ. Comparative anatomic studies of various arterial conduits for myocardial revascularization. *J Thorac Cardiovasc Surg* 1990; **99:** 703–7.
49. Aarnio PTT, Harjula A, Viinikka L, Merikallio EM, Matilla SP. Prostacyclin production in free versus native IMA grafts. *Ann Thorac Surg* 1988; **45:** 380–92.
50. Calafiore AM, Di Giammarco G, Luciani N, Maddestra N, Di Nardo E, Angelini R. Composite arterial conduits for a wider arterial myocardial revascularization. *Ann Thorac Surg* 1994; **58:** 185–90.
51. Cosgrove DM, Loop FD. Techniques to maximize mammary artery length. *Ann Thorac Surg* 1985; **40:** 78–9.
52. Barner HB, Standeven JW, Reese J. Twelve-year experience with internal mammary artery for coronary artery bypass. *J Thorac Cardiovasc Surg* 1985; **90:** 668–75.
53. Jones EL, Lattouf O, Lutz JF, King SB III. Important anatomical and physiological considerations in performance of complex mammary–coronary artery operations. *Ann Thorac Surg* 1987; **43:** 469–77.
54. Rankin JS, Newman GE, Bashore TM. Clinical and angiographic assessment of complex mammary artery bypass grafting. *J Thorac Cardiovasc Surg* 1986; **92:** 832–46.
55. Von Segesser LK. *Arterial grafting for myocardial revascularization.* Springer: Berlin Heidelberg New York, 1990: 48–52.
56. Sarabu MR, Mc Clung JA, Fass A, Reed GE. Early postoperative spasm in left internal mammary artery bypass grafts. *Ann Thorac Surg* 1987; **44:** 199–200.
57. Aris A, Barras X, Ramio J. Patency of internal mammary artery grafts in no-flow situations. *J Cardiovasc Surg* 1987; **93:** 62–4.
58. Dincer B, Barner HB. The 'occluded' internal mammary artery graft: restoration of patency after apparent occlusion associated with progression of coronary disease. *J Thorac Surg* 1983; **85:** 318–20.
59. Kitamura S, Kawachi K, Seki T, Sawataba N, Morita R, Kawata T. Angiographic demonstration of no-flow anatomical patency of internal thoracic-coronary artery bypass grafts. *Ann Thorac Surg* 1992; **53:** 156–9.
60. Puig IB, Neto LF, Rati M. A technique of anastomosis of the right internal mammary artery to the circumflex artery and its branches. *Ann Thorac Surg* 1984; **38:** 533–4.

9 Detection of graft function and patency

Claude Hanet and Robert Dion

The efficacy of coronary artery bypass surgery to prevent myocardial ischaemia supposes that bypass grafts are able to adapt blood flow supply to the metabolic requirements of the underlying myocardium. The functional adaptation of internal thoracic artery (ITA) grafts to the coronary circulation has both qualitative and quantitative aspects. Qualitatively, implantation to the coronary circulation will modify the phasic blood flow pattern through the ITA from a predominantly systolic pattern, characteristic of the peripheral circulation, to a predominantly diastolic flow pattern resulting from systolic compression of intramyocardial coronary vessels. Quantitatively, the adaptation of blood flow through the graft relates to the necessity to accomodate higher blood flow requirements in response to increased myocardial energy demand.

This chapter addresses the technical aspects of angiographic evaluation of ITA graft patency and the results of angiographic follow-up studies, the changes in flow pattern through ITAs resulting from implantation as coronary bypass grafts, the vasoreactivity of ITA grafts and their long-term anatomical adaptation to the coronary circulation.

Angiographic evaluation of ITA graft patency and function: methodological aspects

Graft cineangiography

Contrast angiography is the reference method to assess coronary graft patency. Selective catheterization of the ITA *in situ* can be achieved in most cases through the femoral or the ipsilateral brachial approach using 6F or 8F preformed ITA or right Judkins catheters. Selective catheterization from the femoral approach is sometimes more challenging for the right than for the left ITA; adequate visualization of an ITA graft through the contralateral brachial approach is generally impossible. Given the increasing frequency of bilateral ITA grafting, the femoral approach is most commonly used for angiographic studies. Multiple angiographic projections are necessary to visualize adequately the distal anastomosis of the graft. A full assessment of the anastomotic site and of the distal part of the grafted coronary artery may be difficult when the amount of contrast material injected into the graft is too small because of non-selective catheterization of the ostium. Since any problems that occur usually involve the site of anastomosis with the coronary vessel, great care must be taken to catheterize the graft selectively.

Visual evaluation of angiograms allows assessment of graft patency, the quality of run-off to the distal coronary bed and a comparison of the size of the graft and that of the grafted territory. Although this visual interpretation remains acceptable for clinical and for many research applications, its usefulness is limited in some circumstances by its inherent imprecision and variability. The recent developments of computer-based quantitative angiography which allow accurate quantification of vessel size and of intravascular Doppler flow guide wires has stimulated interest in improving the functional assessment of coronary grafts.

Quantitative angiographic analysis

Several computer-assisted methods have been developed to obtain objective and reproducible measurements of luminal diameters from coronary and graft angiograms. Basically, the principle of these techniques is either contour analysis or densitometric analysis of the selected arterial segment. Most quantitative angiographic studies reported in this section have been done with the computer-based Coronary Angiography Analysis System (CAAS, Pie Data Medical, Maastricht, The Netherlands), using automated contour detection algorithms. The reproducibility of this system was evaluated by comparing the measured dimensions of twelve ITAs opacified twice at 3-min intervals using a non-ionic contrast agent (Iohexol). The difference in mean luminal diameter of the analyzed segment measured from the repeated angiograms averaged 0.03 mm and the standard deviation of the mean difference, i.e. the measurement variability, was 0.05 mm.[1]

Intravascular doppler velocimetry

Measurement of blood flow velocity during routine cardiac catheterization has been made possible through the development of intravascular Doppler ultrasound devices. A limitation of Doppler catheters has been interference with the flow velocity profile in the sample volume due to the size and design of catheters. This problem has been minimized with newly developed 0.014-inch Doppler guide wires (Cardiometrics Inc., Mountain View, CA, USA) which allow measurements of phasic spectral flow velocity across vessels to be made easily. Combination of lumen dimensions with Doppler velocity signals gives an estimation of blood flow using the following previously validated[2] equation:

$$\text{Doppler flow} = \text{CSA} \,.\, \text{APV}/2$$

where CSA equals cross-sectional area derived from quantitative angiography and APV equals time-averaged spectral peak velocity. This equation assumes a parabolic velocity profile where the mean blood flow velocity is half of time-averaged spectral peak velocity (APV/2).

Angiographic follow-up studies

The superiority of the ITA over the traditionally used saphenous vein graft was clearly demonstrated in the early 1980s.[3–5] Several clinical and angiographic follow-up studies have shown that the use of the ITA resulted in improved long-term overall patient survival and event-free survival in parallel with superior graft patency rates.[6–15] Initial studies reported patency rates of 85–90 per cent at 5 years and close to 85 per cent at 10 years. Recent studies of large populations have confirmed the excellent patency rates of ITA grafts. In a consecutive series of 400 patients evaluated after bilateral ITA grafting, angiography was performed in 181 patients 13 months after the operation.[16] Patency rates were similar for pedicled left ITA and right ITA (96.7 vs 95.1 per cent; NS) and were not affected by the grafted vessel. Lower patency rates were however observed for free grafts (79.6 per cent; $P < 0.001$ vs pedicled grafts). Similar results were reported in a consecutive series of 231 patients among whom 157 were recatheterized 6 months after sequential ITA grafting.[17] All but one of 163 sequential grafts (99.4 per cent) and 325 of the corresponding 342 anastomoses (95.0 per cent) were patent. The type of sequential ITA (right, left or free graft) did not influence the patency rate.

Flow-velocity pattern in ungrafted and grafted ITAs

Unlike peripheral vascular beds, the coronary circulation is characterized by cyclic variations of arteriolar resistance resulting from phasic systolic compression of intramyocardial coronary vessels. The resulting changes in flow velocity pattern through ITAs after coronary grafting could theoretically influence the endothelium-dependent control of vasomotor tone, circumferential growth and long-term patency. To assess the changes in blood flow velocity pattern resulting from chronic implantation into the coronary circulation, fourteen chronically implanted pedicled ITA grafts and eight ungrafted ITAs were studied during cardiac catheterization more than 4 months after surgery. Spectral flow velocity signals were recorded in the middle part of the ITA at basal conditions and during a pacing-induced tachycardia at 150 beats/min. Representative signals are shown in Fig. 9.1. Flow velocity pattern in ungrafted ITAs is typical of peripheral

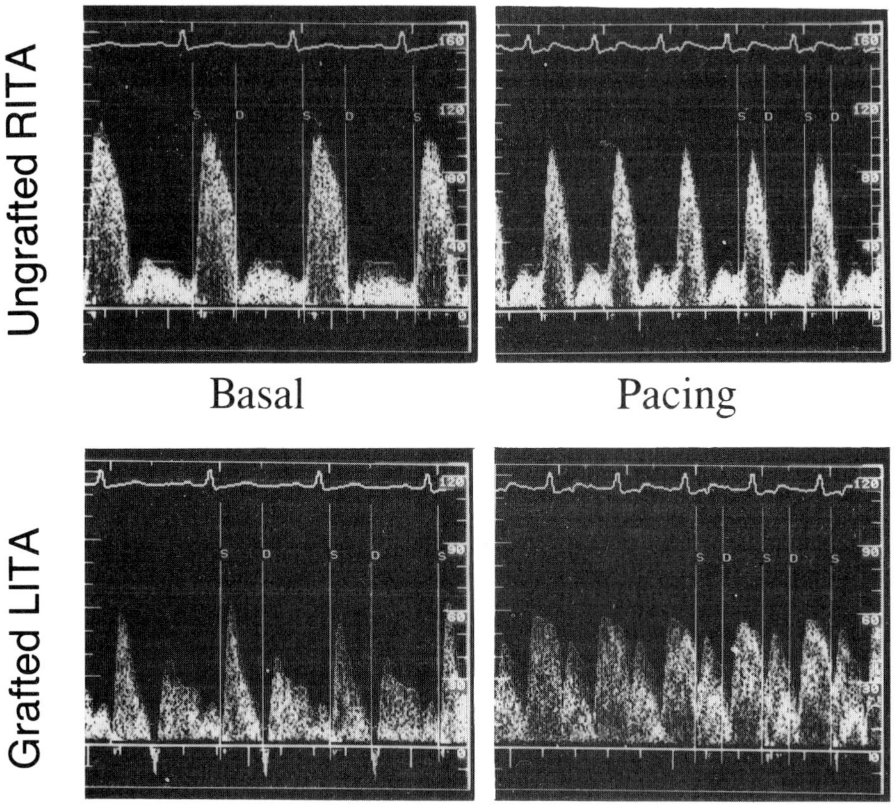

Fig. 9.1 Representative phasic flow velocity signals recorded in the ungrafted right ITA and in the left ITA grafted to the LAD coronary artery in basal sinus rhythm and during pacing-induced tachycardia.

arteries with a predominantly systolic velocity signal reflecting arterial pressure pulses. Only minor changes in signal morphology appeared during tachycardia, the diastolic to systolic velocity ratio remaining lower than unity (0.25±0.08 at baseline to 0.35±11 during tachycardia). Mean blood flow velocity remained unchanged, APV averaging 30.3±5.9 at baseline and 29.1±6.4 cm/sec during tachycardia. Flow velocity signals in grafted ITAs are characterized at baseline by a slower systolic flow and greater diastolic velocities, the diastolic/systolic velocity ratio being close to unity (0.92±0.32; $P<0.001$ vs ungrafted arteries). This pattern reflects the compression of intramyocardial coronary vessels during systole. During tachycardia, the diastolic component of the blood flow velocity signal increased as reflected by a significant rise in the diastolic to systolic velocity ratio to 1.57±0.41 ($P<0.0001$). Mean blood flow velocity increased significantly during tachycardia as a result of increased myocardial metabolic demand (APV: 21.3±8.4 to 27.4±10.8 cm/sec; $P<0.001$).

Vasoreactivity of ITA grafts

Vasomotor response to tachycardia

Animal studies have shown that increasing blood flow through conduit arteries results in a vasodilation that may be abolished by removal of the endothelium.[18,19] This flow-induced vasodilation is mediated by the release from endothelial cells of a relaxing substance that has many characteristics of endothelium-derived relaxing factor recently identified as nitric oxide. In humans, an increase in blood flow induced by rapid atrial pacing is associated with vasodilation of angiographically smooth but not of atherosclerotic coronary arteries.[20] This dilator response of coronary arteries to tachycardia is independent of innervation since it has been observed in transplanted and thus denervated hearts. The flow-mediated vasodilation of normal epicardial coronary arteries may have important physiological implications for maximizing flow rates during increased myocardial oxygen demand. Heterogeneity, however, exists among different vessels in the amount of nitric oxide released in basal conditions and in response to various stimuli. *In vitro* experiments using small vascular rings obtained from patients undergoing coronary artery bypass surgery have demonstrated that endothelium-dependent vasodilation is more prominent in human ITA than in saphenous vein.[21,22] Using quantitative angiography, we demonstrated that this endothelium-dependent mechanism may play a role in the acute adaptation of the luminal diameter of ITAs but not of saphenous vein grafts to an increase in myocardial blood flow demand during tachycardia.[23] Angiograms of ten chronically implanted ITAs and seven saphenous vein grafts were obtained at 3-min intervals in basal conditions and during pacing-induced tachycardia. The cross-sectional area of ITA grafts increased by 14.8±11.5 per cent ($P<0.005$) during tachycardia, this vasodilation being interpreted as reflecting the preserved capacity of the endothelium to modulate the tone of underlying smooth muscle cells in response to vasoactive stimuli. In contrast, the luminal cross-sectional area of saphenous vein grafts remained virtually unchanged (+0.3±5.4 per cent in proportion to basal value) during tachycardia (Figs. 9.2 and 9.3).

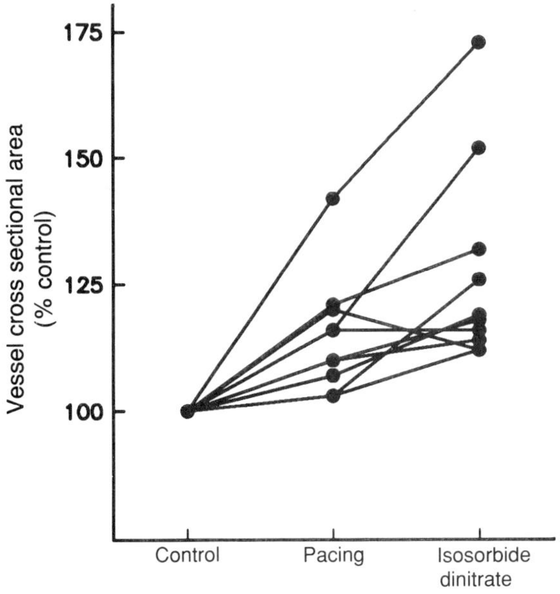

Fig. 9.2 Individual changes in cross-sectional area of ITA grafts in response to atrial pacing and to intragraft infusion of isosorbide dinitrate (ISDN). Reproduced with permission from Hanet *et al.*[23]

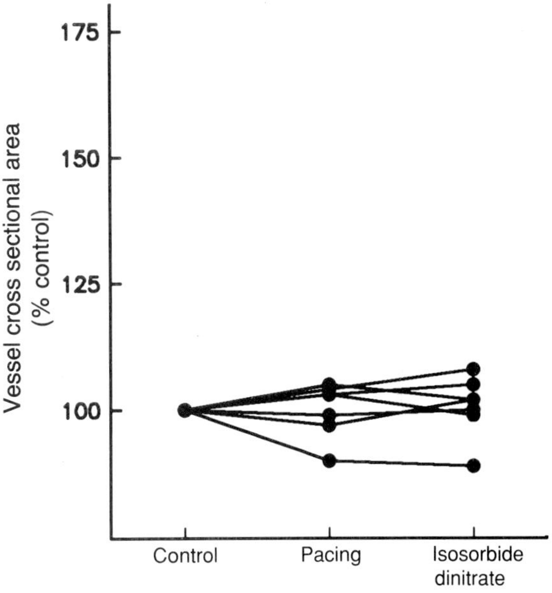

Fig. 9.3 Individual changes in cross-sectional area of saphenous vein grafts (SVG) in response to atrial pacing and to intragraft infusion of isosorbide dinitrate (ISDN). Reproduced with permission from Hanet *et al.*[23]

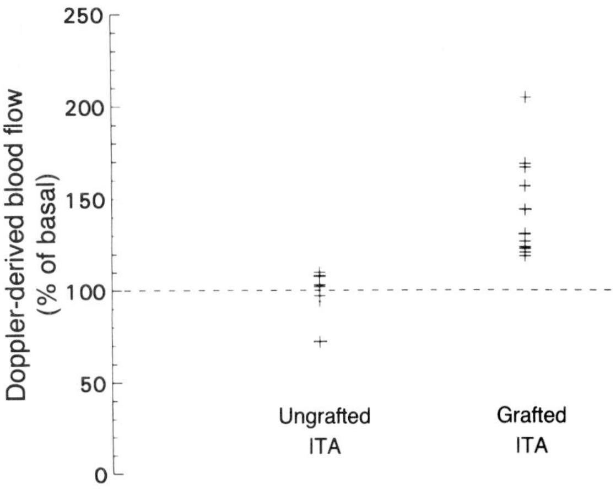

Fig. 9.4 Individual changes in Doppler-derived blood flow through ungrafted and grafted ITA during pacing-induced tachycardia. Changes are expressed as per cent of basal blood flow.

Combining the flow velocity data and the quantitative angiographic data, it was possible to determine the absolute changes in blood flow through fourteen ITA grafts during tachycardia.[24] Doppler-derived flow increased from 30±14 ml/min at baseline to 42±20 ml/min during tachycardia as a combined result of flow acceleration and vasodilation. No change in blood flow through the eight ungrafted ITAs was noted during tachycardia (Fig. 9.4).

Vasomotor response to ergometrine and nitrates

Ergot alkaloids such as ergometrine and ergonovine are routinely used in catheterization laboratories as provocative agents for coronary spasm in patients suspected of suffering from vasospastic angina. In patients with or without coronary artery disease, the administration of ergonovine or ergometrine results in a significant constriction of epicardial coronary arteries. In animal models, these agents induce coronary constriction mainly by activation of serotonergic receptors of smooth muscle cells. Ergonovine also may activate serotonergic receptors on endothelial cells to trigger the release of nitric oxide, thereby attenuating direct constrictor effects.[25] The magnitude of the vasomotor response of a given vascular segment thus depends on the force-generating capacity of the media but also on the capacity of endothelial cells to control the tone of underlying smooth muscle cells through the release of nitric oxide.

We recently reported that, unlike saphenous vein grafts, chronically implanted ITA grafts are protected against the constrictor influence of ergot alkaloids.[26] Changes in luminal diameter were measured using computerized quantitative angiography after intravenous administration of 0.4 mg methylergometrine and after intragraft infusion of 1 mg isosorbide dinitrate. The vasomotor response of fourteen ITA grafts was compared to that of eleven saphenous vein grafts and of eleven grafted coronary arteries. After methylergometrine, a significant constriction of coronary arteries and saphenous vein grafts was observed (9.3±7.2 and 6.9±7.4 per cent, respectively), which contrasted with the inconsistent response of ITA grafts (0.3±5.1 per cent; $P<0.02$ vs venous grafts and $P<0.002$ vs coronary arteries). After intragraft isosorbide dinitrate, the luminal diameter of both grafted coronary arteries and ITA grafts increased significantly beyond basal values (+17.8±9.8 and +5.5±3.3 per cent

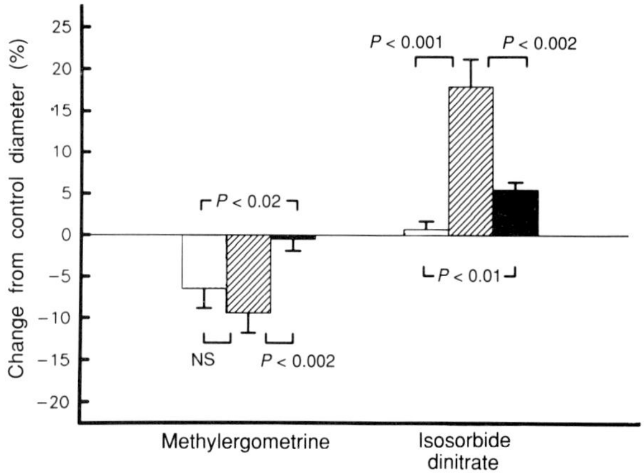

Fig. 9.5 Changes in luminal diameter (mean±SEM) of saphenous vein (SV) grafts (□), ITA grafts (■) and grafted coronary arteries (▨) in percentage of control diameter after intravenous injection of methylergometrine and after intragraft infusion of isosorbide dinitrate. Reproduced with permission from Hanet *et al.*[26]

respectively) and that of saphenous vein grafts returned to control values (+0.7±3.3 per cent in proportion to basal diameter; Fig. 9.5).

This differential response to ergometrine of both types of grafts is consistent with the results of previous *in vitro* studies demonstrating differences in the ability of endothelial cells of both grafts to control the tone of underlying smooth muscle cells in response to vasoactive interventions.[21] Interestingly, the response to nitrates demonstrates in ITA grafts, but not in saphenous vein grafts, the persistence of a vasodilator reserve and thus of some degree of basal vasomotor tone.

Long-term anatomical adaptation of ITA grafts

The ability of the ITA to increase its diameter over time when anastomosed to a severely stenotic coronary artery with good perfusion area was described several years ago. In twelve paediatric patients who underwent ITA grafting for severe coronary lesions secondary to Kawasaki disease, Kitamura *et al.* reported a consistent increase in length and diameter of the graft in the late postoperative period. In contrast, the lengths and diameters of saphenous vein grafts tended to slightly decrease over time.[27] Several authors[28–30] have reported the restoration of patency of previously documented ITA graft occlusions after progression of the disease in the proximal segment of the native coronary vessel. These data demonstrate that the ITA graft is a physiologically active conduit with dynamic adaptive capacity. This growth potential of ITAs was confirmed by comparing the mean diameter of ITAs before and 6 months after implantation as sequential grafts into a large coronary vascular bed. In basal conditions, the mean luminal diameter was significantly larger in grafted than in ungrafted arteries (3.41 ± 0.36 vs 2.97 ± 0.39 mm; $P<0.05$). Intragraft infusion of 1 mg isosorbide dinitrate induced dilatation of ITAs, similar in grafted and ungrafted vessels (to 3.6 ± 0.37 and to 3.12 ± 0.36 mm, respectively). Although this dilation appeared relatively modest when compared to that observed in grafted coronary arteries, it clearly demonstrated that the circumferential enlargement is a real anatomical adaptation and that the vasodilator reserve of the ITA is preserved after coronary artery bypass grafting.

Non-invasive assessment of ITA graft patency

Transcutaneous duplex ultrasound through supraclavicular or parasternal approaches can be used to evaluate ITA graft patency.[31,32] Flow velocity signals are similar to those obtained by intravascular ultrasound devices (*see* Fig. 9.1) with a predominantly systolic flow in ungrafted arteries and a systolic to diastolic velocity ratio close to 1:1 in patent ITA grafts. An estimation of absolute blood flow can be obtained, based on flow-velocity signals and on the cross-sectional area of the vessel. The accuracy of this estimation is, however, limited by the relative imprecision of luminal diameter measurements and by the necessity to correct velocity measurements for the angulation between the axis of the vessel and that of the Doppler transducer. Failure to detect the typical pattern of graft flow cannot be taken as evidence of graft failure since in at least a proportion of patients satisfactory Doppler signals cannot be obtained for technical reasons.[31] In addition, the morphology of the Doppler velocity pattern is of limited value in the assessment of the quality of the anastomosis and of the distal coronary bed. Because of these limitations, the use of transcutaneous ultrasound appears inadequate to evaluate ITA graft patency routinely in follow-up studies. It may, however, be a promising tool for studying the physiology and pathophysiology of ITA grafts, were satisfactory images can be readily obtained.

Conclusion

Several *in vitro* studies conducted on isolated vascular rings have demonstrated that endothelium-dependent relaxant activity is more prominent in ITAs than in saphenous veins.[21–23] Differences have been reported in the capacity of endothelial cells to release both prostacyclin and nitric oxide, two mediators whose potent vasodilator and antithrombotic effects are thought to contribute to long-term vessel patency. The results of quantitative angiographic studies support this concept of a more efficient endothelium-dependent control of vasomotor tone, possibly contributing to the favourable long-term functional results of ITA grafts. They also demonstrate the adaptability of ITAs to chronic and to acute changes in blood flow requirements resulting both from growth potential and from vasomotor properties.

Selective angiography remains at the present time the reference method to assess ITA graft patency. In addition to anatomical information, by using this invasive approach, functional information can be obtained, such as dynamic changes in lumen diameter and flow velocity in response to physiological and pharmacological interventions. Until newer imaging modalities allow a reliable non-invasive evaluation of graft patency and function, the combination of direct and precise measurements of lumen diameter, blood flow velocity and pressure yield important pathophysiological information that will be instrumental in the validation of noninvasive approaches.

Acknowledgements

This work was supported by a grant 'Concerted European Action on Coronary Thrombosis – BIOMED and Health research program PL920055' from the European Communities. The authors wish to thank Magdalena Delgadillo-Redaway for expert secretarial assistance.

References

1. Hanet C, Wijns W, Decoster P *et al.* Angiographic evaluation of vasomotor properties of internal mammary arteries before and after coronary artery bypass grafting. *Am J Cardiol* 1990; **65:** 918–21.
2. Doucette JW, Corl PD, Payne HM *et al.* Validation of a Doppler guide wire for intravascular

measurement of coronary artery flow velocity. *Circulation* 1992; **85:** 1899–911.
3. Grondin CM, Campeau L, Lesperance J *et al.* Comparison of late changes in internal mammary artery and saphenous vein grafts in two consecutive series of patients 10 years after operation. *Circulation* 1984; **70**(Suppl. I): I208–12.
4. Singh RN, Sosa JA, Green GE. Long-term fate of the internal mammary artery and saphenous vein grafts. *J Thorac Cardiovasc Surg* 1983; **86:** 359–63.
5. Okies JE, Page US, Bigelow JC *et al.* The left internal mammary artery: the graft of choice. *Circulation* 1984; **70**(Suppl I): I213–21.
6. Singh RN, Sosa JA, Green GE. Long-term fate of the internal mammary artery and saphenous veins. *J. Thorac Cardiovasc Surg* 1983; **86:** 359–63.
7. Rankin JS, Newman GE, Bashore TM. Clinical and angiographic assessment of complex mammary artery bypass grafting. *J. Thorac Cardiovasc Surg* 1986; **92:** 832–46.
8. Olearchyk AS, Magovern GJ. Internal mammary artery grafting: clinical results, patency rates, and long-term survival in 833 patients. *J. Thorac Cardiovasc Surg* 1986; **92:** 1082–7.
9. Loop FD, Lytle BW, Cosgrove DM. Influence of the internal mammary artery graft on 10-year survival and other cardiac events. *New Engl J Med* 1986; **314:** 1–6.
10. Cameron A, Kemp HG, Green GE. Bypass surgery with the internal mammary artery graft: 15-year follow-up. *Circulation* 1986; **74**(Suppl. 3): 30–6.
11. Johnson WD, Brenowitz JB, Kayser KL. Factors influencing long-term (10- year to 15-year) survival after a successful coronary artery bypass operation. *Ann Thorac Surg* 1989; **48:** 19–25.
12. Green GE, Swistel DG, Cameron AA. Bilateral internal thoracic artery surgery: 17-year experience. *Eur Heart J* 1989; **10**(Suppl. H): 57–60.
13. Galbut DL, Traad EA, Dorman MJ *et al.* Seventeen-year experience with bilateral internal mammary artery grafts. *Ann Thorac Surg* 1990; **49:** 195–201.
14. Fiore AC, Naunheim KSQ, Dean Ph *et al.* Results of internal thoracic artery grafting over 15 years: single versus double grafts. *Ann Thorac Surg* 1990; **49:** 202–9.
15. Naunheim KS, Barner HB, Fiore AC. Results of internal thoracic artery grafting over 15 years: single versus double grafts; 1992 Update. *Ann Thorac Surg* 1992; **53:** 716–18.
16. Dion R, Etienne PY, Verhelst R *et al.* Bilateral mammary grafting. Clinical, functional and angiographic assessment in 400 consecutive patients. *Eur J Cardiothorac Surg* 1993; **7:** 287–93.
17. Dion R, Verhelst R, Rousseau M *et al.* Sequential mammary grafting. Clinical, functional and angiographic assessment 6 months postoperatively in 231 consecutive patients. *J Thorac Cardiovasc Surg* 1989; **98:** 80–9.
18. Rubanyi GM, Romero JC, Vanhoutte PM. Flow-induced release of endothelium-derived relaxing factor. *Am J Physiol* 1986; **250:** H1145–9.
19. Pohl U, Holtz J Busse R, Bassenge E. Crucial role of endothelium in the vasodilator response to increased flow in vivo. *Hypertension* 1986; **7:** 37–44.
20. Nabel EG, Selwyn AP, Ganz P. Paradoxical narrowing of atherosclerotic coronary arteries induced by increases in heart rate. Circulation 1990; **81:** 850–9.
21. Lüscher TF, Diedrich D, Siebenmann R *et al.* Difference between endothelium-dependent relaxation in arterial and in venous coronary bypass grafts. *New Engl J Med* 1988; **319:** 462–7.
22. Schoeffter Ph, Dion R, Godfraind T. Modulatory role of the vascular endothelium in the contractility of human isolated internal mammary artery. *Br J Pharmacol* 1988; **95:** 531–43.
23. Hanet C, Schroeder E, Michel X *et al.* Flow-induced vasomotor response to tachycardia of the human internal mammary artery and saphenous vein grafts late following bypass surgery. Circulation 1991; **84** (Suppl. III); III 268–74.
24. Hanet C, Semaan C, Leblois Th, Dion R. Comparison of flow-velocity pattern in internal mammary arteries before and after coronary artery bypass grafting (abstract). *Eur Heart J* 1994; **15:** 232.
25. Shimokawa H, Flavahan NA, Shepherd JT, Vanhoutte PM. Endothelium-dependent inhibition of ergonovine-induced contraction is impaired in porcine coronary arteries with regenerated endothelium. *Circulation* 1989; **80:** 643–50.
26. Hanet C, Robert A, Wijns W. Vasmotor response to ergometrine and nitrates of saphenous vein grafts, internal mammary artery grafts and grafted coronary arteries late after bypass surgery. *Circulation* 1992; **86** (Suppl. II): II210–16.
27. Kitamura S, Seki T, Kawachi K *et al.* Excellent patency and growth potential of internal mammary artery grafts in pediatric coronary artery bypass surgery. New evidence for a 'live' conduit. *Circulation* 1988; **78** (Suppl. I): I129–39.
28. Dincer B, Barner HB. The 'occluded' internal mammary artery graft. Restoration of patency after apparent occlusion associated with progression of coronary disease. *J Thorac Cardiovasc Surg* 1984; **87:** 936–8.
29. Aris A, Borras X, Ramio J. Patency of internal mammary artery grafts in no-flow situation. *J Thorac Cardiovasc Surg* 1987; **93:** 62–4.
30. Feld H, Navarro V, Kleeman H, Shani J. Early postoperative occlusion of a left internal mammary artery bypass graft with subsequent restoration of patency. *Cath Cardiovasc Diag* 1992; **27:** 280–3.
31. Fusejima K, Takahara Y, Sudo Y, Murayama H, Masuda Y, Inagaki Y. Comparison of coronary

hemodynamics in patients with internal mammary artery and saphenous vein coronary artery bypass grafts. a noninvasive approach using combined two dimensional and Doppler echocardiography. *J Am Cardiol* 1990; **15:** 131–9.
32. Krijne R, Lyttwin RM, Holtgen R, Heinrich KW, Marx R, Sons H. Combined two-dimensional and Doppler echographic examination of internal mammary artery grafts from the supraclavicular fossa. *Int J Cardiol* 1992; **37:** 61–4.
33. Vanhoutte PM. The endothelium-modulator of vascular smooth muscle tone. *New Engl J Med* 1988; **319:** 512–13.

10 Early and late clinical results

Andrew C. Fiore and Hendrick B. Barner

The use of the internal thoracic artery (ITA) for myocardial revascularization was introduced in 1964 by Spencer and promoted by Green in 1968.[1,2] Surgeons were reticent to adopt this conduit because mobilization from the chest wall was time consuming and the ITA anastomosis proved more difficult and demanding. At the close of the first decade of myocardial revascularization there was little objective data to support preferential use of the ITA and most surgeons continued to avoid this conduit. However, a minority of surgeons remained convinced that revascularization with arterial conduits was superior and maintained their belief throughout the early years of coronary artery surgery.[3–7]

Single ITA grafts

In the early 1980s Grondin and associates demonstrated that the saphenous vein graft was prone to progressive intimal proliferation and atherosclerosis.[8] Angiographic studies demonstrated a 2 per cent per year incidence of vein graft attrition between the first and seventh postoperative years. The incidence increased to 5 per cent per year thereafter. As far as the twelfth postoperative year. At 12 years postoperatively, 50 per cent of all vein grafts have occluded and 50 per cent of those remaining patent have obvious atherosclerosis. The gradual rise in the risk of sudden death beginning 3.5 years after saphenous vein bypass grafting is probably due more to vein closure than progressive native coronary artery disease as recently described by Lytle.[9] During this same time period, clinical studies appeared demonstrating that patency of the ITA conduit exceeded that of saphenous veins.

In 1985 Barner reported a 12-year experience consisting of 1000 patients having at least one ITA graft.[10] The incidence of postoperative complications was exceedingly low and included myocardial infarction (3.7 per cent), reoperation for bleeding (2.4 per cent) and mediastinal infection (0.8 per cent). The 30-day mortality was 1.4 per cent. The patency rate for the left ITA was 96 per cent at 1 year, 88 per cent at 5 years and 83 per cent at 10 years. Comparison of patency rates for all ITA grafts versus vein conduits demonstrated nearly identical 1 year patency rates of 95 vs 93 per cent respectively ($P < 0.25$). However, significant differences were found at 5 years with ITA grafts demonstrating superior patency (88 vs 74 per cent $P < 0.001$). At 10 years, the advantage of the ITA was further magnified (83 vs 41 per cent $P < 0.001$). This study demonstrated that single ITA grafting was safe and efficacious, and the patency of the ITA far exceeded that of saphenous vein conduits.

Does the prolonged patency of the ITA influence long-term patient survival and the development of late cardiac events? Loop and his associates examined this question by comparing those patients receiving a left ITA conduit to the LAD coronary artery plus saphenous vein grafts to those receiving only saphenous vein grafts.[11] The 10-year actuarial survival rate among hospital survivors in whom the ITA was used was superior to that of the group in whom only vein grafts were used. The incremental improvement was different for patients with one (93 vs 88 per cent, ($P = 0.05$), two (90 vs 79 per cent ($P = 0.001$) and three (83 per cent vs 71 per cent $P < 0.001$)

vessel coronary disease. Patients receiving only vein grafts had a 1.6 times greater risk of death throughout the 10-year follow-up as compared with those who received an ITA. In addition, patients with only vein grafts demonstrated a significantly greater risk of late myocardial infarction ($P < 0.0001$), hospitalization for cardiac events ($P < 0.001$) and cardiac reoperation ($P < 0.001$) as compared with patients with ITA grafts.

These important observations demonstrated that the long-term patency of the atherosclerosis-resistant ITA translates into superior actuarial survival and improved freedom from all cardiac events at 10 years in the subset of patients with double and triple vessel disease who have the left ITA anastomosed to the LAD coronary artery. These favourable late results were strong incentives for surgeons to use the ITA despite the additional effort required.

Following this report a number of investigators published clinical data supporting the ITA as the conduit of choice for coronary artery bypass surgery.[4,12,13] The largest series was reported by Acinapura and colleagues in which they compared 5121 patients receiving a left ITA to LAD and supplemental saphenous vein grafts with 2345 patients having only saphenous vein conduits.[14] The operative mortality was 1.8 per cent in the ITA group and 2.4 per cent in the vein graft group ($P =$ NS) with a mean follow-up of 8.5 years. The angiographic patency of the left ITA was 96 vs 75 per cent in the saphenous vein grafts ($P < 0.05$). At a mean follow-up of 6.8 years, recurrent angina developed in 31 per cent of vein graft patients compared to 15 per cent of patients with ITA grafts ($P < 0.01$). Reoperation was required in 10 per cent of patients with saphenous veins compared to 1.2 per cent of patients with ITA grafts ($P < 0.001$). Late myocardial infarction and need for subsequent PTCA was significantly lower in patients receiving an ITA graft.

The actuarial 5-year survival was similar in the ITA and saphenous vein graft cohort. However, at 10 years the curves diverged with a significant survival advantage in patients receiving one ITA graft (88 vs 75 per cent $P < 0.001$).

These articles support the routine use of single ITA grafting to the LAD in the vast majority of patients requiring myocardial revascularization. The only contraindications to single ITA grafting are haemodynamic instability following failed PTCA or ongoing ischaemia. Relative contraindications are patients whose life expectancy is believed to be less than 8 years because of advanced age (> 80 years), poor left ventricular function (ejection fraction < 20 per cent), or concomitant medical illnesses (e.g. malignancy).

Double ITA grafts

The results of bilateral ITA grafting were first reported in 1974.[15] This clinical report established the feasibility and safety of employing two ITA grafts for myocardial revascularization. It also demonstrated the superior early patency of both free and *in situ* ITA grafts as compared to saphenous vein conduits. This early publication did note higher operative mortality (8 per cent) and increase in reoperation for bleeding and sternal infection. Ten years later Lytle and associates reported their results in 500 patients having bilateral ITA grafting.[16] Their operative mortality was lower (1.4 per cent) reflecting improvements in operative technique, extracorporeal circulation and myocardial preservation. The authors also observed increased operative morbidity including reoperation for bleeding (7 per cent), requirement for prolonged ventilatory support (5.2 per cent) and sternal wound complications (1.6 per cent). A total of seventy-nine patients (16 per cent) suffered at least one major postoperative complication.

These reports aroused concern in the surgical community that use of both ITAs was technically demanding and associated with increased morbidity. Until clinical data emerged to demonstrate a definitive advantage to harvesting a second ITA, the majority of surgeons avoided this procedure.

Current results of bilateral ITA grafting have been reported by Galbut and colleagues.[17] These authors reviewed their 17-year experience in 1087 patients receiving bilateral ITA grafts with an operative mortality of 2.7 per cent. The hospital complications of reoperation for bleeding (1.7 per cent), sternal infection (1.5 per cent), intubation beyond 48 hours (2.1 per cent), and perioperative myocardial infarction (2 per cent) were lower than any previous report and comparable to patients receiving a single ITA graft with saphenous vein conduits. However, a significantly higher incidence of sternal wound infection was noted in diabetic patients.

Galbut also reported late results with a mean follow-up of 3.2 years in 1041 patients. At the time of follow-up, 959 patients (91 per cent) were alive with a 10-year actuarial survival of 80 per cent; 97 per cent of the hospital survivors were in New York

Heart Association Class I or Class II. Coronary angiography was performed in fifty-three patients at a mean of 53 months postoperatively and demonstrated 92 per cent (58/63) patency of the left ITA to the LAD and 85 per cent (45/53) patency of the right ITA. The saphenous vein graft patency was 65 per cent.

This important study demonstrated that bilateral ITA grafting can be performed with an operative mortality and morbidity similar to patients receiving saphenous vein grafts only. The superior patency of two arterial grafts translated into an excellent 17-year functional improvement, enhanced freedom from late cardiac events and prolonged patient survival. These results were confirmed by Fiore and associates in a report reviewing the clinical results at 15 years in 586 patients who underwent bilateral ITA grafting.[18]

Although Galbut and Fiore noted that the incidence of postoperative morbidity was lower than earlier reports, both authors emphasized that certain patient subsets experienced increased postoperative morbidity following bilateral ITA grafting.

In order to better identify those patients at higher risk for bilateral ITA grafting, Kouchoukos and colleagues compared patients receiving one or two ITAs with those receiving vein grafts only.[19] The use of bilateral ITA grafting was not associated with a greater 30-day mortality compared with single ITA or venous grafting. Early mortality was similar for unilateral and bilateral ITA patients. With the exception of sternal infection, none of the postoperative complications evaluated occurred with greater frequency among patients receiving unilateral or bilateral ITA grafts than among vein graft patients. The prevalence of sternal wound complications was associated with the use of two ITA grafts (single ITA 1.9 per cent vs double ITA, 7 per cent; $P < 0.0007$). Further statistical analysis demonstrated that diabetes, obesity and the need for prolonged ventilatory support were significant predictors of sternal wound infection following bilateral ITA grafting. This important clinical observation has been confirmed by Cosgrove and associates and Buxton and colleagues.[20,21] The analysis by Kouchoukos and co-workers suggests that obese diabetic patients who require prolonged ventilatory support following bilateral ITA grafting have an estimated risk of sternal wound infection that exceeds 10 per cent. This observation has been confirmed by other investigators who have noted an increased risk of sternal wound infection in diabetic vs non-diabetic patients that have two ITAs harvested (Accola: 9.3 vs 2.5 per cent, $P = 0.006$;[22] Dion: 9.0 vs 4.5 per cent;[23] Cosgrove: 16.7 vs 0.7 per cent, $P < 0.001$;[20] Galbut: 5.5 vs 0.5 per cent, $P < 0.001$[17]). The role of double ITA grafting in obese diabetic patients remains controversial. It is the authors opinion that in these high-risk patient subgroups, consideration should be given to avoiding bilateral ITA grafting with alternative arterial conduits employed if clinically indicated.

These studies confirmed the safety of extended arterial grafting with the ITA in selected patients, but as the second decade of myocardial revascularization came to a close, surgeons questioned whether the addition of a second ITA graft would confer a significantly greater long-term clinical benefit than one ITA graft. Fiore and his associates addressed this issue by comparing ninety eight single with ninety one double ITA patients with a mean follow-up of 15 years.[24] The actuarial survival of hospital survivors was nearly identical at 10 years. At 15 years, the two survival curves diverged suggesting a trend in survival advantage in those patients receiving two ITA grafts, but the difference did not achieve statistical significance. The 15-year actuarial freedom from myocardial infarction (fatal and non-fatal), recurrent angina pectoris and all ischaemic events was significantly improved for those patients receiving a second ITA graft. These observations confirmed an isolated earlier report by Cameron and associates in which patients with one or two ITAs were compared with those receiving saphenous vein grafts alone.[25] Patients with two ITA grafts had the best survival rates as well as the lowest recurrence of angina, late myocardial infarction, and the need for reoperation. These two reports demonstrated that the advantage of a second ITA graft did not manifest itself until 8 years had elapsed. Therefore patients in whom life expectancy is less than 10 years because of advanced age, depressed ventricular function, chronic medical illness or malignancy should not be selected to receive two ITA grafts.

Free ITA grafts

Attempting to increase the versatility of the ITA, Barner and Loop independently reported the successful use of free ITA grafting in 1973.[26,27] In Barner's series, the right ITA was detached from its origin and anastomosed to the ascending aorta in five patients and to the hood of a saphenous vein graft in one. Intraoperative flow measurements demonstrated that the maximum flow capacity of the free ITA graft compared favourably with the *in situ* ITA conduit, but was limited in contrast to flow in the saphenous vein graft. Coronary angiography performed 1–6 weeks postoperatively revealed patency of five grafts. Loop and associates reported the use of a free right ITA in four patients with patency demonstrated in all at 10 days to 2 months. These important early contributions established the free ITA as an additional arterial conduit for myocardial revascularization and defined alternative sites for the proximal anastomosis.

In 1975 Schimert and his associates confirmed the above findings with the report of thirty-four free arterial grafts (sixteen right ITAs; fourteen left ITAs; four radial artery) in twenty-five patients with 100 per cent patency documented 2 weeks to 6 months postoperatively.[28]

The long-term results for free ITA grafting were reported by Loop and colleagues in 156 patients having forty-two free left ITA and 124 free right ITA grafts.[29] Postoperative morbidity included prolonged ventilatory support (10 per cent), reoperation for bleeding (8 per cent), stroke (3 per cent), postoperative myocardial infarction (2 per cent), sternal wound infection (1 per cent) and one hospital mortality (1 per cent). Coronary angiography performed after a mean interval of 49 months demonstrated patency in sixty-three of seventy-five free ITA grafts (84 per cent). The closure rate for free ITA grafts was higher among those restudied within the first 18 months postoperatively (thirty-one of forty; 77 per cent). Beyond 18 months, thirty-two of thirty-five (91 per cent) free grafts were patent. Of twenty-six free grafts studied 5 or more years postoperatively, twenty-four (92 per cent) were patent and none showed evidence of graft atherosclerosis. The 87.7 per cent 5-year and 74.7 per cent 10-year actuarial survival rates for seventy-four patients who received one free ITA graft were not significantly different from 94.1 and 69.4 per cent rates, respectively, for eighty-one patients who had received two free ITA grafts. This study demonstrates the durability and relative resistance to atherosclerosis of the free ITA graft.

The above studies support the use of the free ITA graft on the basis of low operative morbidity, effective angina relief and excellent long-term survival, although patency is not as good as for the *in situ* graft.

Free ITA grafting enhances the utility of arterial conduits. The right ITA can be directed to the right or left side of the heart. Because of unwillingness to cross the anterior mid line (risk of graft injury at reoperation) and dissatisfaction with the transverse sinus route (increased incidence of graft closure) we always use the right ITA as a free graft when it is directed to the left coronary circulation.[30] If the aortic wall is healthy, the ITA is anastomosed to it using a 4–5 mm punch and 7–0 Polypropylene. If the aortic wall is thick or diseased then the ITA is anastomosed to the hood of an associated vein graft or, if there is none, to a vein or pericardial patch placed in the aorta.[31]

Sequential ITA grafts

In 1983 McBride and Barner reported the use of sequential ITA grafting to the LAD and diagonal coronary arteries in thirty-nine patients (age range 32–65 years).[32] There was no operative mortality and one non-cardiac late death. Ten patients (26 per cent) had follow-up coronary angiography from 1 month to 5 years postoperatively which demonstrated all twenty ITA sequential anastomoses patent. These excellent early results were confirmed by Kabbani and associates who performed sequential ITA grafting in eight patients with no operative mortality.[33] Follow-up cardiac catheterization performed 2–5 years postoperatively revealed all sequential anastomoses patent.

In 1984 Tector and associates reported sequential ITA grafting in fifty-three patients (left ITA to LAD-diagonal system in fifty-two patients; left ITA to marginal and circumflex coronary artery in one patient).[34] There were no operative deaths and one late non-cardiac death. Perioperative myocardial infarction, sternal wound complication or reoperation for bleeding did not occur. No patient required intra-aortic balloon counterpulsation or inotropic support for low cardiac output. Follow-up angiography was performed in five patients with stenosis of the left ITA beyond the diagonal anastomosis in one patient.

In 1985 Kamath described sequential ITA grafting in eighty-seven patients (Group I, single sequential, forty-nine patients; Group II, single sequential and one end-to-side, thirty-one patients; Group III, double sequential, seven patients) with no operative deaths.[35] Coronary angiography was performed in thirty-five patients within the first postoperative year. In Group I, fourteen patients were found to have all twenty-eight ITA anastomoses patent (100 per cent). Patency rates were also gratifying in 18

Group II (forty-eight of fifty-four ITA anastomoses patent, 89 per cent) and two Group III (eight of eight, 100 per cent) patients. Follow-up between 8 and 52 months postoperatively revealed three late deaths of non-cardiac aetiology and seventy-nine of eighty-seven (91%) asymptomatic patients.

In 1986 Rankin and his associates confirmed the reliability of sequential ITA grafting in 207 patients who underwent angiography 1–32 weeks postoperatively.[36] Patency rates for sequential ITA coronary anastomoses were 100 per cent for circumflex and marginal end-to-side or side-to-side anastomoses, 99 per cent (133/134) for left ITA to the LAD or diagonal coronary artery and 100 per cent (six of six) for three sequential ITA grafts. Dion reported 246 sequential ITA grafts in 231 patients including bilateral sequential ITA grafts and fifteen free sequential ITA grafts. Catheterization at 6 months revealed 95 per cent of the sequential anastomoses patent.[37]

In 1992 Van Sterkenburg extended the use of arterial revascularization by reporting 116 patients undergoing 119 sequential ITA grafts with three or more anastomoses per conduit.[38] There were no operative deaths. Coronary angiography was performed within 1 month postoperatively in seventy-two patients having seventy-four sequential ITA grafts. The success rate of all coronary anastomoses was 96 per cent: left ITA, 96.4 per cent (215/223); right ITA, 92.9 per cent (twenty-six of twenty-eight). The anastomotic patency rate of the seventy-four sequential ITA conduits with three distal anastomoses was 96.1 per cent (220/229). There was one non-cardiac related late death and five cardiac related mortalities. Control exercise testing performed in sixty patients 5–38 months postoperatively demonstrated no signs of ischaemia. These studies confirmed the safety and efficacy of extended arterial revascularization employing sequential ITA grafts.[39]

Complete revascularization with ITA grafts

Tector and co-workers have achieved complete revascularization of the heart using only ITAs in a 'T' configuration as suggested by the work of Sauvage.[40,41] The 'T' graft is formed by anastomosing the proximal end of the free right ITA to the posterior aspect of the attached left ITA. This adds considerable reach to the right ITA, permitting arterial revascularization of the circumflex and terminal branches of the right coronary artery. They reported 287 patients (mean age 64.6 years) who received a mean of 4.4 ITA to coronary artery anastomoses with an average cross-clamp time of 77 min. There were five operative deaths (1.7 per cent). Three deaths were neurological in origin. Two patients experienced cardiac arrest in the ICU and required urgent placement on cardiopulmonary bypass. Supplemental saphenous vein grafts were used in both patients without success. Six additional patients required supplemental saphenous vein grafts at the initial operation because of hypoperfusion and all survived. Sixty-four patients (22 per cent) required inotropes postoperatively and fifteen patients (5 per cent) needed intra-aortic balloon pump support. The incidence of perioperative myocardial infarction, re-exploration for bleeding and sternal wound infections were 1, 5.6 and 2.9 per cent respectively. Twenty-six patients had postoperative angiography. All forty-five left ITA anastomoses were patent. One right ITA was occluded at its proximal anastomosis and six distal (end-to-side) anastomoses were closed; 107 patients had postoperative stress tests of which ninety-six (89 per cent) were negative.

ITA grafts in the reoperative setting

The excellent early and late results with unilateral and bilateral ITA grafting and the successful use of the ITA with sequential and free grafts encouraged surgeons to employ this conduit in the setting of reoperative myocardial revascularization, particularly when atherosclerotic saphenous vein grafts were present.

Loop and his colleagues reviewed their results in 2509 patients having reoperations for coronary atherosclerosis.[42] Of 1313 patients (52.3 per cent) who received ITA grafts, 112 (8.5 per cent) received ITA grafts at the initial and repeat operations while 1201 (91.5 per cent) received ITA grafts at the second operation. The 2429 hospital survivors were followed for a mean of 72 months. These investigators made the important observation that patients with at least one ITA graft performed either at the first or second operation had an improved 10-year survival when compared to patients with vein grafts alone (73 vs 65 per cent, $P < 0.0004$).

Post-reoperative coronary angiography performed in 684 patients demonstrated vein graft patency of 65 per cent and ITA patency of 88 per cent after a mean of 58 months. These results demonstrated the efficacy and durability of single ITA grafting in appropriately selected patients undergoing reoperative myocardial revascularization.

Lytle reviewed 1663 patients having repeat coronary bypass of which 428 patients had a patent ITA graft to the LAD coronary artery from 1988 to 1991.[43] Multivariate analysis identified no ITA graft at either primary surgery or reoperation as a factor for in-hospital mortality. Furthermore, the presence of an atherosclerotic vein graft to the LAD coronary artery, a factor shown to increase in-hospital risk in previous reports from the Cleveland Clinic, did not increase the risk of reoperation during these years. They attributed the observation that patent ITA and atherosclerotic vein grafts do not appear to be factors specifically increasing the risk of reoperation to the use of retrograde cardioplegia and increased surgical experience. This important observation supports the use of ITA grafts at primary operation and at reoperation in appropriately selected patients. In another report, Lytle found that a right ITA crossing the anterior mid line to the left coronary circulation did not increase the risk of reoperation.[44]

Recognizing the importance of single ITA grafting in reoperative coronary artery bypass surgery, Galbut and associates reported their results in eighty-eight patients undergoing reoperative myocardial revascularization using two ITA grafts.[45] This population was compared with a computer-matched reference group of eighty-eight patients having primary bilateral ITA operations. The hospital mortality for the reoperative group (6.8 per cent) and control group (3.4 per cent) were not significantly different. There were no significant differences in the incidence of reoperation for bleeding, sternal infection, postoperative myocardial infarction or stroke. Prolonged mechanical ventilatory support was more frequent in the reoperation group (13.6 vs 3 per cent; $P = 0.01$) as was the need for perioperative intra-aortic balloon counterpulsation (35 vs 15 per cent; $P = 0.001$). The mean hospital stay was longer for the reoperative group (16.9 vs 12.5 days, $P = 0.03$).

The average duration of follow-up was similar in both groups (reoperation, 37.4 months; reference, 44 months; NS) as was the linearized late mortality rate (reoperation, 2.7 per cent per patient year; control, 2.5 per cent per patient year). At 5 years the actuarial survival was slightly higher for the control group (85 vs 91 per cent) but the difference was not significant.

These data support the use of bilateral ITA grafting for reoperative myocardial revascularization in selected patients. The advantages of two arterial grafts in this setting must be balanced against prolonged ventilatory requirements, longer hospital stay and the greater incidence of perioperative intra-aortic balloon counterpulsation observed in reoperative patients receiving two arterial grafts. Although not addressed by the authors, one cannot help but question whether inadequate ITA flow was in part responsible for the relatively high incidence of intra-aortic balloon pump support. In reoperative situations the native coronary disease has progressed with a reduction in antegrade coronary flow and a myocardium that may be graft-dependent. In this setting the immediate flow demand on the ITA might be greater. Consequently, enthusiasm for bilateral ITA grafting in repeat revascularization must be tempered by the recognized possibility of myocardial hypoperfusion due to inadequate regional ITA flow.

Navia and associates demonstrated that if the saphenous vein graft to a totally occluded left anterior descending coronary artery were divided to prevent atherosclerotic embolization and replaced with an ITA graft alone, the incidence of hypoperfusion syndrome is 19 per cent and is associated with an operative mortality of 8 per cent.[46] Emergency treatment for this syndrome is supplemental vein grafting. However, the high flow in a vein graft can compete with ITA graft flow and may result in a 'string sign' angiographically. This unquestionably occurs, but the frequency is unknown and the clinical significance is unclear. Increasing evidence suggests that an atretic appearing ITA may be able to dilate and function normally if competitive flow is decreased and demand increased.[47–49] Therefore, a better alternative to dividing the old saphenous vein graft to the LAD is to leave the stenotic vein graft intact and add the ITA to the distal LAD. Although concern has been raised about the possibility of perioperative atherosclerotic embolization from the stenotic vein graft to the LAD, this complication is not common.[50] Support for this approach has been recently provided by Turner and associates.[51] Ninety patients undergoing coronary reoperation had an ITA graft added to a stenotic vein graft. There were no operative or hospital deaths. Follow-up angiography in twenty two patients at a mean interval of 48 months demonstrated all but one vein graft to be occluded with the ITA fully patent in twenty patients and obstructed in two, indicating that the ITA continues to function while the vein graft occludes. Distal embolization into the LAD was not documented in any patient. We currently support this approach for patients with atherosclerotic vein grafts to the LAD in whom the ITA can be utilized at reoperation.

While current data support the use of bilateral ITA grafting in appropriately selected patients undergoing reoperative myocardial revascularization, conventional wisdom would dictate that patients with severe left ventricular dysfunction (EF < 25 per cent), obesity, diabetes mellitus or the need for prolonged ventilatory support, should not be selected for bilateral ITA grafting.

ITA grafts in left main coronary disease

The use of ITA grafting in the setting of left main coronary artery disease has not been universally accepted because of concern over inadequate flow with hypoperfusion if the left main coronary artery is severely stenotic.

In 1987, Vijayanajar and associates compared the results of myocardial revascularization employing the left ITA in ninety-eight patients having left main coronary artery disease (≥ 70 per cent stenosis) to a matched population of ninety-eight patients receiving saphenous vein grafts only.[52] The left ITA was used for the LAD/diagonal coronary artery in ninety-six patients and for the circumflex in two patients. There were five operative deaths (ITA group 2 per cent vs SVG Group 3 per cent; P = NS). The two deaths in the ITA group were in patients having concomitant valve replacement with myocardial revascularization. The postoperative complications of low cardiac output (ITA 2 per cent vs SVG 3 per cent), stroke (1 vs 1 per cent), prolonged ventilatory support (3 vs 1 per cent), sternal infection (2 vs SVG 4 per cent) and postoperative myocardial infarction (3 vs 2 per cent respectively) were not significantly different. There were nine late deaths at a mean follow up of 21 months with only one cardiac related death in the ITA group. Twenty-five patients having postoperative coronary angiography demonstrated ten of ten ITA grafts patent. In the saphenous vein group, six of eight single grafts and six of nine sequential vein grafts were open. This early study supports the safety and efficacy of using one ITA graft to the left coronary circulation in patients with left main coronary artery disease.

Barner and co-workers extended these results in forty-five patients with left main coronary artery disease.[53] Both ITAs were employed as the only grafts to the left coronary circulation. No saphenous vein graft was used and there were no operative deaths. Postoperative complications of low cardiac output (4 per cent), perioperative myocardial infarction (2 per cent), stroke (2 per cent), reoperation for bleeding (2 per cent), sternal infection (0 per cent) and prolonged ventilatory support (4 per cent) were low and not significantly different from patients having bilateral ITA grafting with supplemental saphenous vein grafts for non-left main coronary artery disease. These data indicate that use of two ITAs alone for revascularization of the left coronary circulation in the setting of left main coronary artery disease is safe and efficacious practice, which is further supported by the work of Paolini *et al.*[54]

Galbut and associates provided long-term follow-up on 263 of 276 patients with left main coronary artery disease who underwent myocardial revascularization with two ITA grafts.[55] At the completion of their follow up (6–94 months; mean 34 months) 88 per cent of the hospital survivors were alive. The linearized late mortality was 2.5 per cent per patient year. There were twenty late deaths, of which eight were cardiac related. The 3- and 5-year actuarial survival was 93 and 87 per cent respectively. No patient required reoperation. With the exception of four of the remaining 238 survivors, all improved by at least one New York Heart Association function class. Exercise stress testing performed in 143 survivors was negative for ischaemia in 92 per cent (131 patients). Eleven hospital survivors underwent coronary angiography at a mean of 26 months postoperatively and all ITA grafts were patent.

These results furnish evidence that single and bilateral ITA grafting can be accomplished with a low operative risk and can provide excellent intermediate term functional results in patients with left main coronary artery disease. One or both ITAs can provide enough flow to meet the demands of the left ventricular circulation and additional data support the concept that the ITA progressively enlarges with time in order to meet the flow requirements placed upon it.[56–58]

ITA grafts in the elderly

The age of patients referred for myocardial revascularization has been steadily increasing. Advanced age is often associated with saphenous vein of inferior quality and a severely atherosclerotic ascending aorta. The ITA becomes an attractive conduit for myocardial revascularization in this setting and enthusiasm for its use in the elderly has increased. Some surgeons have been concerned that ITA grafting in the elderly may be associated with an increase in operative morbidity and provide no substantial survival benefit in patients with a limited lifespan.

Gardner and associates addressed these issues by comparing the results of ITA grafting in 453 patients, 70 years of age or older (mean 73.7 years) with a similar group of 270 patients receiving vein grafts only.[59] Preoperatively the vein graft group had a higher percentage of coronary care unit patients and more frequent need for preoperative intra-aortic balloon counterpulsation. The hospital mortality was significantly greater in the vein graft group, (9.7 vs 4.9 per cent) as was the incidence of stroke (7.5 vs 2.7 per cent) and length of hospital stay (14 vs 12 days). The frequency of sternal wound infection, reoperation for bleeding and postoperative myocardial infarction was not significantly different in both cohorts. Multiple logistic regression analysis demonstrated that unstable angina, need for intra-aortic balloon preoperatively and the absence of an ITA graft was associated with an increased risk of hospital death. When late survival was analyzed the presence of an ITA graft conferred a significant survival advantage at 4 years in those patients (ITA 87 per cent vs no ITA 77 per cent; $P = 0.03$), although this difference was possibly related to patient selection.

Wareing and his colleagues compared the results of ITA grafting in 341 patients beyond 65 years of age to a matched population of patients less than 65.[60] The 30-day mortality was similar in both cohorts (< 65 years, 2.7 per cent; > 65 years, 3.2 per cent; NS). The incidence of reoperation for haemorrhage, perioperative myocardial infarction, neurological deficit, need for postoperative intra-aortic balloon pump support and sternal wound infection were not significantly different. There was a trend towards more frequent prolonged ventilatory support in the elderly subset (6.5 vs 3.6 per cent; $P = 0.06$) and a significantly longer hospital stay. (10.2 vs 11.8 days; $P = 0.02$). Histological comparison of the ITA in both groups did not demonstrate significant differences in wall thickness, luminal diameter or intimal fibrous thickening. Atherosclerosis of the ITA was not observed in either cohort.

Azariades *et al.* used the ITA in 354 patients aged 70 years or greater, and compared them to a matched population of 720 patients receiving only venous conduits.[61] The operative mortality was significantly lower in patients receiving ITA grafts (2.8 vs 7.6 per cent; $P < 0.05$). Six of the ten deaths in the ITA group were cardiac related. The incidence of perioperative myocardial infarction and the mean hospital stay were not significantly different between groups. The actuarial 5-year survival was better for the ITA patients (89 vs 78 per cent; $P = 0.001$) and again possibly related to selection.

Galbut and co-workers extended these results by reporting on 731 elderly patients (mean age 70.9 years) who received bilateral ITA grafts.[62] When they were compared to a matched population of patients receiving one ITA graft (mean age 73.2 years) there were no differences observed in the rate of reoperation for bleeding, sternal infection, respiratory failure, stroke or postoperative myocardial infarction. The operative mortality was higher in the single ITA group (6.4 vs 3.1 per cent; $P < 0.004$) again probably reflecting patient selection. At a mean follow up of 42 months those patients receiving two ITA grafts had a significant improvement in actuarial survival (60.7 vs 68 per cent; $P < 0.03$). This comparative study demonstrates that bilateral ITA grafting can be accomplished in elderly patients with low operative risk and significant reduction in cardiac events with improved early survival.

These results support the use of single or double ITA grafting in selected septuagenarian patients. Performance of an ITA graft improves actuarial survival which probably reflects patient selection and is not associated with a significant increase in postoperative morbidity but may be associated with a longer hospital stay.

ITA grafts in diabetics

Morris and his associates reviewed the comparative results of ITA grafting in 1132 insulin-dependent diabetic and 4522 non-diabetic patients.[63] The diabetic group had a significantly greater female cohort (34 vs 20 per cent), was older (62 years vs 60 years) had a lower ejection fraction (49 vs 51 per cent) and was more likely to have triple vessel coronary artery disease (55 vs 45 per cent). The frequency of ITA grafting was greater in the diabetic group (67 vs 58 per cent).

Multivariate analysis of risk factors demonstrated that failure to use an ITA graft and the presence of diabetes were equally strong predictors of cardiac mortality. Separate multivariate analysis of non-diabetic and diabetic patients identified similar risk factors for mortality. Each of these risk factors identified the adverse effect of diabetes on long-term survival. The use of an ITA graft did convey independent long-term survival benefits to both non-diabetic and diabetic patients. The survival benefit was the same for both groups. Although diabetic patients received more ITA grafts, the incidence of repeat cardiac catheterization, repeat myocardial revascularization and subsequent interventional coronary angioplasty did not differ in non-diabetic and diabetic patients. These data demonstrate that diabetes is an important risk factor for late cardiac mortality after bypass surgery. ITA grafting conveys a similar benefit to diabetic and non-diabetic patients, but does not negate the adverse effects of diabetes on survival. It is unknown whether bilateral ITA grafts, sequential ITA grafts or the use of supplemental alternative arterial conduits (i.e. radial artery, gastroepiploic artery) in diabetic patients followed beyond 8 years can alter the negative influence of diabetes on long-term survival.

ITA grafts following failed coronary angioplasty

The number of coronary angioplasty procedures performed in the United States exceeded 300,000 in 1993. Despite the increased use of this technique, the incidence of emergency coronary artery bypass surgery ranges between 1 and 6 per cent. Although the ITA is the graft of choice for elective myocardial revascularization, surgeons have been reluctant to employ this conduit for the primary target (culprit) artery which has closed or narrowed following failed coronary angioplasty. Recently, the culprit vessel can be stabilized by a guide wire or bailout catheter, which can prevent the regional myocardial ischaemia and haemodynamic instability often associated with failed coronary angioplasty. In this setting some surgeons have been willing to take the added time for ITA harvesting. Others have initiated cardiopulmonary bypass before harvesting the ITA and some have even clamped the aorta and given retrograde cardioplegia (warm or cold) prior to ITA mobilization.

Zapolanski and his associates utilized the left ITA to revascularize the culprit LAD lesion in thirty-six patients and the right ITA for the culprit right coronary artery (RCA) lesion in three patients.[64] There was one operative death in the ITA cohort (right ITA to culprit RCA). Postoperative complications including Q-wave myocardial infarction (9.3 per cent), cerebrovascular accident (3.7 per cent), reoperation for bleeding (5.6 per cent) and need for intra-aortic balloon pump counterpulsation postoperatively (17.6 per cent) were not significantly different in those patients receiving an ITA versus those receiving only saphenous vein grafts. Long-term follow-up was not provided.

Caes and co-workers described using the ITA in twenty-seven of thirty-two patients following angioplasty failure including two cases of double and two cases of sequential ITA grafting.[65] Five patients received only saphenous vein grafts. The mean ejection fraction was 77 per cent. Temporary reperfusion of the culprit artery was achieved using a bailout catheter in twelve patients.

In eleven culprit LAD patients, the left ITA to the LAD was supplemented by a saphenous vein graft to the same territory (nine to diagonal and two LAD. The interval between failed PTCA and opening of the grafts or the end of cardiopulmonary bypass was similar whether the ITA or saphenous vein were used. There were no operative deaths. Fourteen patients (44 per cent) sustained a perioperative myocardial infarction by ECG and enzyme criteria. The use of a reperfusion catheter after failed PTCA was associated with a significant decrease in the use of anti-arrhythmics following myocardial revascularization ($P < 0.05$), but did not influence survival, incidence of myocardial infarction or use of the ITA graft.

Although the report by Caes and associates supports use of the ITA in selected patients following failed coronary angioplasty, two points merit emphasis. First, eleven of the twenty-seven patients (41 per cent) receiving an ITA to the culprit LAD also received a supplemental saphenous vein graft. This suggests that the ITA alone did not provide enough flow to the anterior septal wall in all patients following failed PTCA of the LAD. Second, it has not been established that the early and late beneficial results of ITA grafting apply in the setting of failed coronary angioplasty. Long-term follow-up studies of failed PTCA patients undergoing emergency myocardial revascularization are scarce and it remains uncertain whether the ITA will be the conduit of choice in this setting.

We encourage use of the ITA following failed coronary angioplasty but only in carefully selected haemodynamically stable patients with no ongoing acute myocardial ischaemia or other contraindications to ITA usage.

Conclusion

Since its clinical introduction in the 1960s, the ITA has established itself as the conduit of choice for myocardial revascularization. When placed to the LAD coronary artery, the ITA confers greater longevity and enhanced freedom from all ischaemic events when compared to patients receiving only saphenous vein conduits. Clinical data now supports bilateral ITA grafting in selected patients whose life expectancy is greater than 10 years. The use of one or two ITAs in the setting of left main coronary artery disease and reoperative myocardial revascularization is safe and efficacious in selected patients.

Free and sequential ITA grafting are technically more demanding, but permit greater versatility for complete arterial revascularization and are not associated with increased patient mortality or morbidity. At the present time such complex arterial revascularization is justified on the basis of graft patency since no long-term survival advantage has been demonstrated. The utilization of both ITAs supplemented with the gastroepiploic, radial or inferior epigastric arteries can achieve nearly complete revascularization with arterial conduits in most patients.

It is the authors' opinion that long-term results of myocardial revascularization will be better in those patients having more complete revascularization with arterial conduits.

Acknowledgement

We are grateful to Mrs Terri Wriley for secretarial help in preparation of the manuscript.

References

1. Spencer FC, Yong NK, and Prachuabmoh, K. Internal mammary-coronary artery anastomoses performed during cardiopulmonary bypass. *Cardiovasc Surg* 1964; **5:** 292.
2. Green GE, Stertzer SH and Reppert EH. Coronary arterial bypass grafts. *Ann Thorac Surg* 1968; **5:** 443.
3. Barner, HB., Kaiser GC, Jellinek, M, *et al.* Aortocoronary vein graft and internal mammary-coronary anastomosis, *Arch Surg* 1973; **105:** 908–11.
4. Green GE. Internal mammary-coronary artery anastomosis: Three year experience with 165 patients. *Ann Thorac Surg* 1972; **14:** 260–71.
5. Loop FD, Irazzaval MJ, Bredee JJ. *et al.* Internal mammary artery graft for ischemic heart disease: Effect of revascularization on clinical status and survival. *Am J Cardiol* 1977; **39:** 516.
6. Mills NL, Ochsner JL. Technique of internal mammary-to-coronary artery bypass. *Ann Thorac Surg* 1974; **17:** 237–46.
7. Sergeant P, Lesaffre E, Flameng W, Suy R. Internal mammary artery: Methods of use and their effect on survival after coronary bypass surgery. *Eur J Cardiothorac Surg* 1990; **4:** 72–8.
8. Grondin CM, Campeau L, Lesperance J *et al.* Comparison of late changes in internal mammary artery and saphenous vein grafts in two consecutive series of patients 10 years after operation. *Circulation* 1984; **70** (Suppl. 1): I208–12.
9. Lytle BW, Loop FD, Taylor PC *et al.* Vein graft disease: The clinical impact of stenoses in saphenous vein bypass grafts to coronary arteries. *J Thorac Cardiovasc Surg*, 1992; **103:** 831–40.
10. Barner HB, Standeven JW, Reese J. Twelve-year experience with internal mammary artery for coronary artery bypass. *J Thorac Cardiovasc Surg*, 1985; **90:** 668–75.
11. Loop FD, Lytle BW, Cosgrove DM. Influence of the internal mammary artery graft on 10-year survival and other cardiac events. *New Engl J Med* 1986; **314:** 1–6.
12. Lytle BW, Loop FD, Cosgrove DM, Ratliff NB, Easley K, Taylor PC. Long-term (5 to 12 years) serial studies of internal mammary artery and saphenous vein coronary bypass grafts. *J Thorac Cardiovasc Surg* 1986; **89:** 248–58.
13. Tector AJ, Schmahl TM, Canino VR. Expanding the use of the internal mammary artery to improve patency in coronary artery bypass grafting. *J Thorac Cardiovasc Surg* 1986; **91:** 9–16.
14. Acinapura AJ, Rose DM, Jacobowitz IJ *et al.* Internal mammary artery bypass grafting: Influence on recurrent angina and survival in 2,100 patients. *Ann Thorac Surg* 1989; **48:** 186–91.
15. Barner HB. Double internal mammary-coronary artery bypass. *Arch Surg* 1974; **109:** 627–30.
16. Lytle BW, Cosgrove DM, Loop FD *et al.* Perioperative risk of bilateral internal mammary artery grafting: analysis of 500 cases from 1971 to 1984. *Circulation* 1986; **74** (Suppl. III): III37.
17. Galbut DL, Traad EA, Dorman MJ *et al.* Seventeen-year experience with bilateral internal mammary artery grafts. *Ann Thorac Surg* 1990; **49:** 195–201.
18. Fiore AC, Naunheim KS, McBride LR *et al.*

Fifteen-year follow-up for double internal thoracic artery grafts. *Eur J Cardiothorac Surg* 1991; 5: 248–52.
19. Kouchoukos NT, Wareing TH, Murphy SF *et al.* Risks of bilateral internal mammary artery bypass grafting. *Ann Thorac Surg* 1990; **49:** 210–19.
20. Cosgrove DM, Lytle BW, Loop FD *et al.* Does bilateral internal mammary artery grafting increase surgical risk? *J Thorac Cardiovasc Surg* 1988; **95:** 850–6.
21. Buxton BF, Tatoulis J, McNeil JJ, Fuller JA. Internal mammary artery grafting: Is this a benign procedure? *J Cardiovasc Surg (Torino)* 1988; **29:** 633–8.
22. Accola KD, Jones EL, Craver JM *et al.* Bilateral mammary artery grafting: Avoidance of complications with extended use. *Ann Thorac Surg* 1993; **56:** 872–9.
23. Dion R, Etienne PY, Verhelst R *et al.* Bilateral mammary grafting. *Eur J Cardiothorac Surg* 1993; **7:** 287–94.
24. Fiore AC, Naunheim KS, Dean P *et al.* Results of internal thoracic artery grafting over 15 years: Single verses double grafts. *Ann Thorac Surg* 1990; **49:** 202–9.
25. Cameron A, Kemp HG, Green GE. Bypass surgery with the internal mammary artery graft: 15 year follow-up. *Circulation* 1986; **74** (Suppl. 3): 30–6.
26. Barner HB. The internal mammary artery as a free graft. *J Thorac Cardiovasc Surg* 1973; **66:** 219–21.
27. Loop FD, Spampinato N, Cheanvechai C, Effler DB. The free internal mammary artery graft. *Ann Thorac Surg* 1973; **15:** 50–5.
28. Schimert G, Vidne BA, Lee AB Jr. Free internal mammary artery graft. *Ann Thorac Surg* 1975; **19:** 474–7.
29. Loop FD, Lytle BW, Cosgrove DM *et al.* Free (aorta-coronary) internal mammary artery graft. *J Thorac Cardiovasc Surg* 1986; **92:** 827–31.
30. Rankin JS, Newman GE, Bashore TM *et al.* Clinical and angiographic assessment of complex mammary artery bypass grafting. *J Thorac Cardiovasc Surg* 1986; **92:** 832–46.
31. Kanter KR, Barner HB. Improved technique for the proximal anastomosis with free internal mammary artery grafts. *Ann Thorac Surg 1987;* **44:** 556–7.
32. McBride LR, Barner HB. The left internal mammary artery as a sequential graft to the left anterior descending system. *J Thorac Cardiovasc Surg* 1983; **86:** 703–5.
33. Kabbani SS, Hanna ES, Bashour TT *et al.* Sequential internal mammary-coronary artery bypass. *J Thorac Cardiovasc Surg* 1983; **86:** 697–702.
34. Tector AJ, Schmahl TM. Techniques for multiple internal mammary artery bypass grafts. *Ann Thorac Surg* 1984; **38:** 281–8.
35. Kamath ML, Matysik LS, Schmidt DH, Smith LL. Sequential internal mammary artery grafts. Expanded utilization of an ideal conduit. *J Thorac Cardiovasc Surg* 1985; **89:** 163–9.
36. Rankin JS, Newman GE, Bashore TM *et al.* Clinical and angiographic assessment of complex mammary artery bypass grafting. *J Thorac Cardiovasc Surg* 1986; **92:** 832–46.
37. Dion R, Verhelst R, Rousseau M *et al.* Sequential mammary grafting. Clinical, functional, and angiographic assessment 6 months postoperatively in 231 consecutive patients. *J Thorac Cardiovasc Surg* 1989; **98:** 80–9.
38. VanSterkenburg SM, Ernst SMPG, Aart Brutel de la Rivière *et al.* Triple sequential grafts using the internal mammary artery. An angiographic and short-term follow-up study. J *Thorac Cardiovasc Surg* 1992; **104:** 60–5.
39. Palatianos GM, Bolooki H, Horowitz MD *et al.* Sequential internal mammary artery grafts for coronary artery bypass. *Ann Thorac Surg* 1993; **56:** 1136–40.
40. Sauvage LR, Wu H-D, Kowalski TE. Healing basis and surgical techniques for complete revascularization of the left ventricle using only the internal mammary arteries. *Ann Thorac Surg* 1986; **42:** 449–65.
41. Tector AJ, Amundsen S, Schmahl TM *et al.* Total revascularization with T grafts. *Ann Thorac Surg* 1994; **57:** 33–9.
42. Loop FD, Lytle BW, Cosgrove DM *et al.* Reoperation for coronary atherosclerosis: Changing practice in 2,509 consecutive patients. *Ann Surg* 1990; **212:** 378–86.
43. Lytle BW, McElroy D, McCarthy PM *et al.* The influence of arterial coronary bypass grafts on the mortality of coronary reoperations. *J Thorac Cardiovasc Surg* 1994; **107:** 675–83.
44. Lytle BW, Loop FD, Taylor PC *et al.* The effect of coronary reoperation on the survival of patients with stenoses in saphenous vein to coronary bypass grafts. *J Thorac Cardiovasc Surg* 1993; **105:** 605–14.
45. Galbut DL, Traad EA, Dorman MJ *et al.* Bilateral internal mammary artery grafts in reoperative and primary coronary bypass surgery. *Ann Thorac Surg* 1991; 52: 20–8.
46. Navia D, Cosgrove DM III, Lytle BW *et al.* Is the internal thoracic artery the conduit of choice to replace a stenotic vein graft? *Ann Thorac Surg* 1994; **57:** 40–4.
47. Dincer B, Barner HB. The 'occluded' internal mammary artery graft. Restoration of patency after apparent occlusion associated with progression of coronary disease. *J Thorac Cardiovasc Surg* 1983; **85:** 318–20.
48. Aris A, Borras X, Ramio J. Patency of internal mammary artery grafts in no flow situations. *J Thorac Cardiovasc Surg* 1987; **93:** 62–4.
49. Kitamura S, Kawacki K, Seki T *et al.* Angiographic demonstration of no-flow anatomical patency of internal thoracic-coronary artery bypass grafts. *Ann Thorac Surg* 1992; **53:** 156–9.

50. Keon WJ, Heggtveit HA, Leduc J. Perioperative myocardial infarction caused by atheroembolism. *J Thorac Cardiovasc Surg* 1982; **84:** 849–55.
51. Turner FE, Lytle BW, Navia D *et al.* Coronary reoperation: Results of adding an internal mammary artery graft to a stenotic vein graft. *Ann Thorac Surg* 1994; **58:** 1353–5.
52. Vijayanagar R, Bognolo D, Eckstein P *et al.* Safety and efficacy of internal mammary artery grafts for left main coronary artery disease. *J Cardiovasc Surg* 1987; **28:** 576–80.
53. Barner HB, Naunheim KS, Willman VL, Fiore AC. Revascularization with bilateral internal thoracic artery grafts in patients with left main coronary stenosis. *Eur J Cardiothorac Surg* 1992; **6:** 66–71.
54. Paolini G, Zuccari M, Di Credico G *et al.* Myocardial revascularization with bilateral internal thoracic artery in patients with left main disease: an incremental risk? *Eur J Cardiothorac Surg* 1994; **8:** 576–9.
55. Galbut DL, Traad EA, Dorman MJ *et al.* Bilateral internal mammary artery grafts in patients with left main coronary artery disease. *J Card Surg* 1993 ;**18:** 18–24.
56. Johnson AM, Kron IL, Watson DD *et al.* Evaluation of postoperative flow reserve in internal mammary artery bypass grafts. *J Thorac Cardiovasc Surg* 1986; **92:** 822–7.
57. Schmidt DH, Balu F, Hellman C *et al.* Isoproterenol induced flow responses in mammary and vein bypass grafts. *J Thorac Cardiovasc Surg* 80: 319–26.
58. Siegel W, Loop FD. Comparison of internal mammary artery and saphenous vein bypass grafts for myocardial revascularization: Exercise test and angiographic correlations. *Circulation* 1976; **54 (Suppl. 3):** 1–30.
59. Gardner TJ, Greene PS, Rykiel MF, RN *et al.* Routine use of the left internal mammary artery graft in the elderly. *Ann Thorac Surg* 1990; **49:** 188–94.
60. Wareing TH, Saffitz JE, Kouchoukos NT. Use of single internal mammary artery grafts in older patients. *Circulation* 1990; **82** (Suppl. IV): IV224–8).
61. Azariades M, Fessler CL, Floten HS, Starr A. Five-year results of coronary bypass grafting for patients older than 70 years: Role of internal mammary artery. *Ann Thorac Surg* 1990; **50:** 940–5.
62. Galbut DL, Traad EA, Dorman MJ *et al.* Coronary bypass grafting in the elderly. Single versus bilateral internal mammary artery grafts. *J Thorac Cardiovasc Surg* 1993; **106:** 128–36.
63. Morris JJ, Smith LR, Jones RH *et al.* Influence of diabetes and mammary artery grafting on survival after coronary bypass. *Circulation* 1991; **84** (Suppl. III): III275–84.
64. Zapolanski A, Rosenblum J, Myler RK *et al.* Emergency coronary artery bypass surgery following failed balloon angioplasty: Role of the internal mammary artery graft. *J Cardiac Surg* 1991; **6(4):** 439–48.
65. Caes FL, Van Nooten GJ. Use of internal mammary artery for emergency grafting after failed coronary angioplasty. *Ann Thorac Surg* 1994; 57: 1295–9.

Part III
Right gastroepiploic artery

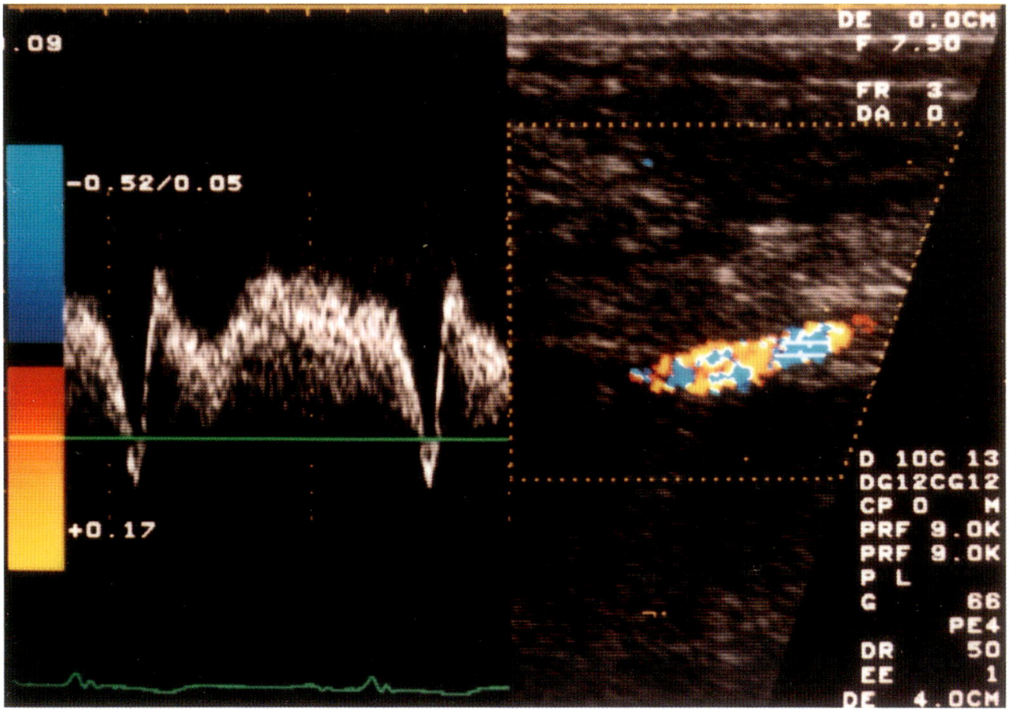

Plate 1 Blood flow in the GEA graft is confirmed non-invasively either by colour- or continuous-wave Doppler ultrasound.

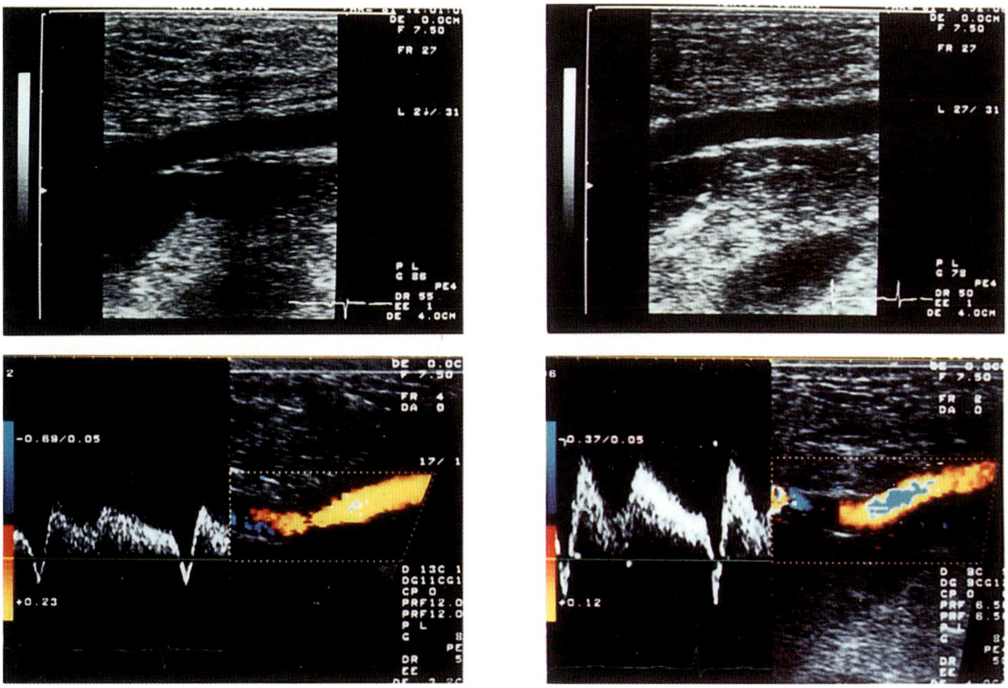

Pre-Prandial: arterial calibre, 4.0 mm; HR, 78 beats/min; flow vol, 235 ml/min.

Post-Prandial: arterial calibre, 4.2 mm; HR, 79 beats/min; flow vol, 252 ml/min.

Plate 2 Percutaneous Doppler echo of the GEA graft before (left) and after (right) a meal in 75-year-old woman. The GEA is clearly visualized (above) and its flow is detectable (below) by ultrasonography (Toshiba SSH-270 HD, linear probe 7.5 MHz). Note that the GEA calibre is about the same at pre- and post-prandial period, but flow velocity is increased after meal, so that the GEA graft flow seems to be increased with meal.

11 Surgical techniques

Hisayoshi Suma

Mobilization of GEA

The right gastroepiploic artery (GEA) is a branch of the gastroduodenal artery which arises from the common hepatic artery. It runs posterior to the duodenum and along the greater curvature of the stomach together with the right gastroepiploic vein. To harvest a GEA graft, the median sternotomy incision is extended to midway between the xiphoid process and the umbilicus, and the peritoneum is opened. The stomach is delivered into the wound, and the GEA is palpated along its greater curvature. It is important that the vessel is handled gently while evaluating its thickness, length and pulsatility, because manipulation readily induces spasm in the artery. The GEA and surrounding tissue is detached from the greater curvature as a pedicle. The branches to the omentum are usually small and easily divided by electrocautery or the LDS stapler® (United States Surgical Corporation, Norwalk, CT, USA). Branches to the stomach, however, should be ligated individually with a silk ligature or absorbable clip (Absolock®, Johnson and Johnson, Arlington, TX, USA) before they are divided because they are thick and short. (Fig. 11.1). If haemostasis at this site is not secure, a haematoma will develop in the pedicle. Mobilization of the GEA should begin at the lower margin of the pylorus and need not include the posterior aspect of the duodenum. Detachment then proceeds to include a half to two thirds of the greater curvature (Fig. 11.2). The GEA pedicle

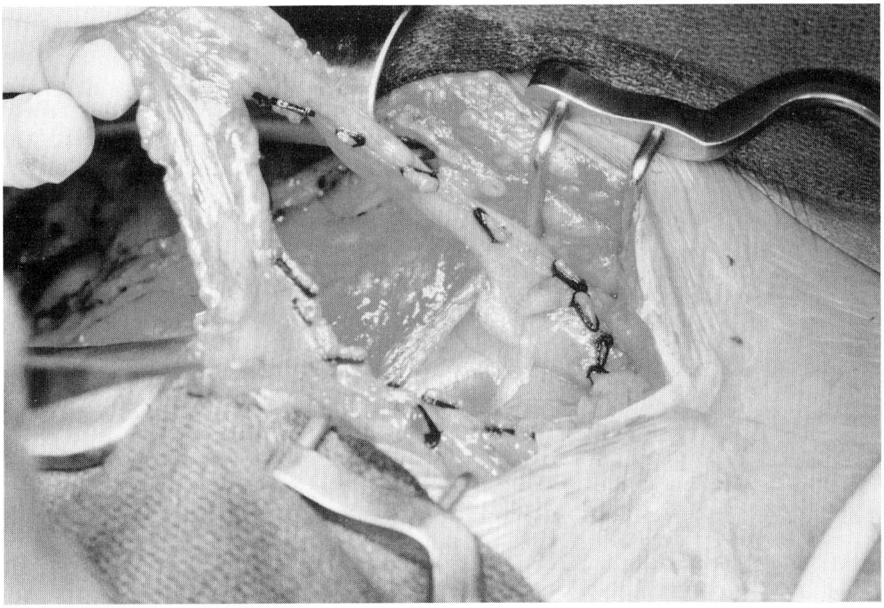

Fig. 11.1 GEA pedicle freed from the greater curvature of the stomach. GEA branches to the stomach were clipped with Absolock ® Clips and divided. Note extension of the skin incision down to the abdomen is minimal.

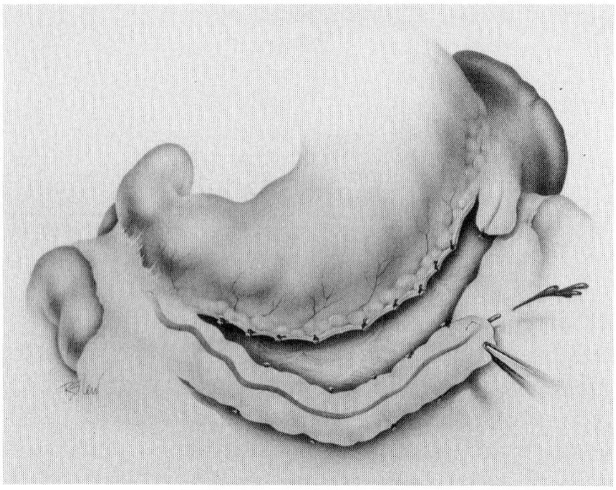

Fig. 11.2 Division of GEA pedicle at the left end of its dissection. Dissection of the proximal (right) GEA is ended at beneath the duodenum. No further dissection is necessary. Reproduced with permission from Suma *et al.*[1]

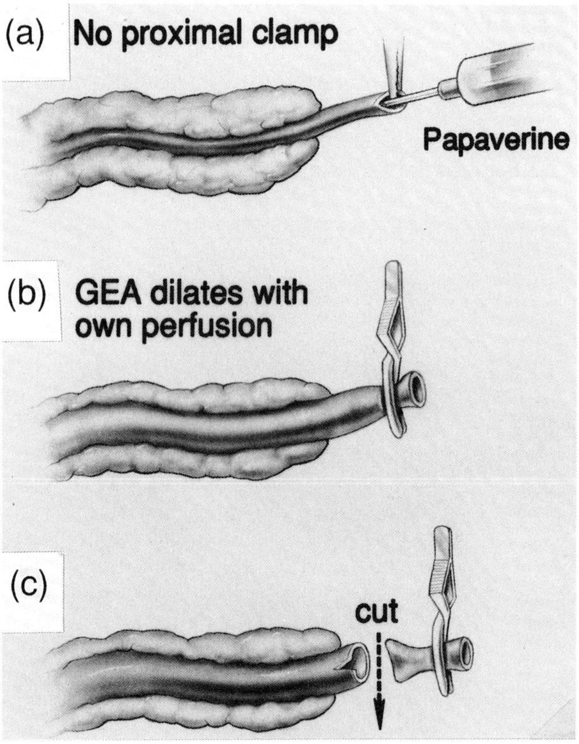

Fig. 11.3 (a) Dilute papaverine is injected into the GEA from the cut end without a proximal clamp to avoid excessive hydrostatic dilatation. (b) Leaving the GEA with a distal clamp, allows dilatation of the GEA by its own perfusion pressure. (c) Finally, the dilated distal end of GEA is trimmed for anastomosis.

should be made as long as possible, based on preservation of strong pulsation. Detachment of the GEA from the greater curvature, performed in the manner described, carries no risk of gastric ischaemia.[2]

The GEA is divided distally, and 3 to 4 ml papaverine hydrochloride (40 mg diluted in 10 ml of physiologic saline) is injected intraluminally to relieve spasm without clamping the graft proximally (Fig. 11.3). The distal end is then clamped so that the artery is dilated by both the pharmacologic effect of the papaverine and distended by its own blood pressure. Leaving the proximal end unclamped during injection prevents intimal damage due to excessive hydrostatic pressure. With the distal end of GEA clamped, the pedicle is checked for bleeding. The distance to the site of the anastomosis is measured to determine the length of the graft. The tissue surrounding the GEA adjacent to the site of anastomosis is ligated, and 2 to 3 cm of the artery is skeletonized. The right gastroepiploic vein running along with the right GEA is also ligated. The many direct communications between the artery and veins in the pedicle may lead to a significant amount of bleeding unless the vein is ligated securely. The distal end of the skeletonized GEA is transected, cut back a few millimeters in preparation for the anastomosis, and checked to ensure free flow.

Anastomosis

Following institution of cardiopulmonary bypass an opening one to two fingers breadth in diameter is made in the diaphragm, using electrocautery and the GEA is delivered into the pericardial space avoiding any twisting of the pedicle. Only a simple incision in the anterior diaphragm is required for GEA grafting to the left anterior descending artery.[3] The GEA pedicle can reach the pericardial space by traversing the anterior surface of the stomach and liver (anterior route), the posterior surface of stomach and liver (posterior route), or along the posterior surface of the stomach and the anterior surface of the liver (crossing route).[4] I always use the anterior route, because it is easier to check for twisting and bleeding of the pedicle following completion of the anastomosis.

I believe that the GEA is long enough to bypass the circumflex artery via the anterior route and have not appreciated a significant difference in the length of pedicle required between the anterior and posterior routes. To obtain a clear view of the anastomotic site, while creating the graft–coronary artery anastomosis, the heart is retracted upward, (anteriorly) and the distal portion of the circumflex or right coronary artery is displaced anteriorly. In this situation, a pedicle traversing the posterior route requires additional length to reach the target site because the opening in the diaphragm is very deep (posterior) in the wound. Additional length is usually not required when the anterior route is chosen because the opening in the diaphragm is more anterior. (Fig. 11.4). Only when the anastomosis is performed deep within the pericardial space, with the heart nearly in its natural position, does the posterior route permit a shorter pedicle. After the GEA pedicle has been introduced into the pericardial space, the distal end of the pedicle is fixed at the anterior margin of the diaphragm with forceps (Fig. 11.5).

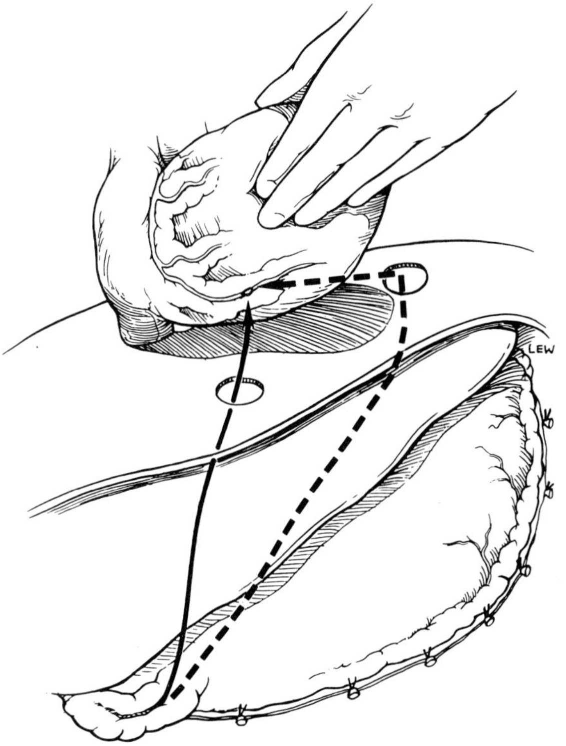

Fig. 11.4 Required length of the *in situ* GEA pedicle for the anterior and posterior route at the time of anastomosis. The target coronary artery comes up anteriorly by retraction of the heart upward (anteriorly): the pedicle through the posterior route needs additional length whereas the anterior route does not. Reproduced with permission from Suma.[5]

The GEA–coronary artery anastomosis is performed during cardioplegic arrest using a 7–0 or 8–0 polypropylene suture. The suture is placed in the heel of the graft using two to three stitches and then traction is applied to approximate the GEA to the coronary artery. The anastomosis is then completed using a single continuous suture. After three quarters of the anastomosis has been carried out a graduated probe is introduced through the anastomosis to confirm patency, and if satisfactory the rest of the suture line is completed.

As shown in Fig. 11.6, the direction of the anastomosis depends upon its site. When the target is the posterior descending or distal main right coronary artery, the GEA is anastomosed in an antegrade fashion, placing the heel of the graft on the proximal end of the arteriotomy. A retrograde anastomosis can be created by placing the heel of the graft on the distal aspect of the arteriotomy, when the target is the anterior descending or, rarely, the proximal right main coronary artery. I prefer an antegrade anastomosis for the circumflex artery (Fig. 11.7).

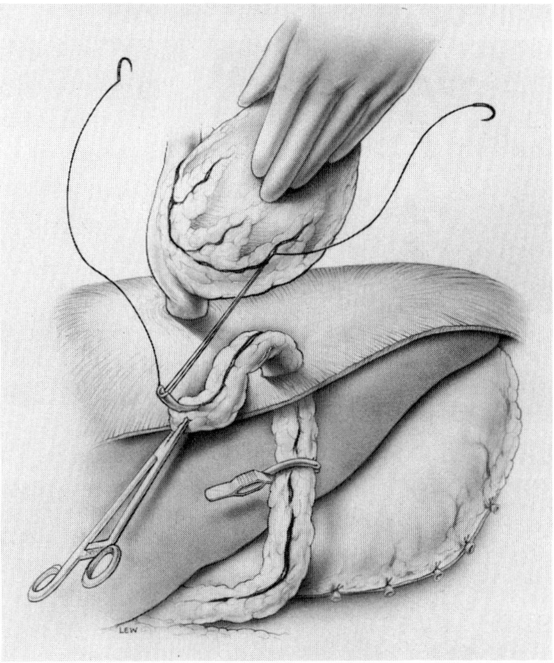

Fig. 11.5 The GEA pedicle introduced into the pericardial cavity through an opening in the diaphragm passing the liver and the stomach anteriorly (anterior route). The distal end of the pedicle is fixed to the anterior margin of the diaphragm to facilitate the anastomosis. The GEA is anastomosed to the coronary artery with a single polypropylene continuous suture.

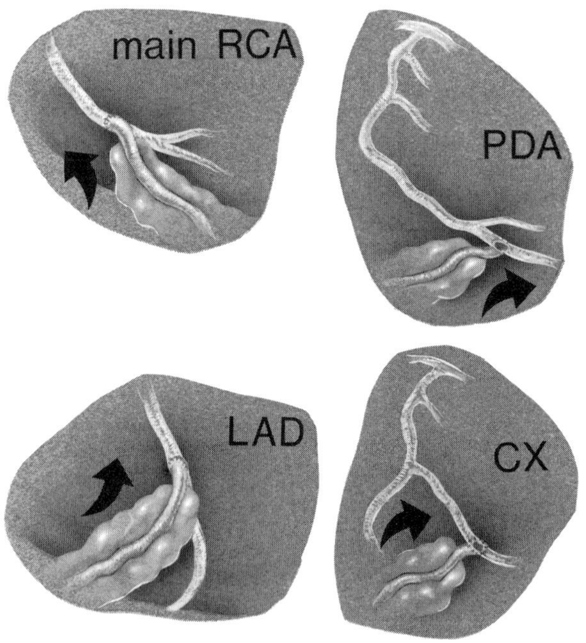

Fig. 11.6 The GEA is anastomosed to the posterior descending artery and the posterolateral branch in the same direction to the native coronary flow (antegrade anastomosis), but is anastomosed in the opposite direction to the native coronary flow when the target is a relatively proximal part of the main right coronary artery or the left anterior descending artery. Main RCA = main right coronary artery; PDA = posterior descending artery; LAD = left anterior descending; CX = circumflex. Reproduced with permission from Suma *et al.*[6]

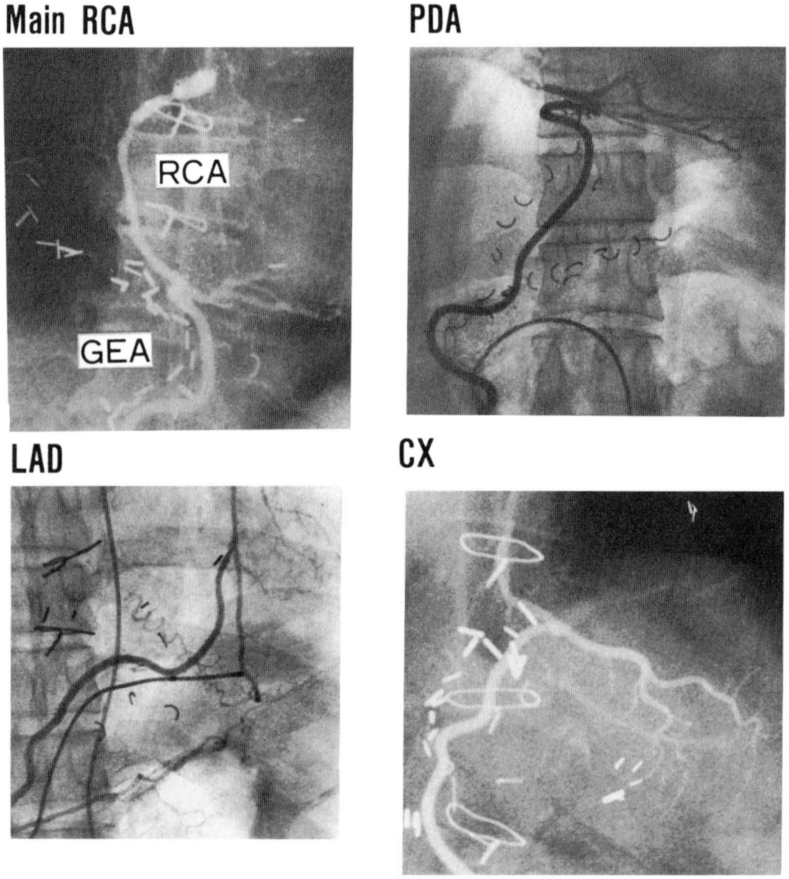

Fig. 11.7 Postoperative angiograms of the anastomosis in Fig. 11.6: main right coronary artery (RCA); posterior descending artery (PDA); left anterior descending (LAD); circumflex (CX). Reproduced with permission from Suma *et al.*[6]

Once the anastomosis has been completed, the GEA is unclamped, and anastomotic haemostasis is checked before the aortic cross-clamp is released. The GEA pedicle is then fixed to the epicardium near the site of the anastomosis. At this time, great care must be taken to avoid kinking or twisting the skeletonized distal GEA in the area of the anastomosis. (Fig. 11.8). After the pedicle has been sutured to the epicardium, blood flow through the GEA frequently induces beating of the heart or coarse ventricular fibrillation. This is good evidence of satisfactory perfusion. Release of the aortic cross-clamp allows the heart to return to its normal size. The pedicle is inspected carefully to make sure that blood flow is unimpeded. The point of fixation should not distort the anatomy. Excess pedicle, if present, is pulled back into the abdominal cavity. The patient is weaned off cardiopulmonary bypass, and the operative fields are again checked for bleeding. Once haemostasis is secure, chest and abdominal wounds are closed. It is usually not necessary to place a drainage tube in the abdominal cavity.

Sequential GEA grafting is technically feasible when the artery is large enough (Fig. 11.9). The free GEA graft is also an attractive alternative although late angiographic follow-up is as yet unavailable (Fig. 11.10). The choice of inflow site for the free GEA graft is either by direct anastomosis to the

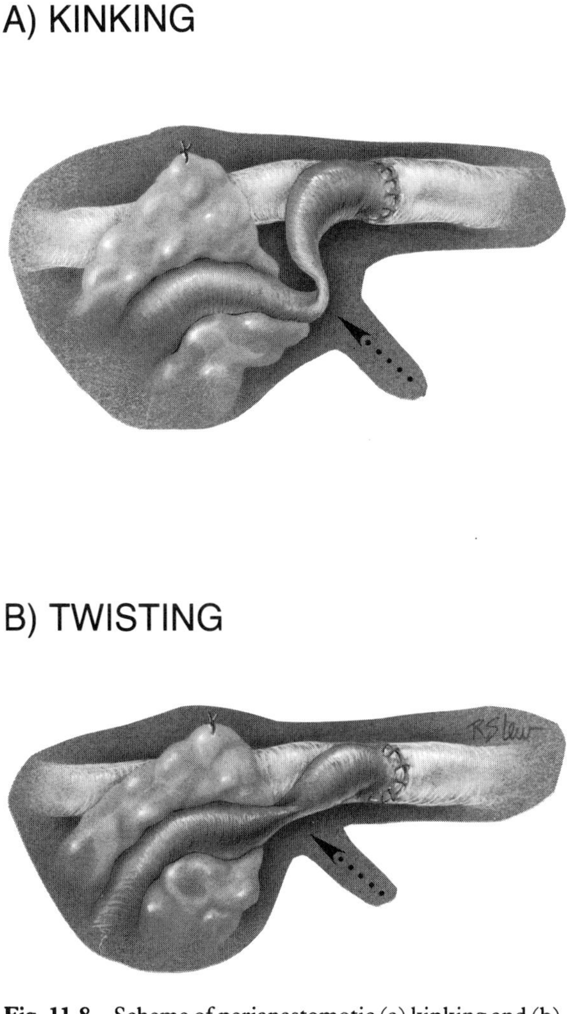

Fig. 11.8 Scheme of perianastomotic (a) kinking and (b) twisting caused by inappropriate fixation of the GEA pedicle to the epicardium. Reproduced with permission from Suma *et al.*[3]

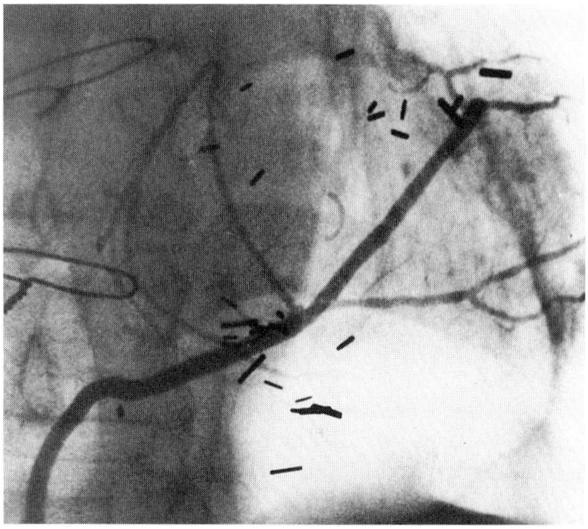

Fig. 11.9 Angiogram of a sequential GEA graft (64 k 50 m).

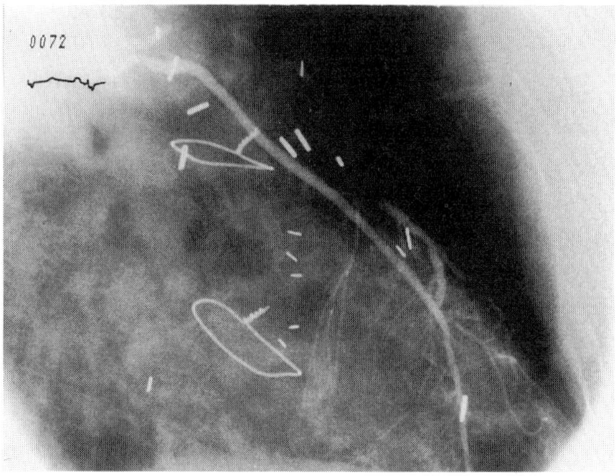

Fig. 11.10 Angiogram of a free GEA graft. Reproduced with permission from Suma *et al.*[3]

ascending aorta, with an interposed pericardial or saphenous vein patch, or to a concomitant saphenous vein graft or internal thoracic artery graft as a Y-graft, or to the proximal right coronary artery using a coronary–coronary artery end-to-side anastomotic technique.

References

1. Suma H, Fukumoto H, Takeuchi A. Coronary artery bypass grafting by utilizing in situ right gastroepiploic artery: basic study and clinical application. *Ann Thorac Surg* 1987; **44:** 394–7.
2. Suma H, Wanibuchi Y, Furuta S, Takeuchi A. Does use of gastroepiploic artery graft increase surgical risk? *J Thorac Cardiovasc Surg* 1991; **101:** 121–5.
3. Suma H, Amano A, Fukuda S *et al.* Gastroepiploic artery graft for anterior descending coronary artery bypass. *Ann Thorac Surg* 1994; **57:** 925–7.
4. Mills NL, Everson CT. Technical considerations for use of the gastroepiploic artery for coronary artery surgery. *J Cardiac Surg* 1989; **4:** 1–9.
5. Suma H. Length of the insitu right gastroepiploic artery for coronary artery bypass (Reply). *Ann Thorac Surg* 1992; **54:** 1244–5.
6. Suma H, Wanibuchi Y, Furuta S, Isshiki T, Yamaguchi T, Takanashi R. Comparative study between the gastroepiploic and the internal thoracic artery as a coronary bypass graft. Size, flow, patency, histology. *Eur J Cardiothorac Surg* 1991; **5:** 244–7.

12 Detection of graft patency

Takaaki Isshiki

The increased use of the right gastroepiploic artery (GEA) as a third conduit for coronary bypass surgery[1–5] has brought another challenge in postoperative graft evaluation. In this chapter, methods for detecting the patency of GEA grafts are presented.

Anatomy of the visceral vessels

When evaluating *in situ* GEA grafts postoperatively, one must be aware of the anatomy of the visceral vessels and their variations (Fig. 12.1). The coeliac trunk divides into the splenic and common hepatic arteries. These arteries travel in opposite directions; the splenic artery to the left and the common hepatic artery to the right. The common hepatic artery runs posterior to the stomach and then divides into the proper hepatic artery, which travels superiorly to the liver, and the gastroduodenal artery, which runs inferiorly towards the stomach, duodenum and pancreas. The gastroduodenal artery then divides into the right GEA and anterior and posterior superior pancreaticoduodenal arteries.

Previous reports have described the origin of the gastroduodenal artery from the coeliac artery system in nearly 96 per cent of cases.[6] At Mitsui Memorial Hospital, we performed 188 postoperative angiograms of GEA grafts between 1989 and 1993. In all but nine patients (95 per cent) normal anatomy was found, but in these nine patients the gastroduodenal artery originated from the superior mesenteric artery. Adachi *et al.* have reported similar findings in a post-mortem study[7] and they also found that the coeliac and superior mesenteric arterial systems were anastomosed via the superior and inferior pancreaticoduodenal arteries. Thus, although the GEA originated from the coeliac artery in the majority of patients, it is important to remember that occasionally it can originate from the superior mesenteric artery.

The route of the GEA graft should also be noted. Two different routes have been employed: in front

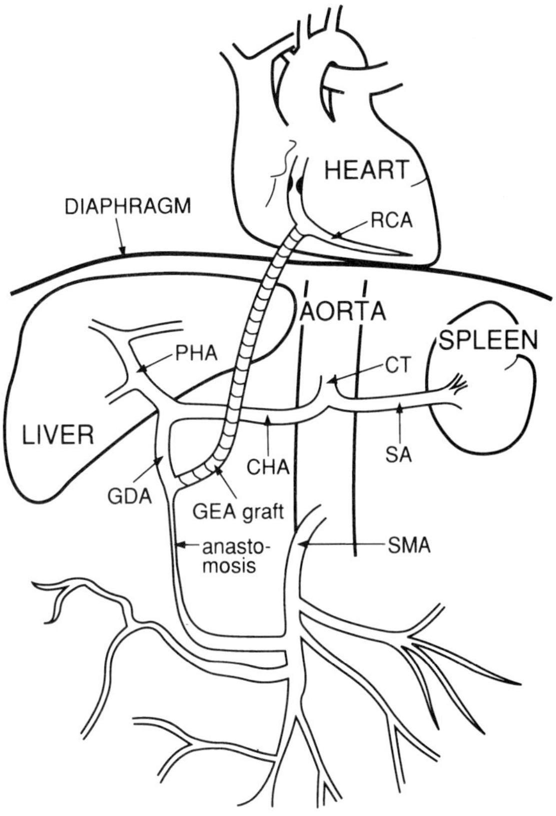

Fig. 12.1 Schematic illustration of the GEA graft and its related vessels. RCA=right coronary artery, CT=coeliac trunk, SA=splenic artery, CHA=common hepatic artery, PHA=proper hepatic artery, GDA=gastroduodenal artery, GEA=gastroepiploic artery, SMA=superior mesenteric artery.

(anterior) or behind (posterior) the liver and stomach. For the purposes of postoperative evaluation, the technique employed must be recorded at the time of surgery.

Angiography of GEA grafts

Angiography is the most accurate method to detect graft patency. The whole graft is visualized including its route, diameter, configuration and blood flow.[8–10] When performing postoperative angiography, there are three principles:

1. all related vessels including the native coronary arteries and grafts should be opacified during the same angiographic procedure;
2. the grafts should be opacified to allow minute evaluation and visualization from different angles;
3. the amount of contrast material should be minimized to avoid complications.

The simplest way to visualize the GEA graft is via coeliac arteriography. If it is necessary to opacify the graft most clearly, selective gastroduodenal arteriography can be employed, although this requires special techniques. When the GEA graft is perfused via the superior mesenteric artery, superior mesenteric arteriography is necessary.

Coeliac arteriography

Using either the brachial or femoral approach, a 5F cobra-shaped catheter is advanced into the abdominal aorta. The catheter tip is inserted into the coeliac trunk, which arises from the anterior wall of the abdominal aorta at the level of the first lumbar vertebral body. Then, 15–20 ml of contrast are injected using a mechanical injection device. Using this manoeuvre, the GEA graft can be visualized with forward blood flow.

With coeliac arteriography, however, opacification of the GEA graft may not be sufficient for detailed evaluation. Since many visceral organs in the upper abdomen are perfused via the coeliac artery, the amount of contrast entering the GEA graft may be less than expected, resulting in substandard opacification. On occasion, a patent GEA graft cannot be visualized with coeliac arteriography. This may be due to slow or reversed flow since these grafts can usually be opacified via selective gastroduodenal arteriography.

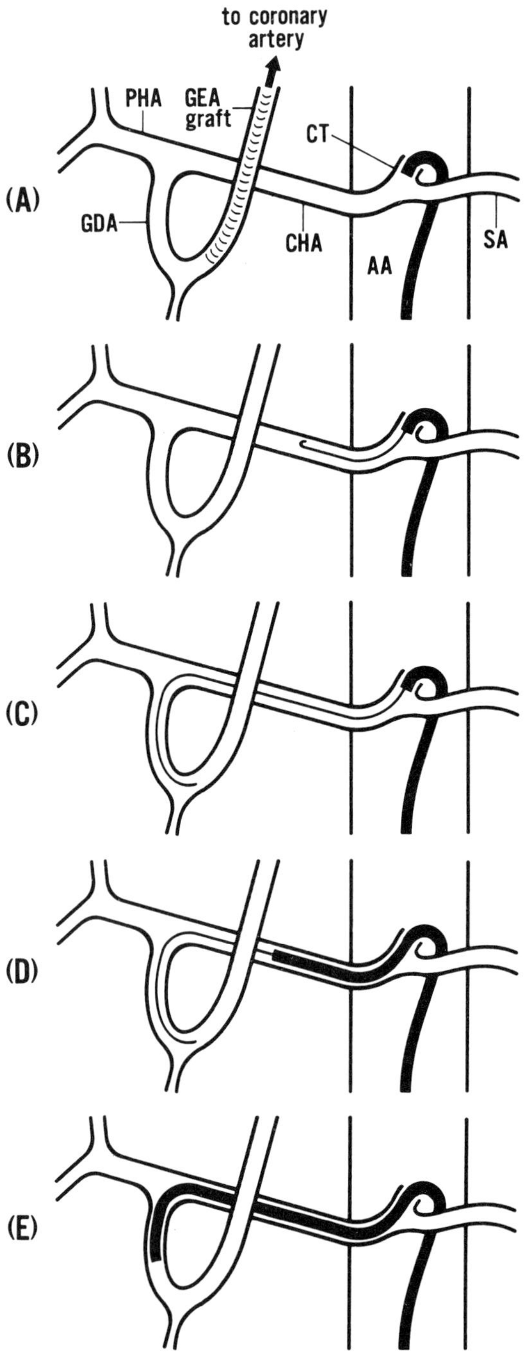

Fig. 12.2 Procedure of selective catheterization into the GDA (schematic illustrations – see text for full explanation). AA = abdominal aorta; CT = celiac trunk; SA = splenic artery; CHA = common hepatic artery; PHA = proper hepatic artery; GDA = gastroduodenal artery; GEA = gastroepiploic artery. Reproduced with permission from Isshiki T *et al.*[10]

A comparatively large quantity of contrast material is needed for a single injection during coeliac arteriography. Since numerous images are required from different angles using repeated 20 ml contrast injections, the routine use of coeliac arteriography is clinically limited.

Selective gastroduodenal arteriography

In contrast to coeliac arteriography, selective gastroduodenal arteriography offers clear visualization of the GEA graft.[10] Once a catheter is placed into the gastroduodenal artery (GDA), the graft can be opacified with only a few millilitres of contrast medium. This technique is fundamentally an over-the-wire method (Figs 12.2 and 12.3) Using the femoral approach, preparation is made as for coronary angiography with Judkins' technique. A 5F cobra-shaped catheter is advanced into the abdominal aorta. The catheter tip is inserted into the coeliac trunk (Figs 12.2(a), 12.3(a). A small amount of contrast is injected manually to obtain a route map of related arteries and to identify the GDA. Then, a 0.025- or 0.035-inch guide wire (plastic-coated is preferable since it becomes smoother when wet) is advanced slowly into the coeliac trunk through the common hepatic artery until the tip of the wire is securely placed in the GDA (Figs 12.2(b–c), 12.3(b–c)). The catheter is fed along the guide wire until its tip reaches the GDA (Fig. 12.2(d)). The guide wire is then removed (Figs 12.2(e), 12.3(d)) and the catheter tip adjusted with test injections to obtain good opacification of the GEA graft. An appropriate amount of contrast is injected manually using the same methods employed to study coronary arteries (Fig. 12.3(e)).

When the coeliac trunk originates at an acute angle from the abdominal aorta, a cobra-shaped

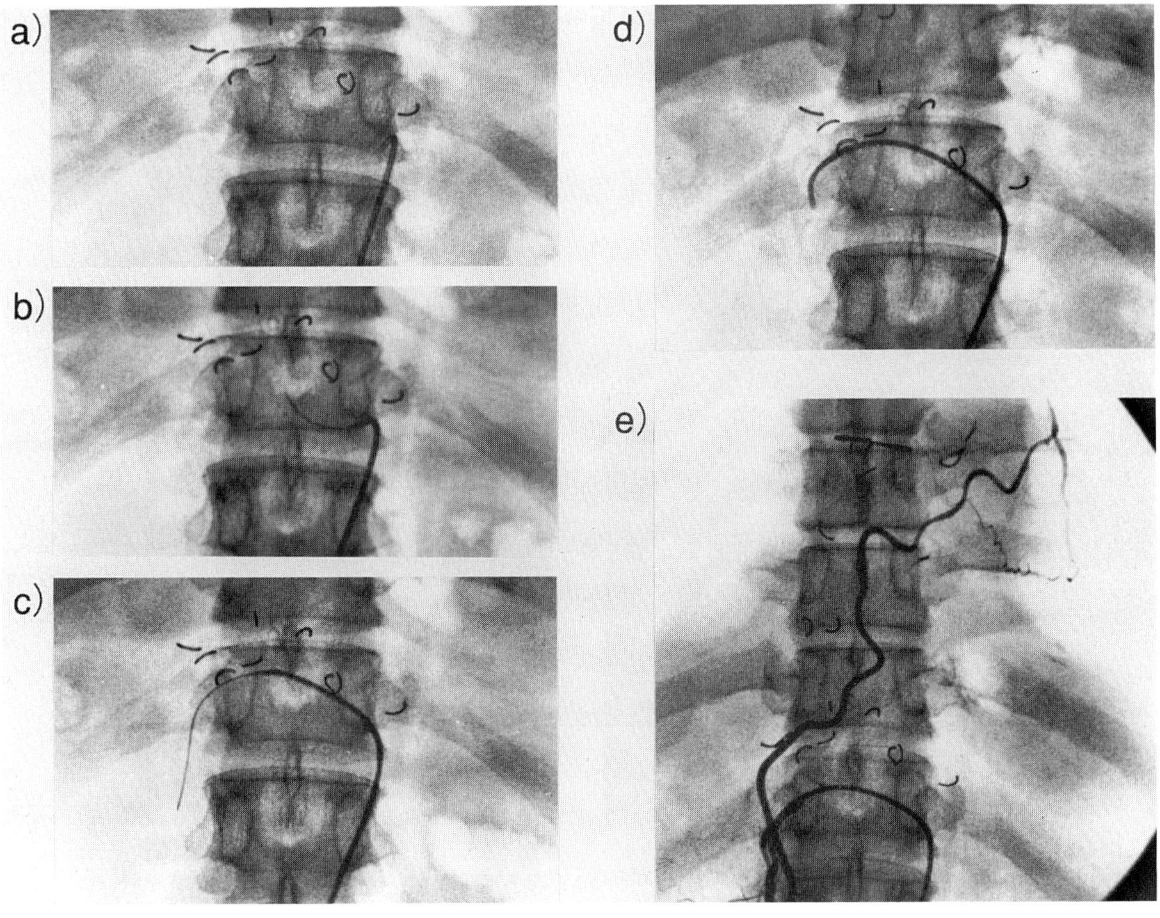

Fig. 12.3 Procedure of selective catheterization into the GDA.

catheter is often difficult to advance into the artery even after successful insertion of the guide wire. In such instance, a set of two coaxial catheters consisting of a 7F external guiding catheter (sheath) and a thin 4F internal catheter are used (Fig. 12.4). The technique is similar to that for PTCA. First, the guiding catheter is inserted into the coeliac trunk, then the guide wire is placed into the GDA. The thin internal catheter is advanced along the guide wire to the GDA and contrast is injected manually.

Using these techniques, we have successfully imaged GEA grafts in 170 of 188 patients (91 per cent). Since only a small quantity of contrast (approximately 5 ml per injection) is sufficient to opacify the GEA graft, it is possible to obtain images from several different angles. Postero-anterior (PA) and lateral anterior oblique (LAO) cranial views are essential. On the PA view, an overview of the route of the graft is obtained. This information may be useful when other non-invasive interventions are to

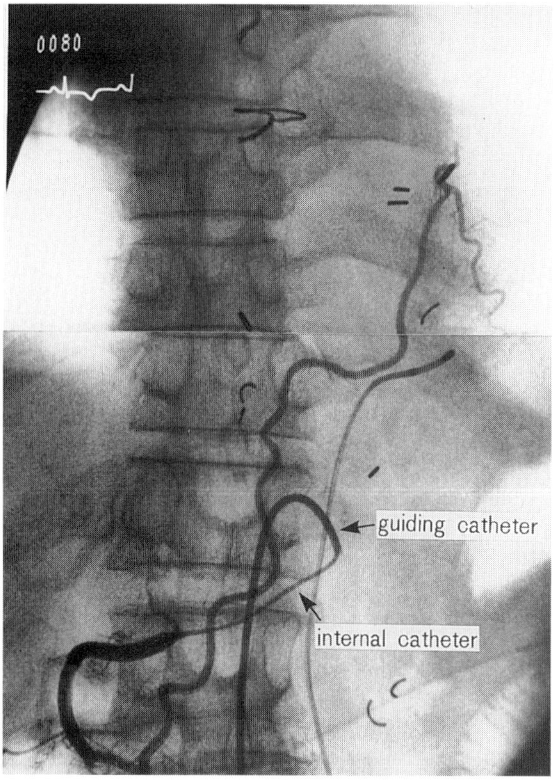

Fig. 12.4 Selective gastroduodenal arteriogram in a 62-year-old man showing a GEA graft, which was anastomosed to the left anterior descending coronary artery. The 4F internal catheter was advanced through the 7F external sheath which was inserted into the coeliac trunk.

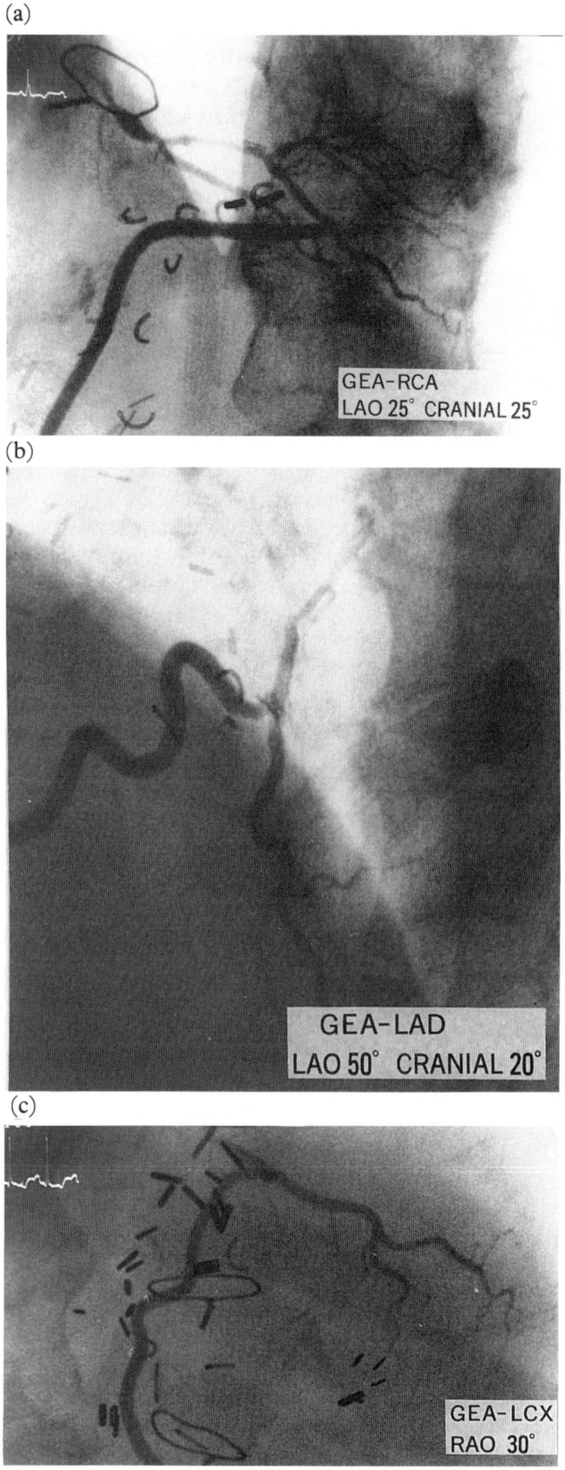

Fig. 12.5 Selective gastroduodenal arteriograms showing anastomosis sites between the GEA graft and (a) the right coronary artery (RCA); (b) the left anterior descending (LAD), and (c) the left circumflex (LCX) coronary arteries.

be employed. On the LAO cranial view, the anastomotic site between the GEA graft and the recipient coronary artery is easily identified (Figs 12.5(a) and (b)). A right anterior oblique view may provide added definition when the graft is anastomosed with the left circumflex artery, although this reconstruction is rare (Fig. 12.5(c)).

Selective GDA catheterization can be performed via the brachial artery using either Judkin's (puncture) or Sone's (cut-down) technique. Ishimura *et al.* have reported excellent success with selective GDA catheterization using Sone's technique.[11] Although this technique is not very complicated, there are some difficulties which can result in complications. In our eighteen patients who failed selective GDA catheterization, ten grafts were perfused via the superior mesenteric artery. These were visualized with superior mesenteric arteriography. The other eight patients had extremely tortuous vessels either in the abdominal aorta or in the coeliac arteries and were evaluated by coeliac arteriography.

GDA catheterization resulted in a few major vascular complications. In two patients the GDA occluded as a result of injury sustained during catheterization.[12] This could be fatal if it occurred in another type of graft. Fortunately, neither patient showed signs of chest pain or ECG changes of ischaemia. These GEA grafts were both shown to be perfused via the superior mesenteric artery. The anastomoses between the two arterial systems (the coeliac and superior mesenteric arteries) is of particular relevance in situations of this nature. Although this does not justify aggressive catheterization manoeuvres which may lead to vascular injury, it provides a certain degree of safety. Thus, superior mesenteric arteriography should be performed when occlusive vascular injury has occurred in the coeliac arterial system.

Vasospasm occurs frequently during GDA catheterization.[10,13,14] In these cases, intra-arterial injection of nitroglycerine is usually effective, although it may take several minutes for the spasm to subside.

Superior mesenteric arteriography

Superior mesenteric arteriography is performed when the GDA or the GEA graft is not visualized with coeliac arteriography (Fig. 12.6).[10] Superior mesenteric arteriography is not technically difficult. The superior mesenteric artery arises from the anterior wall of the abdominal aorta just below the orifice of the coeliac trunk. In most cases, a cobra-shaped catheter can be easily inserted into the orifice of the superior mesenteric artery and the whole tree can be opacified with a single 15–20 ml mechanical contrast injection.

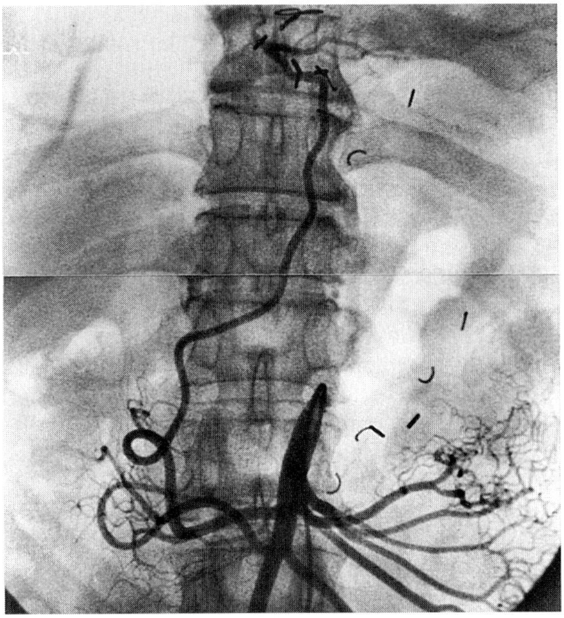

Fig. 12.6 Superior mesenteric arteriogram in a 59-year-old man. The GEA graft originates from the superior mesenteric artery. Reproduced with permission from Isshiki T.[15]

Non-invasive evaluation of GEA graft patency

Doppler ultrasound

The GEA graft, when it runs anteriorly to the stomach and the liver, is close to the abdominal wall, and therefore may be detected using Doppler ultrasound. It is impossible to visualize the lumen if the graft runs along the posterior hepatic route to the heart. Oei *et al.* evaluated the patency of the GEA graft using a colour Doppler system in twenty-one patients.[14] They were able to identify colour signals inside a tubular lumen running longitudinally between the abdominal wall and the left lobe of the liver. Postoperative angiography was used to confirm patency in ten patients. However, they failed to detect signals in grey-scale.

We tried similar techniques in several patients, and were also able to identify Doppler signals in the tubular lumen using a 7.5 MHz transducer (see Plate 1 at the beginning of Part III). However, in about half of the patients, it was difficult to distinguish these flow signals from noise. Moreover, these images were influenced by the thickness of the abdominal wall and intra-abdominal fat. Thus, Doppler ultrasound may contribute to the detection of blood flow in GEA grafts, but further evaluation of this method is still required. At the present time, Doppler ultrasound evaluation is meaningful only if flow signals are demonstrated, which confirms graft patency. However, absence of a flow signal does not necessarily indicate graft occlusion. Currently, Doppler ultrasound evaluation can only be considered supplementary to angiography.

Thallium-201 myocardial scintigraphy

Although ^{201}Tl myocardial scintigraphy does not visualize blood flow, it detects graft patency by showing effective myocardial perfusion. Kusukawa *et al.* have reported the efficacy of this procedure in eight patients with multiple bypass grafts including GEA grafts.[16] An increase in the washout rate in the inferior region has been noted, as well as recovery of the SPECT images. Thus, patency of the GEA graft can be inferred from this method, especially in patients who show marked recovery after surgery. However, it is inadvisable to rely on this method alone, since scintigraphic images can be influenced by other factors such as collaterals or native coronary blood flow.

MRI

Nishimura *et al.* have reported that GEA grafts were clearly visualized with MRI in fourteen postoperative patients.[17] Using cine-MRI techniques, blood flow was confirmed in grafts by observation of a high-intensity signal. As with other non-invasive methods, MRI may be employed for postoperative screening. These findings are surprising since previous studies have failed to detect blood flow in ITA grafts. The reason for this discrepancy remains obscure, but may be related to differences between types of grafts.

Conclusion

The reliability of angiography to detect patency of GEA grafts is superior to that of non-invasive methods. Currently, therefore, angiography is recommended unless specifically contraindicated. In view of the increasing number of patients receiving arterial bypass conduits, a more efficient, cost-effective strategy for evaluation of graft patency using a combination of invasive and non-invasive methods must be developed.

References

1. Suma H, Fukumoto H, Takeuchi A. Coronary artery bypass graft by utilizing in situ right gastroepiploic artery: Basic study and clinical application. *Ann Thorac Surg* 1987; **44:** 394–7.
2. Mills NL, Everson CT. Right gastroepiploic artery: A third arterial conduit for coronary artery bypass. *Ann Thorac Surg* 1989; **47:** 706–11.
3. Lytle BW, Cosgrove DM, Ratliff NB, Loop FD. Coronary artery bypass grafting with the right gastroepiploic artery. *J Thorac Cardiovasc Surg* 1989; **97:** 826–31.
4. Suma H, Wanibuchi Y, Furuta S, Isshiki T, Yamaguchi T, Takanashi R. Comparative study between the gastroepiploic and internal thoracic artery as a coronary bypass graft:: Size, flow, patency, histology. *Eur J Cardiothorac Surg* 1991; **5:** 244–7.
5. Suma H, Wanibuchi Y, Terada Y, Fukuda S, Takayama T, Furuta S. The right gastroepiploic artery graft: Clinical and angiographic mid-term results in 200 patients. *J Thorac Cardiovasc Surg* 1993; **105:** 615–23.
6. Lipper H, Pabst R. *Arterial variations in man: Classification and frequency*. Verlag Munchen: JF Berbmann, 1985.
7. Adachi T. Variation of truncus coeliacus (in Japanese). In: *Human anatomy* Ura R ed. Nankodo: Tokyo, 1940; 1130–3.
8. Black AJR, Gibbons F. Angiographic visualization of a right gastroepiploic artery-left circumflex coronary artery graft. *Cath Cardiovasc Diag* 1987; **13:** 121–4.
9. Tanimoto Y, Matsuda Y, Fujii B *et al.* Angiography of right gastroepiploic artery for coronary bypass graft. *Cath Cardiovasc Diag* 1989; **16:** 35–8.
10. Isshiki T, Yamaguchi T, Nakamura M *et al.* Postoperative angiographic evaluation of gastroepiploic artery grafts: Technical considerations and short-term patency. *Cath Cardiovasc Diag* 1990; **21:** 233–8.
11. Ishimura T, Funauchi T, Umezawa T, Wakabayashi A, Suma H. Mid-term results of right gastroepiploic artery grafts: Sequential angiographic follow-up. *J Am Coll Cardiol* 1992; **19** (Suppl. A): 160A (abstract).
12. Hashimoto H, Isshiki T, Ikari Y *et al.* A dual blood

supply protects the right gastroepiploic arterial graft: report of two cases (submitted).
13. Suma H. Spasm of the gastroepiploic artery graft. *Ann Thorac Surg* 1990; **49:** 168–9.
14. Oei KT, Sie HT, Penn OCKM, van Engelshoven JJMA. Colour Doppler imaging of the right gastroepiploic artery as an in situ coronary artery bypass graft. *Eur J Radiol* 1992; **15:** 37–9.
15. Isshiki T. Postoperative coronary arteriography. In: Haze K ed. *Coronary arteriography*. Tokyo: Medical View, 1993 (in Japanese).
16. Kusukawa J, Hirota Y, Kawamura K *et al.* Efficacy of coronary bypass surgery with gastroepiploic artery. Assessment with thallium-201 myocardial scintigraphy. *Circulation* 1989; **80** (Suppl. I): I135–40.
17. Nishimura F, Yoshino Y, Ichikawa S, Hayama Y, Toyama M. MRI of the gastroepiploic artery used as a bypass graft. *J Comput Assist Tomogr* 1992; **16:** 549–52.

13 Clinical results

Hisayoshi Suma

Initial successful clinical reports of the right gastroepiploic artery (GEA) graft for direct myocardial revascularization were presented in 1987 by Pym, Suma, Carter and their co-workers.[1–3] Following these reports the GEA graft has become increasingly used worldwide.

Clinical outcome

In 1987, Pym *et al.*[1] first reported nine patients in whom a GEA graft was used to bypass the right coronary artery combined with other graft conduits without operative mortality. Suma *et al*[2] reported the use of the GEA to the left anterior descending coronary artery (LAD) in two patients at reoperation, with no deaths, and Carter[3] reported thirty patients using the GEA to bypass the circumflex or the right coronary arteries with one operative death. All these GEAs were used as *in situ* grafts. In 1989 Verkkala *et al.*[4] reported eleven patients using the GEA to bypass the right coronary artery without operative mortality. Mills and Everson[5] presented their experience in thirty-nine patients with three (7.7 per cent) early deaths. Lytle *et al.*[6] reported thirty-six patients with GEA grafts with two (5.6 per cent) early deaths. In these latter two reports the higher mortality rate may be attributed to the use of the artery in more complex cases, including reoperations and patients with an atherosclerotic ascending aorta. Most of the GEA grafts, both free and *in situ*, were used for the circumflex or the right coronary arteries.

In 1990, Beretta *et al.*[7] reported patients who underwent coronary artery bypass using free GEA grafts without operative mortality. Pym *et al.*[8] presented their extended results of the GEA graft in fifty-seven patients with one early death. All but one artery was used as an *in situ* graft to bypass mostly the right coronary artery and less frequently the circumflex artery. From Japan, Takeuchi *et al.*[9] and Isomura *et al.*[10] have both reported successful use of the *in situ* GEA graft in small children with Kawasaki disease.

In 1991, we compared the early surgical results in matched groups of seventy patients with and without GEA grafts.[11] There was no increase in perioperative morbidity or mortality with use of this graft, and we noted that there was no gastric ischaemia following detachment of the artery from the greater curvature of the stomach detected by endoscopic Doppler velocimetry (Fig. 13.1). We also compared the size, flow and patency of the GEA with the internal thoracic artery (ITA).[12] The mean free flow after intraluminal injection of papaverine was 91 ml/min in the GEA and 81 ml/min in the ITA, and the patency rate was 96 per cent in ninety-two GEA and 98 per cent in 322 ITA grafts, respectively.

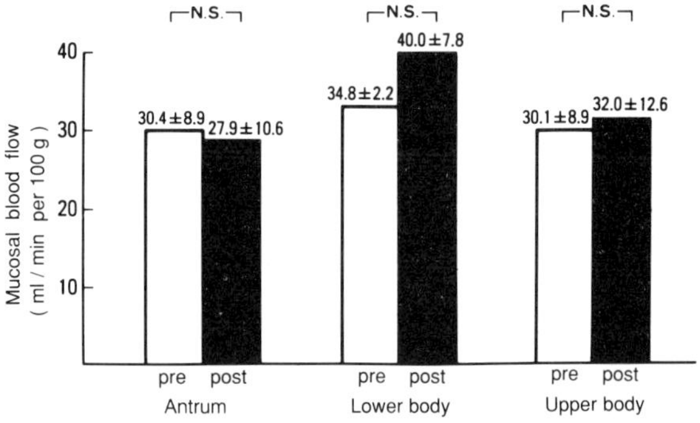

Fig. 13.1 Gastric mucosal blood flow measured by laser Doppler velocimetry showing no reduction of blood flow after division of the right GEA in five patients. Gastric mucosal blood flow before GEA takedown (□) and after right GEA detachment from the greater curvature of the stomach (■). Reproduced with permission from Suma *et al.*[11]

In 1993, we reported the mid-term results of the GEA graft in 200 patients, followed up from 6 to 70 months with a mean of 27 months:[13] 182 *in situ* and eighteen free GEA grafts were anastomosed to eleven LAD, three diagonal, twenty-six circumflex and 160 right coronary arteries. With concomitant use of the ITA graft in 192 (95 per cent) patients, early mortality was 3 per cent and late mortality 2 per cent. Grandjean *et al.*[14] presented their experience of GEA grafts combined with the ITA in 300 patients, with an early mortality of 3.3 per cent and no late deaths.

Mills *et al.*[15] reported ninety consecutive *in situ* GEA grafts performed from 1989 to 1991 in which the artery was anastomosed predominantly to the right coronary system with two early deaths (2.2 per cent), with free flow after intraluminal papaverine injection ranging from 42 to 660 ml/min (mean 180 ml/min).

Our most recent data in 400 patients with GEA grafts, included 327 males with an age range from 6 to 80 years old (mean 59 years). The extent of coronary artery disease was single vessel disease in four patients, double vessel disease in fifty-one patients, triple vessel disease in 283 patients and left main disease in sixty-two patients. Previous myocardial infarction was noted in 208 patients, and preoperative unstable angina in seventy-two patients. There were forty patients with a previous coronary artery bypass operation. The GEA was anastomosed to forty-three LAD, six diagonal, seventy-one circumflex and 287 right coronary arteries. Most of the GEA grafts were used as an individual *in situ* graft except twenty-four free grafts and seven sequential grafts. The mean number of bypass grafts was 3.2 and 2.3. Coronary arteries were bypassed with arterial grafts by concomitant use of the ITA in 388 patients (97 per cent) and the inferior epigastric artery (IEA) in thirty patients (8 per cent). Combined cardiac and non-cardiac procedures were: aortic valve replacement in three patients, mitral valve replacement in six patients, left ventricular aneurysmectomy in five patients, grafting of abdominal aortic aneurysm in three patients, lower limb revascularization including femoro–femoral bypass or aorta–bifemoral bypass in seven patients, cholecystectomy in fourteen patients and splenectomy for associated idiopathic thrombocytopenic purpura in two patients. There were eight (2 per cent) early and four (1 per cent) late deaths. New Q waves were noted in six patients.

Overall, given the experience reported from a number of institutions, it may be concluded that early to mid term clinical outcome with use of the GEA is excellent and there is no evidence that perioperative morbidity or mortality is increased. The impact of this graft on long-term outcome after coronary artery bypass has not yet been clearly defined

(a)

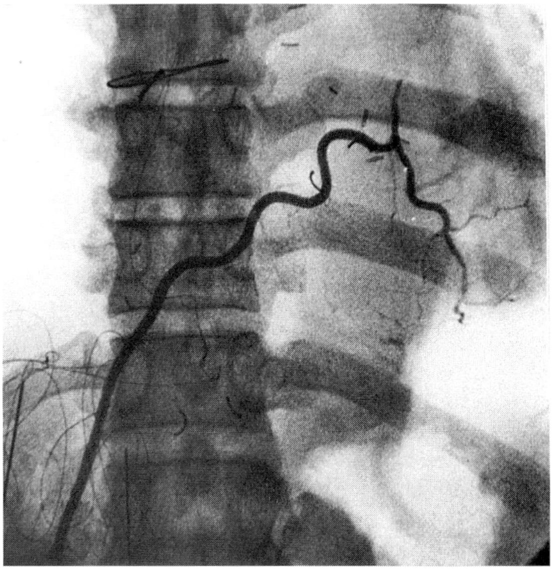

(b)

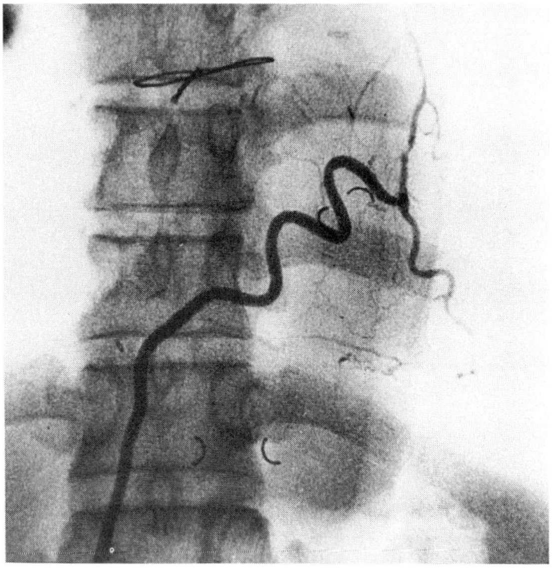

Fig. 13.2 Postoperative angiogram of a GEA graft anastomosed to the LAD in a 54-year-old man at (a) 10 days postop. and (b) 26 months post op.

because most such grafts have been used to bypass the circumflex or the right coronary artery which are of secondary importance when compared to the LAD. From our experience, however, the GEA is a suitable conduit to bypass the LAD when the ITA is not available.[16]

Graft patency

Postoperative angiographic patency rate of the GEA graft varies from 78 to 100 per cent.[1–15] Grandjean *et al.*[14] reported an improvement in patency rate from 77 to 94 per cent with increasing experience. In our experience the early patency rate (mean 2 months) was 95 per cent (241/253) for *in situ* grafts and 80 per cent (12/15) for free grafts. Mid term (mean 2 years up to 5 years), angiographic patency rate was 94 per cent (47/50) in 400 GEA grafts (Figs. 13.2 and 13.3). Focal stenoses were rarely found in the GEA trunk on mid term postoperative angiography and no significant intimal hyperplasia was observed in the graft obtained from a single autopsy specimen at 2 years after surgery (Fig. 13.4). The early patency rate of the free GEA graft is inferior to the *in situ* graft probably because of the technically difficult proximal anastomosis to the aorta, and late angiographic data with respect to its use as a free graft is still lacking at present.

Whilst most reports have demonstrated favourable results regarding patency, little attention has been paid to the problem of spasm in the GEA.[5,17] Because the GEA is a muscular artery which contains many smooth muscle cells in the media, it becomes spastic easily with surgical manipulation or catheter stimulation.[17] Fortunately, however, clinically evident myocardial ischaemia or angina pectoris due to spontaneous spasm in the GEA graft postoperatively has not been described. Nakao and Kawaue[18] showed angiographically that this graft changes its diameter in relation to competitive flow or distal run off in a similar manner to the ITA. As Nishida *et al.*[19] have demonstrated, percutaneous Doppler ultrasound is a useful method to detect the patency of the *in situ* GEA when it is located in front of the liver, and this technique may be applied to the investigation of physiological and pharmacological reactivity of this conduit noninvasively (see Plate 2 at the beginning of Part III).

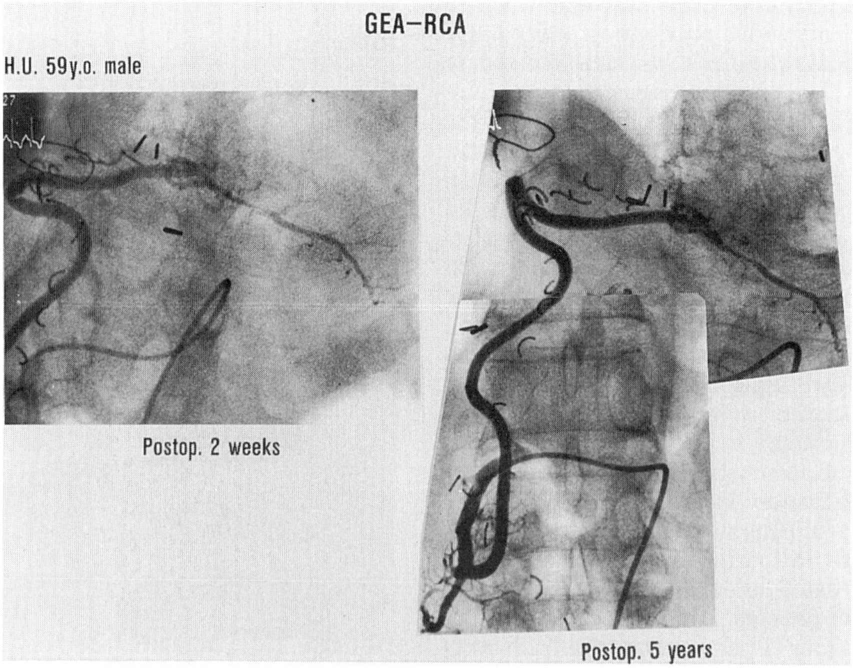

Fig. 13.3 GEA graft anastomosed to the right coronary artery in a 59-year-old man. Postoperative angiograms were taken at 2 weeks (left) and 5 years (right) after surgery.

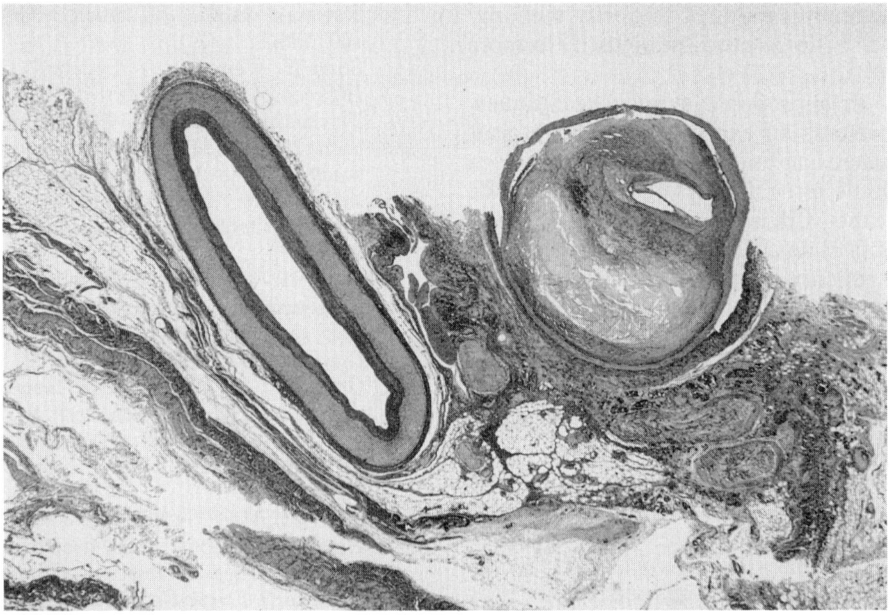

Fig. 13.4 Pathology of GEA (left) and the right coronary artery (right) taken at autopsy. The patient died of pneumonia 2 years after coronary artery reoperation. There is no significant intimal hyperplasia in the GEA graft while the right coronary artery shows prominent arteriosclerosis.

Functional capacity

Using stress myocardial scintigraphy, Kusukawa *et al.*[20] have shown that the *in situ* GEA graft has sufficient flow capacity under maximal stress. Thallium-201 washout rate significantly improved in the area grafted with the GEA. In our mid-term study,[13] washout rate improved from 35±10 per cent preoperatively to 45 ±15 per cent in the early postoperative period and remained at 43 ± 6 and 48 ± 15 per cent at 1 and 2 years after surgery, respectively. Isomura *et al.*[21] demonstrated that the mean regional ejection fraction of the myocardial area grafted with the GEA increased from 28 per cent before operation to 43 per cent after operation in fourteen patients who had a GEA graft to the right coronary system. In their twenty patients who underwent coronary artery bypass grafting with the GEA and ITA grafts, the results of an exercise test using a bicycle ergometer was improved from 3.6±1.9 metabolic units preoperatively to 7.8±1.3 at 6–12 weeks after surgery. In our thirty-eight patients whose GEA was anastomosed to the LAD, twenty-five patients underwent postoperative exercise study after angiographic patency was confirmed. Twenty three patients showed a negative stress test and two patients showed a positive test. Causes of a positive test in those two patients were a stenosed vein graft to the circumflex artery and a residual stenosis in a large diagonal branch of the LAD respectively.[16] From these investigations it would seem that the functional capacity of the *in situ* GEA graft exhibits sufficient flow capacity under conditions of exercise stress.

Conclusion

The GEA is an excellent alternative conduit for myocardial revascularization. Precise indications for use of this graft have not yet been clearly established. While mid-term angiographic patency is excellent in the *in situ* GEA graft, the free GEA graft is still unproven. Concerns remain in patients who undergo abdominal surgery after successful GEA grafting or require coronary artery reoperation with patent GEA grafts, although successful clinical outcomes have been reported individually. A further period of evaluation is required to clarify the long-term patency and clinical outcome to justify its more liberal use.

Already, with appropriate surgical techniques, the GEA represents an excellent alternative graft particularly where conduit is scarce, in reoperations or when multiple arterial grafts are indicated. We may speculate that with increasing use the GEA may be seen not only as an alternative but considered as an important primary conduit for myocardial revascularization.

References

1. Pym J, Brown PM, Charrette EJP *et al.* Gastroepiploic-coronary anastomosis: a viable alternative bypass graft. *J Thorac Cardiovasc Surg* 1987; **94:** 256–9.
2. Suma H, Fukumoto H, Takeuchi A. Coronary artery bypass grafting by utilizing in situ right gastroepiploic artery: basic study and clinical application. *Ann Thorac Surg* 1987; **44:** 394–7.
3. Carter MJ. The use of the right gastroepiploic artery in coronary artery bypass grafting. *Aust NZ J Surg* 1987; **57:** 317–21.
4. Verkkala K, Jarvinen A, Keto P *et al.* Right gastroepiploic artery as a coronary bypass graft. *Ann Thorac Surg* 1989; **47:** 716–19.
5. Mills NL, Everson CT. Right gastroepiploic artery: a third arterial conduit for coronary bypass. *Ann Thorac Surg* 1989; **47:** 706–11.
6. Lytle BW, Cosgrove DM, Ratliff NB *et al.* Coronary artery bypass grafting with the right gastroepiploic artery. *J Thorac Cardiovasc Surg* 1989; **97:** 826–31.
7. Beretta L, Lemma M, Vanelli P *et al.* Gastroepiploic artery free graft for coronary bypass. *Eur J Cardiothorac Surg* 1990; **4:** 323–8.
8. Pym J, Parker JO, West RO. The right gastroepiploic artery as a coronary artery bypass graft. Abstract from 27th Annual Meeting of The Society of Thoracic Surgeons; 1990; San Francisco, Calif.: 68.
9. Takeuchi Y, Gomi A, Okamura Y *et al.* Coronary revascularization in a child with Kawasaki disease: Use of right gastroepiploic artery. *Ann Thorac Surg* 1990; **50:** 294–6.
10. Isomura T, Hisatomi K, Asoh S *et al.* Revascularization with the right gastroepiploic artery in Kawasaki disease. *J Thorac Cardiovasc Surg* 1990; **100:** 796–8.
11. Suma H, Wanibuchi Y, Furuta S *et al.* Does use of gastroepiploic artery graft increase surgical risk? *J Thorac Cardiovasc Surg* 1991; **101:** 121–5.
12. Suma H, Wanibuchi Y, Furuta S *et al.* Comparative study between the gastroepiploic and the internal thoracic artery as a coronary bypass graft. Size, flow, patency, histology. *Eur J Cardiothorac Surg* 1991; **5:** 244–7.
13. Suma H, Wanibuchi Y, Terada Y *et al.* The right gastroepiploic artery graft. Clinical and angiographic mid-term results in 200 patients. *J Thorac Cardiovasc Surg* 1993; **105:** 615–23.
14. Grandjean JG, Boonstra PW, Heijer PD, Ebels T. Arterial revascularization with the right gastroepiploic artery and internal mammary arteries in 300 patients. *J Thorac Cardiovasc Surg* 1994; **107:** 1309–16.
15. Mills NL, Hockmuth DR, Everson CT, Robert CC. Right gastroepiploic artery used for coronary artery bypass grafting. Evaluation of flow characteristics and size. *J Thorac Cardiovasc Surg* 1993; **106:** 579–86.
16. Suma H, Amano A, Fukuda S *et al.* Gastroepiploic artery graft for anterior descending coronary artery bypass. *Ann Thorac Surg* 1994; **57:** 925–7.
17. Suma H. Spasm of the gastroepiploic artery graft. *Ann Thorac Surg* 1990; **49:** 168–9.
18. Nakao T, Kawaue Y. Effect of coronary revascularization with the right gastroepiploic artery. comparative examination of angiographic findings in the early postoperative period. *J Thorac Cardiovasc Surg* 1993; **106:** 149–53.
19. Nishida H, Endo M, Koyanagi H *et al.* Coronary artery bypass grafting with the right gastroepiploic artery and evaluation of flow with transcutaneous Doppler echo. *J Thorac Cardiovasc Surg* 1994; **108:** 532–9.
20. Kusukawa J, Hirota Y, Kawamura K *et al.* An assessment of the efficacy of aorta-coronary bypass surgery using gastroepiploic artery with thallium-201 myocardial scintigraphy. *Circulation* 1989; **80** (Suppl I): 135–40.
21. Isomura T, Hisatomi K, Hirano A *et al.* Clinical evaluation with exercise performance in twenty patients who underwent coronary artery bypass grafting with both the gastroepiploic and internal thoracic arteries. *J Thorac Cardiovasc Surg* 1993; **105:** 1088–94.

Part IV
Inferior epigastric artery

14 Surgical anatomy and operative technique

Michel Buche

Complete arterial myocardial revascularization in patients with three-vessel disease using only ITA grafts remains a challenge.[1,2] This has prompted a search for other arterial conduits which could have the same properties as the ITA. The inferior epigastric artery (IEA) is one of these alternative arteries. In this chapter, the anatomy and surgical technique of IEA grafting are presented.

Anatomy

The IEA originates from the medial side of the external iliac artery almost immediately posterior to the inguinal ligament just opposite to the deep circumflex iliac artery. At first, it pursues a tortuous course along the medial side of the deep inguinal ring, hooking around the vas deferens in the male or the round ligament in the female. Thereafter, it ascends obliquely towards the umbilicus (Fig. 14.1). On this course it lies on the transversalis fascia as far as the arcuate line; afterwards it progresses between the rectus muscle and its posterior sheath up to the umbilicus where it usually divides into several terminal branches which form intramuscular anastomoses with the terminal branches of the superior epigastric artery.[3] Exceptionally, these distal branches may be large enough to be used as a natural Y graft (Fig. 14.2). Three collateral branches usually arise from the proximal IEA. These are the external spermatic artery, the pubic branch artery, and the anastomotic branch to the obturator artery or in some patients the obturator artery itself. This third branch, if it is adequately sized, can provide additional length to the IEA as a coronary artery bypass conduit (Figs 14.3–14.6).

In a preliminary study undertaken in our institution, selective angiography of the right IEA *in situ* was performed in 100 consecutive patients with proven coronary artery disease during routine cardiac catheterization. Selective opacification of the left ITA was also obtained in ninety-eight of these patients. No atherosclerotic lesion of either the IEA nor the ITA was observed. Ninety six of the hundred IEA were considered suitable for CABG whereas four were considered of insufficient calibre or length. Quantitative angiography was performed

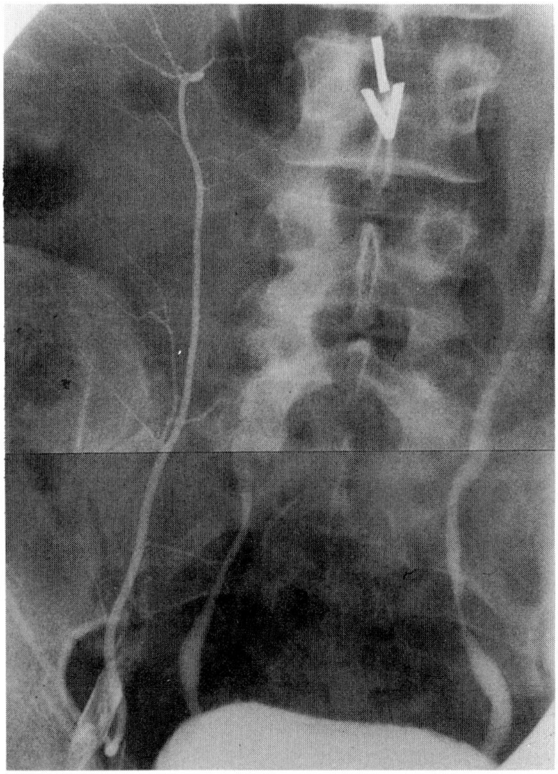

Fig. 14.1 Selective angiography of a right IEA *in situ*. The arrow points out the umbilicus.

in twenty of the patients with an adequate IEA. The mean length of the IEA *in situ* from its iliac origin to its distal bifurcation was 13.1±1.3 cm and its size at 5 cm from its ostium was 2.4±0.4 mm. In comparison all the ninety-eight left ITA grafts were suitable for use in coronary artery surgery, and observing similar landmarks, their mean length and size were 20.3±1.9 cm and 2.8±0.4 mm respectively.[4]

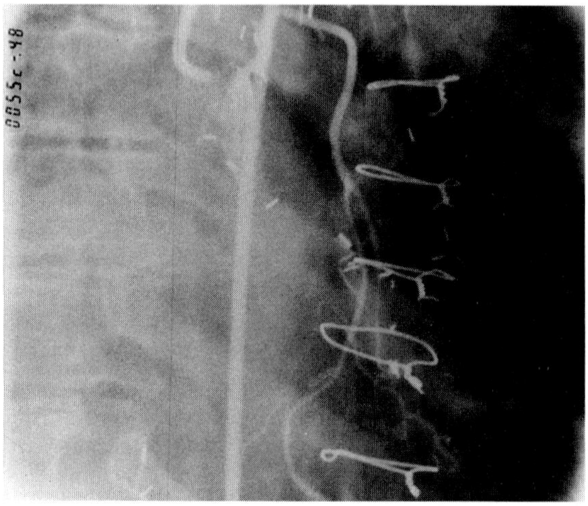

Fig. 14.2 Postoperative angiogram of a natural IEA Y graft anastomosed to two obtuse marginal branches of the circumflex artery.

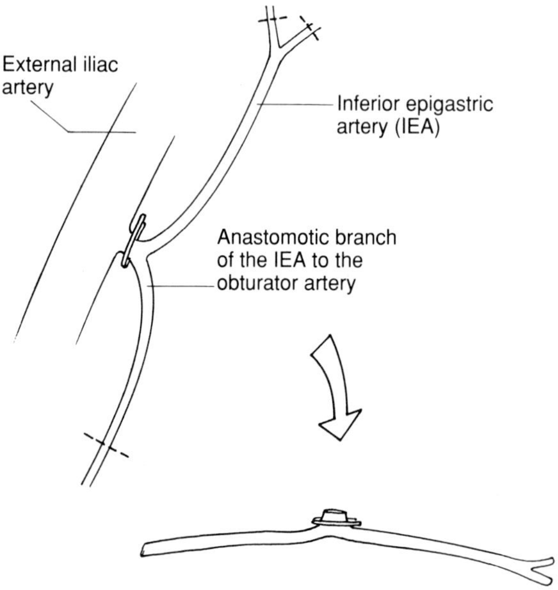

Fig. 14.3 Technique of extension of the IEA with the obturator artery.

Operative technique

Selective opacification of one IEA (most commonly the right IEA) and if needed both IEA is routinely performed before surgery, usually during the diagnostic catherization. The IEA is harvested only when its length and size seem to be adequate to reach and match the target coronary artery. It has been our practice to harvest the IEA through a paramedian infraumbilical incision.[5,6] Bilateral symmetrical abdominal incisions may be used when both IEAs are needed.[7,8] The skin incision starts from the level

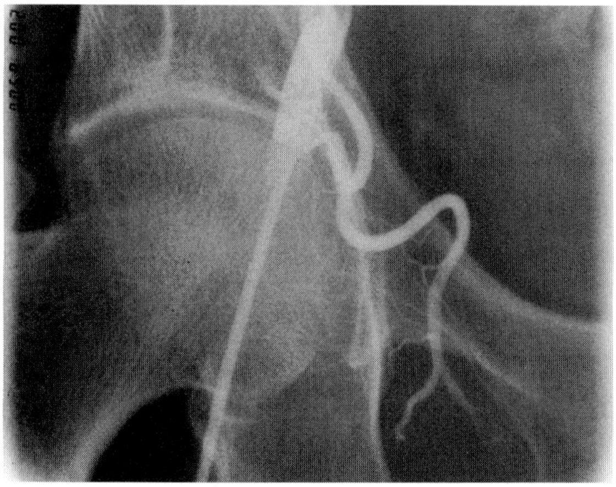

Fig. 14.4 Preoperative angiogram of a right IEA *in situ* showing a large obturator artery originating from the proximal IEA.

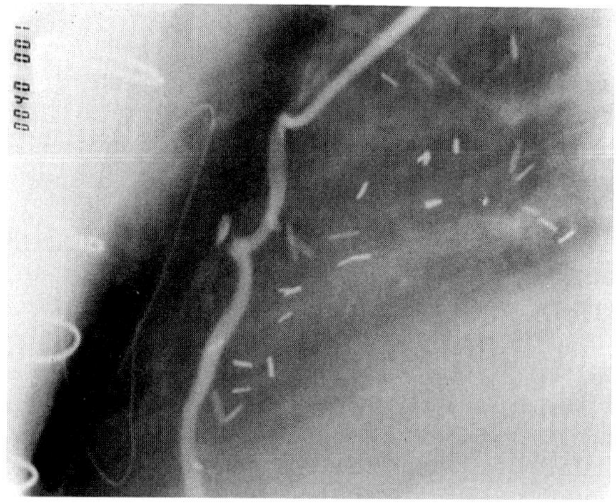

Fig. 14.5 Postoperative angiogram at 10 days: the IEA is extended with the obturator artery which is directly anastomosed onto the aorta.

of the umbilicus. It first follows the external edge of the rectus muscle, then it is angled slightly down towards the femoral vessels in a hockey stick fashion ending 3 cm above the inguinal ligament (Fig. 14.7). The anterior sheath of the rectus muscle is divided and the rectus muscle is retracted medially (Fig. 14.8). The IEA is mobilized with its two satellite veins and the surrounding preperitoneal fat. Its collateral branches are clipped and divided at some distance from the main IEA in a manner similar to ITA harvesting. The IEA is mobilized from its origin from the external iliac artery to its terminal division usually close to the umbilicus.

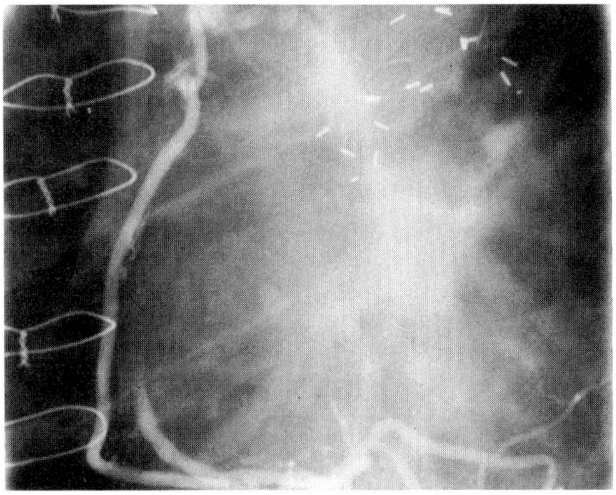

Fig. 14.6 Postoperative restudy at 12 months of the same composite conduit anastomosed to the right coronary artery.

(a)

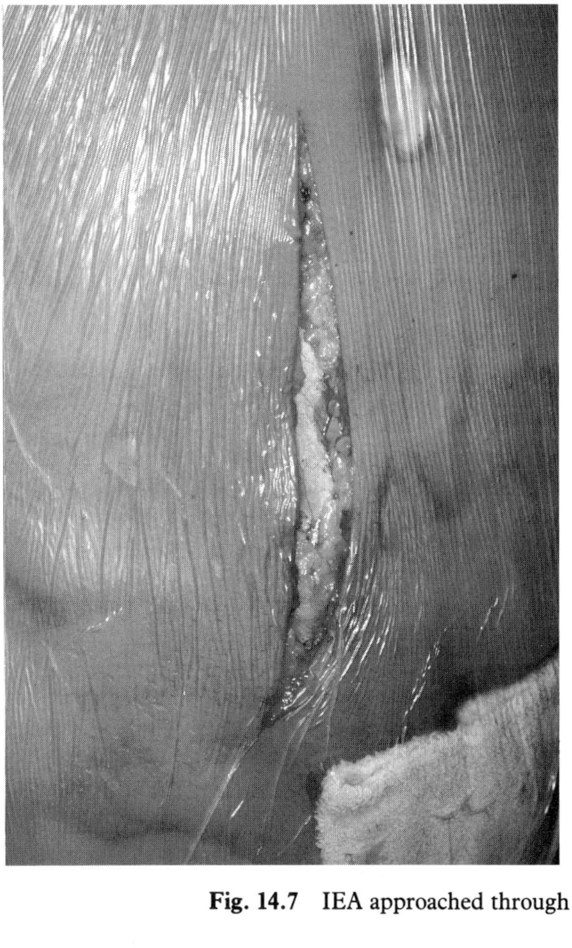

(b)

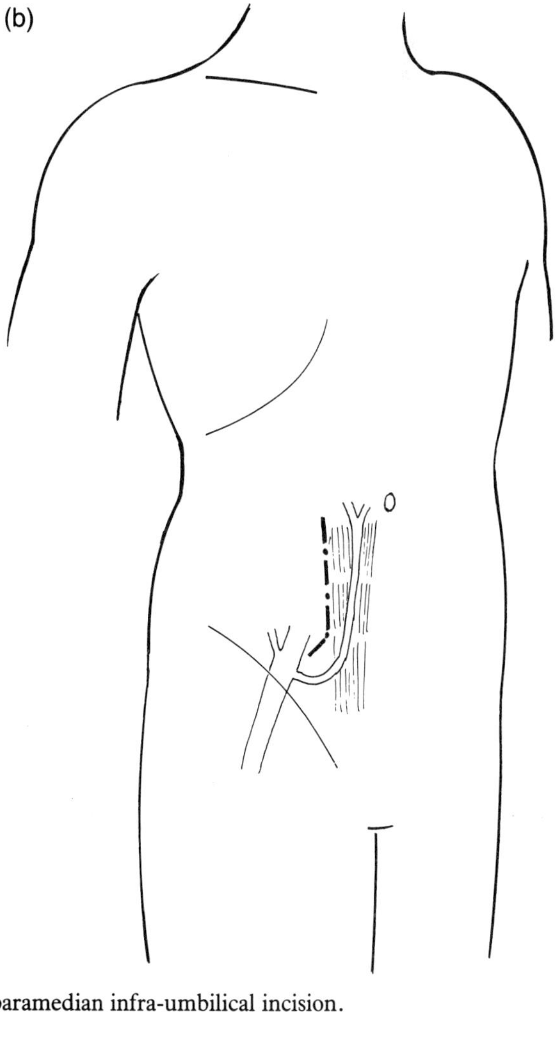

Fig. 14.7 IEA approached through a paramedian infra-umbilical incision.

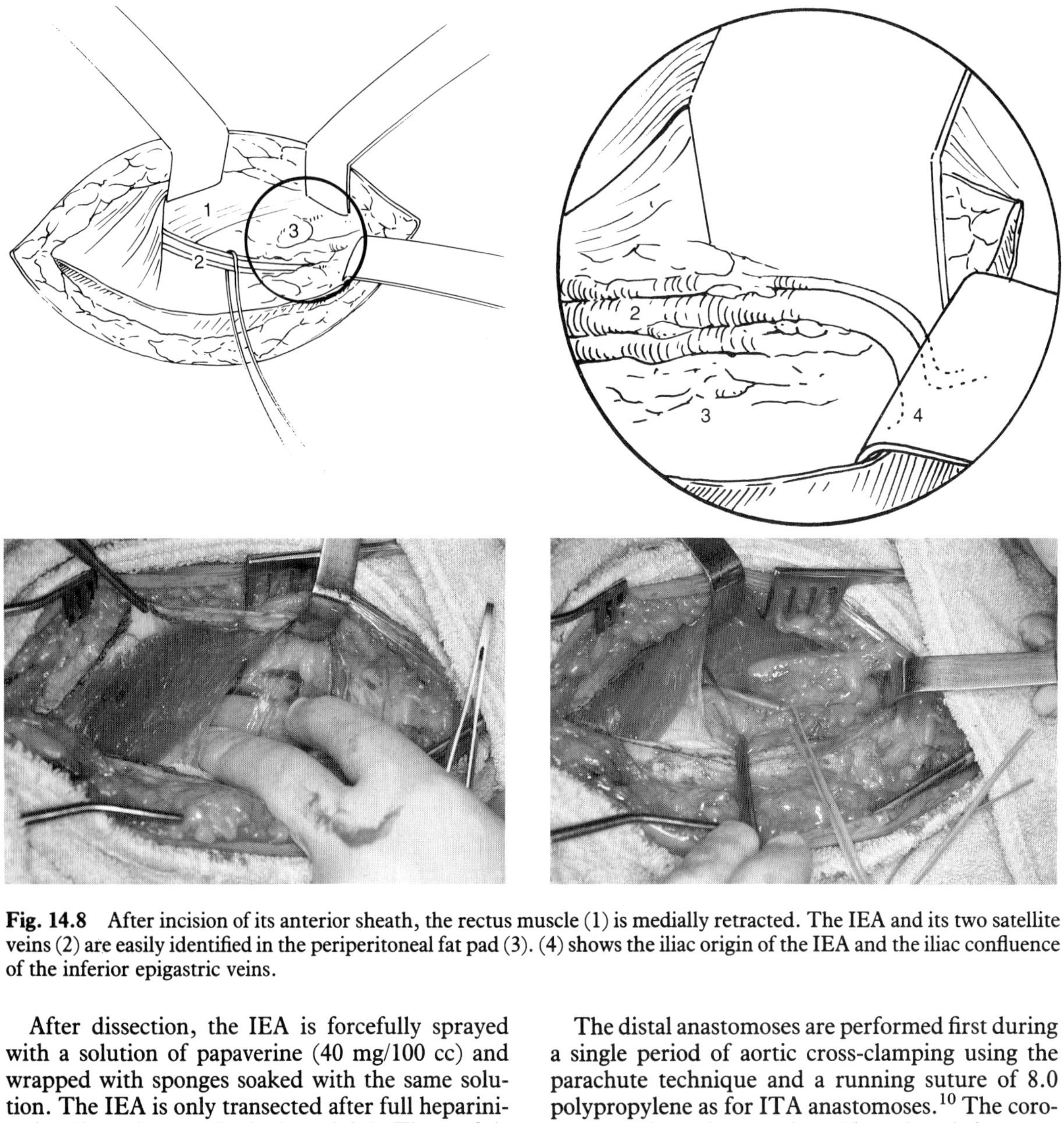

Fig. 14.8 After incision of its anterior sheath, the rectus muscle (1) is medially retracted. The IEA and its two satellite veins (2) are easily identified in the periperitoneal fat pad (3). (4) shows the iliac origin of the IEA and the iliac confluence of the inferior epigastric veins.

After dissection, the IEA is forcefully sprayed with a solution of papaverine (40 mg/100 cc) and wrapped with sponges soaked with the same solution. The IEA is only transected after full heparinization (heparin 3 mg/kg body weight). The graft is then gently flushed with and preserved in a medium consisting of warm heparinized blood with added papaverine (40 mg/100 ml) and dipyridamole (20 mg/100 ml).[9] The abdominal wound is packed with gauze during cardiopulmonary bypass. At the end of the procedure, after administration of protamine, it is closed in two layers with continuous polyglycolic acid (Dexon, Davis and Geck) sutures. A single suction drain is positioned behind the rectus muscle which can usually be removed within 48 hours.

The distal anastomoses are performed first during a single period of aortic cross-clamping using the parachute technique and a running suture of 8.0 polypropylene as for ITA anastomoses.[10] The coronary arteriotomies are short (5 mm) and the proximal anastomoses are performed using a partial exclusion clamp placed on the ascending aorta. A 4.5-mm circular aperture is punched in the ascending aorta to which the IEA is directly anastomosed when the aortic wall is free of atheroma and the IEA is large. When the aortic wall is diseased the proximal ITA may be anastomosed either end to end to a interposed segment of saphenous vein or end to side to the proximal portion of another vein graft. The hood of an old saphenous vein graft at its aortic

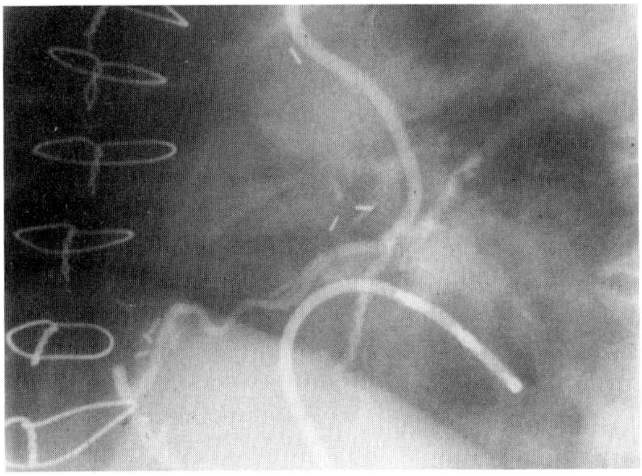

Fig. 14.9 IEA anastomosed end-to-end to a pedicled left ITA: left ITA is anastomosed to LAD, and IEA to right coronary artery (left lateral oblique angiogram, 13 months postoperatively).

anastomosis can also be used for the proximal IEA anastomosis in reoperations. The IEA graft can also be anastomosed to an ITA graft, end to side or end to end. (Fig. 14.9)[11,12] Optical magnification (× 3.5) is used to perform all the anastomoses.

References

1. Gold JP, Shemin RJ, DiSesa VJ, Cohn LH, Collins JJ. Multiple-vessel coronary revascularization with combined in situ and free sequential internal mammary arteries. *J. Thorac Cardiovasc Surg* 1985; **90:** 301–8.
2. Bakay C, Akçevin A, Süzer K *et al.* Combined internal mammary artery graft for coronary artery revascularization. *Ann Thorac Surg* 1990; **50:** 553–6.
3. Rouvière H *Anatomie humaine: descriptive et topographique*, 10th edn.: Masson et Cie Editeurs, Paris 1970: 172–4.
4. Schroeder E, Chenu P, Buche M *et al.* Angiographic data of the epigastric artery: a new conduit for myocardial revascularisation. *J Am Coll Cardiol* 1990; **15:** 116A.
5. Buche M, Schoevaerdts JC, Chalant CH Multiple-vessel coronary revascularization using both *in situ* mammary arteries and a free inferior epigastric artery. *J Thorac Cardiovasc Surg* 1990; **99:** 754–5.
6. Buche M, Schoevaerdts JC, Louagie Y *et al.* Use of the inferior epigastric artery for coronary bypass. *J Thorac Cardiovasc Surg* 1992; **103:** 665–70.
7. Amrani M, El Khoury G, Dion R. Complete myocardial revascularization with arterial grafts without using the mammary artery. *Eur J Cardiothorac Surg* 1994; **8:** 283–4.
8. Louagie Y, Buche M, Schroeder E, Schoevaerdts JC. Coronary bypass with both internal mammary and inferior epigastric arteries. *Ann Thorac Surg* 1992; **53:** 1117–19.
9. Dion R, Lavenne-Pardonge E, Scheiff JM, Verhelst R, Baele Ph, Moriau M. A novel preservation medium protecting prostacyclin production and endothelial integrity of the human saphenous vein graft. *Thromb Res* 1990; **XII:** 81–6.
10. Dion R, Verhelst R, Rousseau M *et al.* Sequential mammary grafting. Clinical, functional and angiographic assessment 6 months postoperatively in 231 consecutive patients. *J Thorac Cardiovasc Surg* 1989; **98:** 80–9.
11. Buche M, Schroeder E, Devaux Ph, Louagie Y, Schoevaerdts JC. Right internal mammary artery extended with an inferior epigastric artery for circumflex and right coronary bypass. *Ann Thorac Surg* 1992; **54:** 381–3.
12. Calafiore AM, Di Giammarco G, Luciani N, Maddestra N, Di Nardo E, Angelini R. Composite arterial conduits for a wider myocardial arterial revascularisation. *Ann Thorac Surg* 1994; **58:** 185–90.

15 Detection of graft function and patency

Erwin Schroeder, Oliver Gurné, Patrick Chenu

Since the relatively recent introduction of the inferior epigastric artery (IEA) as a free aortocoronary bypass graft, only limited early angiographic follow-up data are available in the literature.[1–4]

Since our first procedure in December 1988, we have undertaken a prospective angiographic study, which at present consists of opacification of the *in situ* IEA before bypass surgery and repeat angiography at day 10 and 1 year after the surgical procedure. Preoperative angiography was aimed at detecting IEAs of insufficient size or length, approximately 5 per cent of the screened arteries.[5] A qualitative assessment can be obtained by injection of the common femoral artery; quantitative measurements can only be obtained by selective injection of the IEA.

Angiographic data obtained in 187 patients operated on between December 1988 and May 1994 are reported here. The target coronary vessels were the right coronary artery in 155, the circumflex artery in thirty-five and diagonal branches in seven cases. In ninety-eight cases, the graft was anastomosed directly to the ascending aorta and, in eighty-one cases, via a short piece of saphenous vein. In eight cases, a composite arterial graft was constructed by extending a pedicled internal thoracic artery (ITA) graft with the IEA.

This angiographic study allowed us to assess not only the early (± day 10 after surgery) and the mid term patency (± 12 months) but also changes in calibre and vasomotor tone of this graft during follow-up by using quantitative angiography.

Methods

All angiograms were performed using a standard femoral approach. Vasoactive medications were withheld 24 hours before the angiographic study, except before the diagnostic procedure during which the patients were kept on antianginal therapy including nitrates, calcium blockers and β-blockers. Selective injections of the native coronary arteries, the IEA and ITAs were performed using 6F diagnostic catheters. All patients gave their informed consent for the early and late angiographic study.

Among the first sixty patients, a cerebrovascular accident occured in three at early postoperative angiography. In two patients, the neurological symptoms were transient, but one patient developed a persistent hemiparesis. No complications occurred during those late studies.

The angiographic appearance of the graft after nitrate infusion was assessed qualitatively as:

- perfect appearance
- focal irregularities (diameter stenosis of ≤ 60 per cent)
- significant stenosis (diameter stenosis of ≥ 70 per cent)
- string-like appearance
- graft occlusion.

This terminology is proposed for use in all postoperative angiograms in order to allow an adequate comparison between different grafts.

Furthermore, the severity of the coronary artery stenosis has to be taken into account since arterial grafts can adapt their calibre to flow demand.[6]

In order to obtain a quantitative assessment of the IEA, a single view with optimal visualization in the centre of the image intensifier field (17.5 cm) was chosen for serial measurements of the graft. All graft injections were performed according to the standards of quantitative coronary angiography.

Angiographic data were obtained at baseline and after intra-arterial infusion of 1 or 2 mg of isosorbide dinitrate. Quantitative analysis of the IEA was performed with the use of a computer-assisted coronary angiographic analysis system (CAAS®, Pie Data Medical, Maastricht, The Netherlands). The proximal vessel diameter – identified with the help of anatomical reference points, such as side branches or vascular clips placed at surgery – was measured using automated contour detection algorithms. The precision and the short-term variability of vascular dimensions have been reported.[7]

Results

Early patency

An early control angiogram was obtained in 154 (82 per cent) of the 187 patients on the day before discharge (mean interval: 10.14 ± 4.4 days).

Four (2.1 per cent) IEA grafts were occluded at early angiography. Furthermore, three grafts showed a string-like appearance (1.9 per cent). In one case, this string-like graft was anastomosed to a right coronary artery with a 50 per cent stenosis. In five cases, a significant (> 70 per cent) stenosis of the graft was observed. The stenosis was observed in three cases at the aortic anastomosis and in two cases at the distal anastomosis.

The overall patency rate in the early postoperative period was 97.4 per cent (150/154). Among these 154 patients, a perfect result (a widely patent graft without significant stenosis and no string-like appearance) of the IEA graft was observed in 142 patients (perfect patency rate: 92 per cent).

Mid-term patency

Out of 153 patients eligible for late angiographic restudy, eighty-seven patients (57 per cent) consented to the procedure at a mean interval of 12.5 ± 6.6 months after bypass surgery. Nine of these patients experienced recurrent angina. Eight IEA grafts were occluded, of which four had been anastomosed to a moderately stenotic coronary artery (≤ 60 per cent). The overall patency rate of the IEA graft at 12 months was therefore 91 per cent, in contrast with the 99 per cent patency rate of pedicled ITA grafts in the same group of patients ($P < 0.0001$). A string-like appearance was observed in eleven cases; of these, eight grafts had been anastomosed to a moderately stenotic coronary artery (≤ 60 per cent). A significant stenosis was found in four cases. In one patient, this stenosis was located at the mid point of the graft and in three cases at the distal anastomosis. In three cases, however, the angiographic appearance improved over time (Figs 15.1 and 15.2). Thus, a perfect angiographic result was observed in sixty-four (74 per cent) of the eighty-seven patients. All of the cases with a string-like appearance or graft occlusion were not documented at early angiography. In twelve cases, with poor angiographic results (four occlusions and eight string-like grafts), the anastomosis had been constructed to a moderately stenotic coronary artery and the myocardial flow was predominantly provided by the native coronary artery. If these twelve patients are

(a)

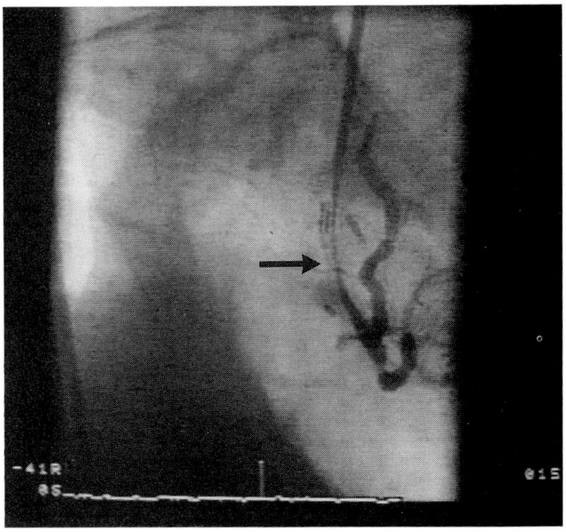

(b)

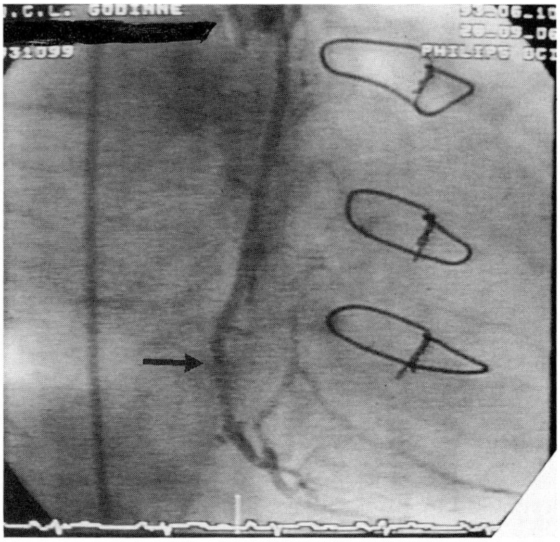

presence of a long concentic stenosis (arrow), unresponsive to nitrates, of an IEA graft anastomosed to the right coronary artery (a); late control angiogram at 12 months after bypass surgery: resolution of the stenosis (b).

excluded, a perfect angiographic appearance was observed in 66 (88 per cent) of the seventy-five patients. These patency rates (ranging from 74 to 91 per cent depending on the definition of patency) at 1 year seem comparable to those of free ITA grafts and saphenous vein grafts.[8,9]

The overall patency rate of the IEA in patients restudied between 6 to 12 months was similar to that in patients restudied between 13 and 43 months after surgery. The patency rates did not seem to be influenced by the type of proximal anastomosis. We believe that, beyond this early attrition rate, the

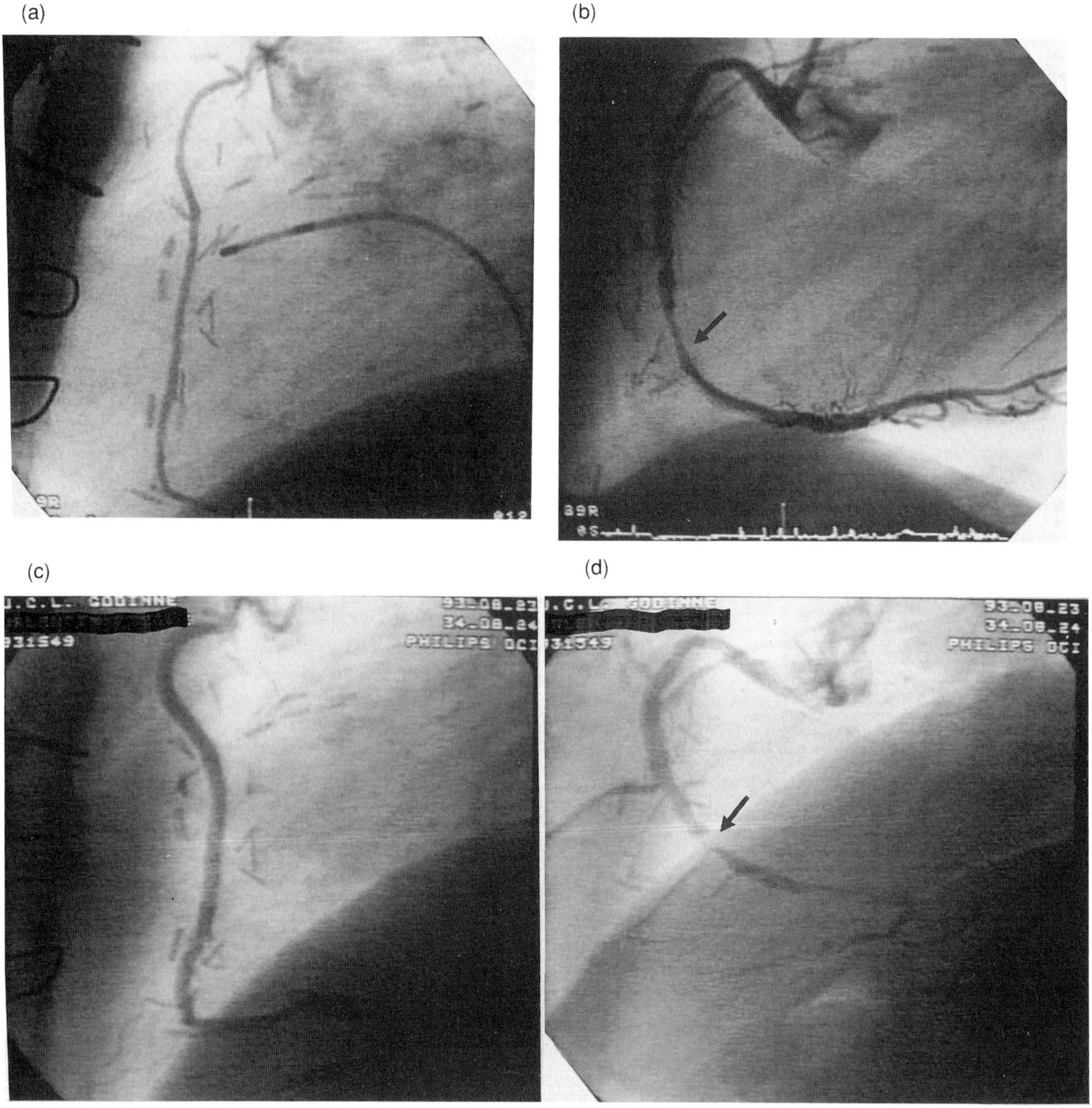

Fig. 15.2 Early control angiogram (left lateral projection) showing a patent IEA graft (a) anastomosed to the right coronary artery presenting moderate stenosis (arrow) (b); the dimension of the IEA graft after nitrate infusion is 2.50 mm; late control angiogram at 24 months showing widely patent IEA graft (c), whereas the right coronary artery now has a severe stenosis at its mid point (arrow) (d); the dimension of the IEA graft after nitrates is 3.01 mm.

patency of the IEA graft will be comparable to that of the free ITA graft.[8,10] Indeed, all IEA grafts were patent in the six patients who consented to a third angiographic restudy after more than 3 years.

Changes of graft dimensions during follow-up

In sixty-nine patients, adequate diameter measurements of the *in situ* IEA could be obtained before surgery. Mean vessel diameter was 2.24 ± 0.40 mm. After 'coronary implantation', the vessel size increased significantly to 2.61 ± 0.50 mm ($P < 0.0001$; n = 119). These results were also found in the patients in whom serial quantitative angiographic data were available before and after bypass surgery.[7] This early increase in graft diameter may be due to the harvesting technique during bypass surgery or to the maximal vasodilation resulting from an increased shear stress in the setting of increased flow demand or anaemia. However, at 12 months, the mean graft diameter came down to 2.21 ± 0.41 mm (vs early control $P < 0.0001$; vs preoperative data: NS).

The progressive reduction of graft dimensions over time may be the result of increased basal vasomotor tone, changes in flow velocity or vessel wall thickening. This is currently under investigation by intravascular ultrasound.

Vasomotor responses

Before surgery, significant vasodilation was observed after intra-arterial infusion of 1 or 2 mg of isosorbide dinitrate (mean diameter change: 0.32 ± 0.20 mm, $P < 0.0001$; n = 67). Overall, the free grafts did not to respond to nitrates early after bypass surgery (mean diameter change 0.03 ± 0.14 mm, NS; n = 119).

However, in a subgroup of fifty-one patients, vasodilation was observed after intra-arterial infusion of nitrates (Fig. 15.3). Only two parameters were different between the two groups of patients (nitrates responders (ISDN +): n = 51; nitrates non-responders (ISDN -); n = 68): the responders had a smaller basal diameter at early control (2.47 ± 0.49 mm vs 2.67 ± 0.54 mm; $P < 0.05$) and a poor runoff (2.18 ± 0.62 vs 2.71 ± 0.51; $P < 0.01$) as assessed by the following scoring system. For instance in the right coronary area:

- poor runoff: the posterior descending artery
- intermediate runoff: the posterior descending artery plus one posterolateral branch
- good or large runoff: dominant right coronary artery with several posterolateral branches.

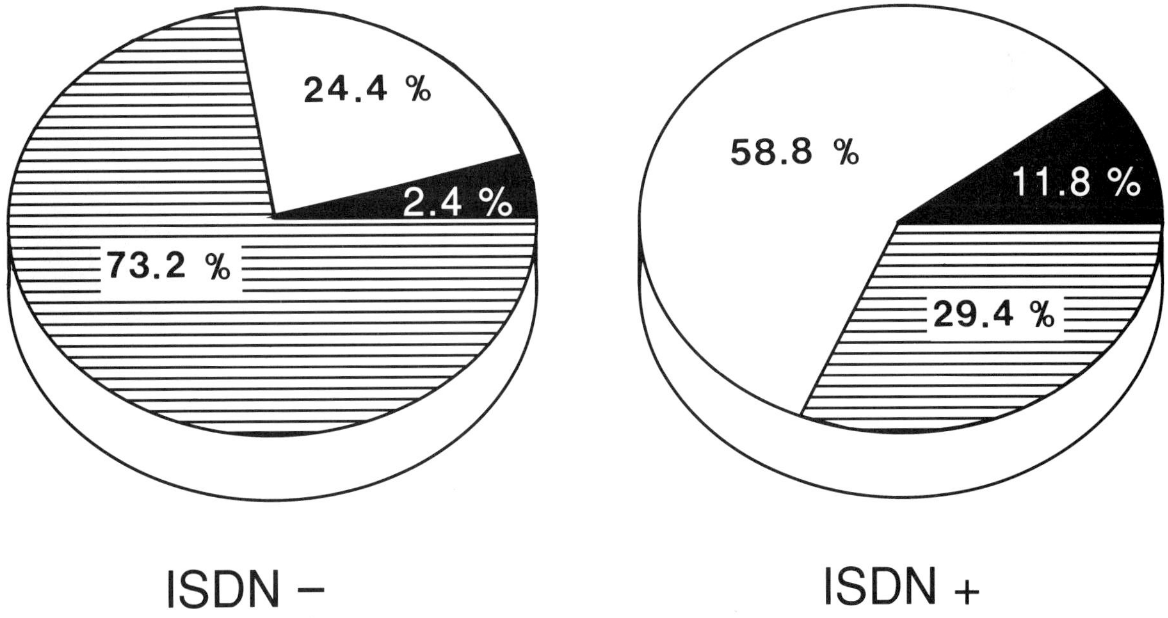

Fig. 15.3 Distribution of different sizes of areas at risk depending on the grafted coronary vessel, according to vasomotor response of the IEA graft to nitrates infusion. Runoff is poor (■), intermediate (□) or good (▤). $P < 0.001$.

The influence of the runoff on the graft's response to ISDN is depicted in Fig 15.3. IEA grafts with a poor run-off keep a vasodilator reserve, in contrast with those with a good runoff. Recovery of vasomotor tone was detected at the late control with nitrate infusion (mean diameter change: 0.20 ± 0.17 mm; $P < 0.0001$; $n = 49$).

Conclusion

IEA grafts have lower early patency rates compared to pedicled ITA grafts. However, the mid-term patency rate of this new graft is comparable to that of free ITA and saphenous vein grafts. We believe that, beyond an early attrition phase, the patency rates of the IEA graft will tend to stabilize and later results similar to those of free ITA grafts are anticipated. Serial quantitative angiographic studies have shown recovery of vasomotor tone at mid-term restudy. In order to establish precisely the place of this new arterial graft among other available arterial conduits, long-term clinical, functional and angiographic restudies beyond 5 years are currently under way in our institution.

References

1. Puig LB, Ciongolli W, Cividanes GVL *et al.* Inferior epigastric artery as a free graft for myocardial revascularisation. *J Thorac Cardiovasc Surg* 1990; **99:** 251–5.
2. Buche M, Schoevaerdts JC, Louagie Y *et al.* Use of the inferior epigastric artery for coronary bypass. *J Thorac Surg* 1992; **103:** 665–70.
3. Cremer J, Mugge A, Schulze N, Liesmann T, Haverich A, Borst HJ. The inferior epigastric artery for CABG: functional assessment and clinical results. *Eur J Cardiothorac Surg* 1993; **7:** 423–7.
4. Perrault LP, Carrier M, Hebert Y, Cartier R, Leclerc Y, Pelletier LC. Early experience with the inferior epigastric artery in CABG. *J Thorac Cardiovasc Surg* 1993; **106:** 928–30.
5. Schroeder E, Chenu P, Buche M *et al.* Angiographic data of the epigastric artery – a new conduit of myocardial revascularization. *JACC* 1990; **15:** 116A.
6. Dincer B, Barner HB The 'occluded' internal mammary artery graft: restoration of patency after apparent occlusion associated with progression of coronary disease. *J Thorac Cardiovasc Surg* 1983; **5:** 318–22.
7. Gurne O, Buche M, Chenu P *et al.* Quantitative angiographic follow-up study of the free inferior epigastric coronary bypass graft. *Circulation* 1994; **90** (II): 148–154.
8. Loop FD, Lytle BW, Cosgrove DM, Golding CAR, Taylor PC, Stewart RW. Free aorto coronary internal mammary artery grafts: late results. *J Thorac Cardiovasc Surg* 1986; **92:** 827–31.
9. Dion R, Etienne PY, Verhelst R, *et al.* Bilateral mammary grafting: clinical, functional and angiographic assessment in 400 consecutive patients. *Eur J Cardiothorac Surg* 1993; **7:** 287–94.
10. Grondin CM, Campeau L, Lesperance J, Enjelbert M, Bourassa MG. Comparison of late changes in internal mammary artery and saphenous vein grafts in two consecutive series of patients 10 years after operation. *Circulation* 1984; **70** (I): I208–12.

16 Early and late results

Hendrick B. Barner and Andrew C. Fiore

Interest in the so called 'alternative arterial conduits' has been generated through the success of the internal thoratic artery (ITA), because of need for additional conduit when the ITA was not available, and because of the desire to achieve complete revascularization with only arterial conduits. Some surgeons have not been comfortable with complex configurations of both ITAs to achieve complete arterial revascularization[1] and have sought to use one or more alternative arterial conduits to attain such a goal. One of these alternative conduits is the inferior epigastric artery (IEA) and it is the purpose of this chapter to discuss early and late results with the use of this conduit.

The IEA is the most recent addition to the surgical armementarium of arterial conduits, having been first reported by Puig in 1990.[2] Depending on the definition of early and late it could be argued that with a 5-year period of observation all results are early and there is no late information on performance of this conduit. Nevertheless, for the purposes of this chapter early results will be those of the perioperative interval, namely within 1 month of operation and late results will be those beyond 1 month to the maximum interval of follow-up, which in one report extends to 5 years.

Early results

Operative mortality

Table 16.1 summarizes data from seven reports in which sufficient information was included to allow meaningful interpretation of some or all clinical material presented. This table comprises 411 patients. In Table 16.2 the last report[3] from Table 16.1 has been omitted leaving 325 patients because information pertinent to the eighty-six patients having IEA grafting was not separated from data on the total of 130 patients having radial artery grafting. Thus, it is not clear whether one death in the 130 patients occurred in the eighty-six patients with IEA grafting or in the remaining forty-four patients.

In Table 16.2 there were ten deaths to give an operative mortality of 3.1 per cent. The two largest series[5,8] comprise 265 patients with seven deaths for a mortality of 2.6 per cent.

Table 16.1 Reports of patients having utilization of inferior epigastric artery

			Number of Conduits							*Grafts/Patient*	
Author	*Year*	*Patients*	*1 IEA*	*2 IEA*	*1 ITA*	*2 ITA*	*GEA*	*RA*	*SV*	*Artery*	*Total*
Puig[2]	1990	22	20	2	3	3			8	1.5	1.9
Mills[3]	1991	18	17	1							
Milgalter[4]	1992	38	34	4	7	31			51	2.9	4.3
Barner[5]	1993	108	91	17	21	87	12		21	3.1	3.3
Cremer[6]	1993	50	50		40	8			38	3.1	2.9
Perrault[7]	1993	18	18			17	3		1	3.1	3.1
Buche[8]	1994	157	157		285[a]				6	3.4	3.4
Calafiore[9]	1994	86	86		*b*	*b*	*b*	*b*	*b*	*b*	*b*

[a] Data provided for total number of ITA grafts.
[b] Data not provided for 86 patients with IEA grafts but for all (130) the patients in the report.
IEA = inferior epigastric artery; ITA = internal thoracic artery; GEA = gastroepiploic artery; RA = radial artery; SV = saphenous vein.

Table 16.2 Mortality and morbidity for 325 patients

Author	*Deaths*	*Periop MI*	*Reop bleeding*	*Med inf*	*Abdominal incision*		
					Infection	*Haematoma*	*Necrosis*
Puig[2]	1			1	1		
Mills[3]	0				1	1	1
Milgalter[a4]	0	1	2	2	5		
Barner[5]	3	7	2	2	1		2
Cremer[6]	1	1	1		5		1
Perrault[7]	1					3	
Buche[8]	4	3	2			6	
	10(3.1%)	12(3.9%)	7(2.2%)	5(1.5%)	13(4.1%)	10(3.19%)	4(1.2%)

[a] One patient not included in the table had bleeding from the proximal stump of the IEA requiring wound exploration for control.
Periop MI = perioperative myocardial infarction; Reop = reoperation for; Med inf = mediastinal wound infection.

Table 16.3 Preoperative risk factors

Author	*Mean age*	*Age range*	*IDDM*	*Prior CAB*
Puig[2]		40–72		
Milgalter[4]	58	29–74		14/38
Barner[5]	58.6	39–75	6/108	27/108
Cremer[6]	54.9	30–68	6/50	3/50
Perrault[7]	52	38–69		
Buche[8]	60.2	37–78		

IDDM = insulin dependent diabetes mellitus; CAB = coronary artery bypass.

It can be argued that this mortality is excessive in as much as operative mortalities of 1–2 per cent have been reported for large series of patients having coronary bypass grafting. Sufficient details are not included in reports of patients with IEA grafting to perform risk-factor analysis. The mean age at operation is perhaps five to eight years younger (Table 16.3) than that noted for the total population of patients having coronary bypass grafting during the same time frame.[10] The incidence of patients having reoperation for failed coronary bypass grafts is somewhat higher than in the total institutional experience in several instances,[4,5] but this is not true for all the reports (Table 16.3). The reported incidence of insulin-dependent diabetes mellitus is low. There is also a learning curve for each new procedure and although death was not attributed in any specific instance to the learning curve, it is possible that this was a factor in operative mortality.

Detailed analysis of the deaths (Table 16.4) indicates that five were related to low cardiac output in

Table 16.4 Perioperative deaths

Author	*Deaths*	*Cause(s) of death*
Puig[2]	1	Impaired LV, low output, COPD
Barner[5]	2	Impaired LV, low output, periop MI, prior CAB
	1	CVA, multiorgan failure, LVAD, died day 65
Cremer[6]	1	Periop MI, low output, IABP, LVAD, died day 26
Perrault[7]	1	Acute renal failure
Buche[8]	2	Low output
	1	Ventricular fibrillation
	1	Tamponade due to bleeding from IEA–aortic anastomosis

LV left ventricle; COPD = chronic obstructive pulmonary disease; Periop MI = perioperative myocardial infarction; CAB = coronary bypass; CVA = cerebral vascular accident; IABP = intra-aortic balloon pump; LVAD = left ventricular assist device.

the postoperative interval. The authors do not indicate in all instances that these patients had impaired ventricular function preoperatively but several did. Two of these five were having their second coronary bypass procedure and the same two sustained a perioperative myocardial infarction.[5]

Two additional patients suffered a perioperative myocardial infarction; one was thought to have closure of a vein graft to a posterolateral branch of the circumflex artery, resulting in lateral myocardial infarction. This was treated with an intra-aortic balloon pump followed by a left ventricular assist device which was successfully weaned but with eventual death from cerebral embolization.[6] The other patient with a major myocardial infarction died suddenly after anterior infarction secondary to failure of an ITA graft to the left anterior descending coronary artery.[8] One patient had a perioperative stroke followed by multi-organ failure and died on postoperative day 65.[5] One patient died from aortic haemorrhage at the site of anastomosis of the IEA[8] and one patient died from renal failure occurring in the postoperative interval.[7]

The only pattern that can be made of these postoperative deaths is that five were related to low cardiac output. At least two of these patients were having reoperative coronary bypass grafting and at least two had perioperative myocardial infarction. The authors have indicated that there was no evidence that the low output or the associated infarction was related to the IEA graft, but this opinion was not always confirmed by angiography or autopsy. In two instances it was felt that death was directly related to perioperative infarction. Neither of the infarctions were related to the IEA graft (one was related to a vein graft and one to a left ITA graft). The one patient who died because of haemorrhage from the anastomotic site of the IEA to the aorta had a 'very fragile aortic wall'.

Two patients who died on postoperative days 33 and 34 after transfer to other hospitals on postoperative days 6 and 13 (respirator-dependent) should, strictly speaking, be included as perioperative deaths.[4] This would raise mortality for the collected patients to twelve from ten (Table 16.2) or 3.7 per cent.

Wound complications

Morbidity specific to the IEA has been that of wound complications (Table 16.2). Haematoma of the abdominal incision required surgical drainage in six patients,[6] drained spontaneously in one,[3] and should be avoidable by delaying wound closure until after reversal of the heparin. A closed wound drainage system is favoured by some but we have not used it. One patient required abdominal wound exploration for bleeding from the iliac stump of the IEA.[4] The occurrence of wound infection has been greater than the 1–2 per cent incidence expected in clean surgical incisions but the majority (ten) of these were superficial rather than deep. A specific problem we have encountered is that of abdominal wall necrosis in two of seventeen patients with both ITAs and both IEAs harvested.[10] The skin, subcutaneous tissue, anterior rectus sheath and rectus muscle became necrotic and were eventually debrided. The tissue posterior to the rectus muscle remained viable and both wounds had delayed closure of the skin over a granulating wound without other intervention. One of these two patients had evidence of a vasculitis by history and pathological loss of digital pulse amplitude in response to cold stimulation of the fingers while the other did not. We must conclude that there is some risk of this complication with harvest of these four conduits which has been rarely done by others than ourselves (*see* Table 16.1). Isolated rectus muscle necrosis is frequently mentioned as a potential complication of IEA mobilization but this only occurred in one patient.[6] We believe that it may occur more often, but go unrecognized. Other potential wound complications have been suggested as being possible but have not been specifically reported. These include injury to the ductus deferens, the genitofemoral nerve, the external iliac artery or vein, or the anomalous obturator artery which arises from the proximal 1–1.5 cm of the IEA.

Mediastinal wound infection or dehiscence (*see* Table 16.2) in 5/325 (1.3 per cent) has not occurred more frequently than anticipated in patients having ITA mobilization and at least 275/325 patients had bilateral ITA mobilization (*see* Table 16.1). Thus, the use of the IEA does not increase the likelihood of mediastinal wound complications.

Other morbidity

Reoperation for bleeding (*see* Table 16.2) has been infrequent in the reported cases (7/325, 2.2 per cent). Perioperative myocardial infarction has similarly been infrequent (12/325, 3.7 per cent). Stroke has only been specifically reported by us (2/108, 1.9 per cent).[5] Low cardiac output requiring the intra-aortic balloon pump has only been reported by us

(4/108, 3.8 per cent).[5] (The other use of the intra-aortic balloon which is reported under operative mortality was for perioperative infarction due to vein graft closure.)[6]

Hypoperfusion by the IEA

The specific problem of myocardial hypoperfusion by the IEA graft has not been addressed in the reports in Table 16.1 or in reports not included in Table 16.1. This could be related to use of the IEA in that it was frequently, but not always, placed to vessels of secondary importance. However, in one experience,[6] twenty-four of fifty IEAs were grafted to the left anterior descending artery and in another,[10] seventeen of forty-seven patients had an IEA supplying the left anterior descending coronary. Thus, a modest number of patients have had the IEA grafted to the left anterior descending coronary without the development of recognized hypoperfusion.

Other data supporting the adequacy of the IEA flow are the intraoperative measurements of graft flow. Internal thoracic artery flow (49 ± 31 ml/min) was identical to IEA flow (50 ± 34 ml/min) after discontinuation of bypass.[5] These observations suggest that hypoperfusion is unlikely, but obviously do not preclude its occurrence. This is always a possibility with any arterial conduit and may be secondary to the small diameter of the conduit, spasm, conduit injury or technical anastomotic error.

Use of the intra-aortic balloon pump must be considered a flag for hypoperfusion related to arterial conduits. Obviously there are other causes for low cardiac output or haemodynamic deterioration and it is not always possible to determine the aetiology. In our report four patients were so treated and we could not identify inadequate conduit flow as the cause.[5]

Graft patency

Graft patency at less than one month postoperatively has ranged from 57 to 100 per cent (Table 16.5). In the largest series in which 135 grafts were studied, three were occluded (97.8 per cent patent) and twelve had segmental irregularities or anastomotic stenosis (88.8 per cent widely patent).[8] The poorest patency rate (57 per cent) was in the numerically smallest group (eighteen cases) and may well represent the learning curve.[4] The best patency (100 per cent) is from a series in which none of the IEAs was anastomosed to the aorta, but rather to an *in situ* ITA.[7] When the early results from Table 16.5 are combined, the overall early graft patency (stenotic, irregular, or 'string sign' grafts are considered occluded) is 88.5 per cent (177/200).

Late results

Late follow-up data on patients having IEA grafting are very limited and almost anecdotal in nature with the exception of one report.[8]

Mortality

Buche and associates have followed 157 patients from 6 to 62 months (average 32 months) with four late deaths, two of which were sudden and two non-cardiac.[8]

Table 16.5 Angiographic assessment of graft patency

		Widely patient grafts/grafts studied postop		
		Postoperative interval (months)		
Author	*<1*	*1–6*	*6–12*	*13–43*
Puig[2]	15/17			
Mills[3]		3/8[a]		
Perrault[7]	8/14			
Cremer[6]		19/23		
Buche[8]	120/135		36/48	25/29
Calafiore[9]	34/34		20/21[b]	
Total	177/200(88.5%)	22/31(71.0%)	56/69(81.2%)	25/29(86.2%)

[a] Postoperative interval, 10 days–14 months.
[b] Postoperative interval, 6–14 months.

Angina, infarction, reintervention

Angina recurred in nine of 157 all within the first year and all had coronary angiography.[8] In four it was related to closure of the IEA graft and in two it was secondary to closure of an ITA graft. Stenosis occurred in two old saphenous vein grafts (one patient) and stenosis developed distal to two ITA grafts in two patients. One myocardial infarction (non-Q wave) occurred in these 157 patients in an area not bypassed by the IEA two years after operation. Cremer and coworkers have followed fifty patients 1–18 months without evidence of recurrent ischaemic events.[6] Milgalter and associates performed stress testing on thirty-two patients 6–17 months after IEA grafting also without evidence of myocardial ischaemia.[4]

Reintervention for recurrent ischaemia was required in four of nine with two having coronary angioplasty, one having vein graft angioplasty, and one having repeat coronary bypass.[8]

Graft patency

Four groups have reported IEA patency beyond 1 month (*see* Table 16.5) but in one the interval spanned was 10 days to 10 months and only eight patients were studied with three of eight (37.5 per cent) grafts patent.[11] Cremer *et al.* have studied twenty-three patients between 1 and 6 months postoperatively with nineteen (82.6 per cent) patent grafts.[6] Calafiore and coworkers have obtained a 95.2 per cent (twenty of twenty-one) graft patency 6–14 months postoperatively.[9]

In the longest and largest angiographic follow-up, seventy-seven patients were studied 6–43 months postoperatively:[8] forty-eight grafts were studied 6–12 months (mean 11.5) after operation with forty-four patent but eight had diffuse narrowing so that thirty-six of forty-four (81.8 per cent) were widely patent. Between 13 and 43 months (mean 25) twenty-eight of twenty-nine IEAs were patent but three had diffuse narrowing for an 86 per cent patency (twenty-five of twenty-nine). Five patients had a third angiogram 16 – 60 months (average 39) after operation with five patent grafts.[8] A majority of the occluded or diffusely narrowed grafts were placed to coronary arteries having mild stenosis on the control angiogram. Narrowing of arterial conduits has been related to competitive flow through the coronary artery having a less than critical stenosis.[12] Also a majority of these failed grafts occurred in the first half of this experience.

There is little doubt that a learning curve exists for arterial conduits in general as well as for each of the individual conduits. We also do not know the ultimate fate of grafts exhibiting diffuse narrowing or the 'string sign'. Anecdotal reports indicate that some of these grafts have full patency restored when

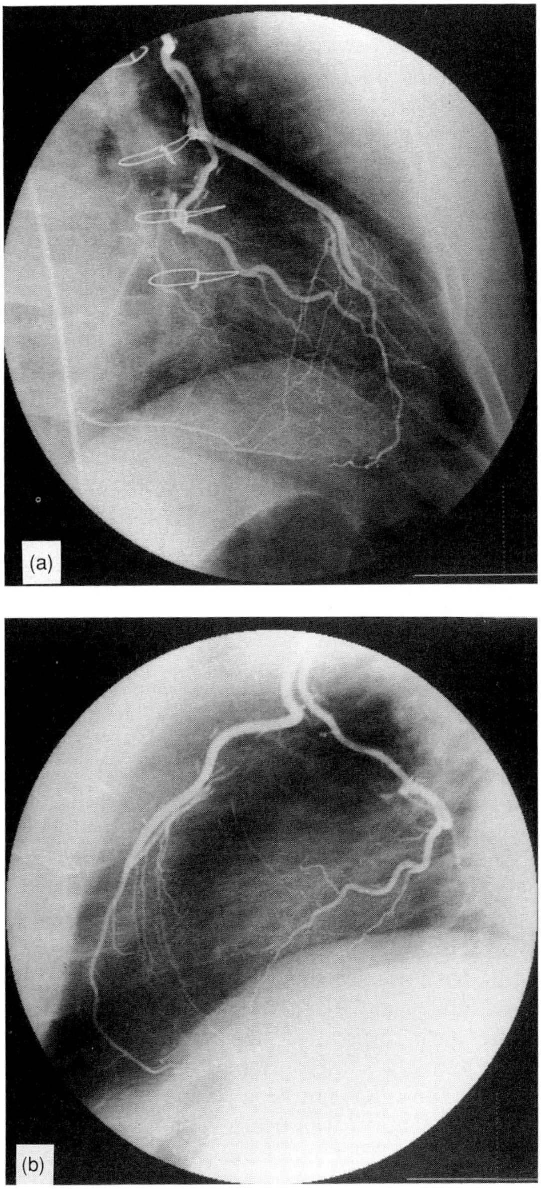

Fig. 16.1 A 32-month postoperative angiogram showing IEA anastomosed to left ITA proximally and the left anterior descending coronary artery in the right anterior oblique projection (a) and in the left anterior oblique projection (b) (Courtesy Prof. AM Calafiore).

the coronary lesion progresses from a subcritical stenosis to a critical one, but this cannot be said to occur in all or even a certain percentage of such apparently compromised conduits.

Importantly, in the experience of Buche and associates,[8] IEA patency remains stable after the first year and is comparable to that for the free internal thoracic artery graft.[13]

The best IEA patency was reported by Calafiore.[9] Because of the small numbers it is unclear whether these differences in patency are significant. However, it is worthwhile noting that all of the proximal IEA anastomoses were to an *in situ* ITA (one of eighty-six was to saphenous vein). Calafiore believes that anastomosis of any arterial conduit to the aorta results in haemodynamic stress to the conduit based on wall stretching with intimal injury and secondary intimal hyperplasia related to the abrupt rise in pressure in the ascending aorta with each cardiac cycle. Figure 16.1 shows a 32-month postoperative angiogram of the IEA anastomosed proximally to the left ITA and distally to the left anterior descending artery in which the IEA has increased in diameter when compared to the early control angiogram (Calafiore personal communication, July 1994).

Conclusions

Experience with all of the alternative arterial conduits is extremely limited relative to that with the ITA. The IEAs are paired, like all but one of the putative arterial conduits, but are the shortest of the arterial conduits. Conduit length in our experience (11.9 ± 2.6 cm) is less than that of the ITA (16.5 ± 1.0 cm) whereas both the radial artery and gastroepiploic artery can be harvested in lengths of 20–22 cm in many instances. Complications related to harvesting have been few and the commonest, wound haematoma, can be avoided by delaying wound closure until reversal of heparin with protamine and/or using a closed drainage system. Rectus muscle necrosis has not been recognized as a problem and abdominal wall necrosis has only occurred in the setting of bilateral harvesting of IEAs and the ITAs.

Enhanced long-term patency has been the primary driving force in the search for new arterial conduits as well as additional conduits when usual conduits are unavailable or their use limited by insulin-dependent diabetes mellitus. Unfortunately graft patency data for the IEA are limited and come from five sites with three reporting fifty or fewer patients. The learning curve for utilization of arterial conduits has never been numerically defined, but clearly exists. We believe it must be fifty to 100 per surgeon. Although IEA patency does not compare with that for *in situ* ITA or right GEA it more appropriately must be compared with the use of these conduits as free grafts. These data for use as a free graft of the GEA are non-existent and for the ITA they are limited numerically and for the most part were generated from experience in the 1970s.[13] Virtually all angiographic follow up for the IEA is with use of an aortic anastomosis except for that of Calafiore, and he reports the best graft patency. Not only may conduit-to-conduit anastomosis be a better technique from the standpoint of patency, but it also facilitates use of a shorter conduit (he commonly harvests 6 cm of the IEA which is one half or less of the length harvested by most surgeons). Tector is now utilizing conduit-to-conduit anastomosis exclusively in his 'T' graft configuration of the right ITA grafted to the left with 96 per cent patency of this anastomosis in the twenty-five patients having angiography.[1] Tector has utilized the 'T' graft in 500 patients (personal communication, March 1994) and he is obviously confident with conduit-to-conduit anastomosis which has hithertofore troubled many surgeons because of fear of jeopardizing flow through the donor conduit to its coronary anastomosis, or of finding that the proximal donor conduit provides inadequate flow to all the grafted coronaries, leading to myocardial hypoperfusion.

Thus, at this juncture the optimal utilization and ultimate usefulness of the IEA has not been defined. Patency will most likely improve with increasing experience and perhaps with conduit-to-conduit grafting. Limited length can be overcome by conduit-to-conduit anastomosis which will allow access to more distal sites or subtotal harvesting for more proximal sites.

References

1. Tector AJ, Amundsen S, Schmal TM, Kress DC, Peter M. Total revascularization with T-grafts. *Ann Thorac Surg* 1994; **57**: 33–9.
2. Puig LB, Ciongolli W, Cividanes GVL *et al*. Inferior epigastric artery as a free graft for myocardial revascularization. *J Thorac Cardiovasc Surg* 1990; **99**: 251–5.
3. Mills NL, Everson CT. Technique for use of the

inferior epigastric artery as a coronary bypass graft. *Ann Thorac Surg* 1991; **51:** 208–14.
4. Milgalter E, Pearl JM, Laks H *et al.* The inferior epigastric arteries as coronary bypass conduits. *J Thorac Cardiovasc Surg* 1992; **103:** 463–5.
5. Barner HB, Naunheim KS, Peigh PS, Willman VL, Fiore AC. Inferior epigastric artery for myocardial revascularization. *Eur J Cardiothorac Surg* 1993; **7:** 478–81.
6. Cremer J, Mugge A, Schulze M *et al.* The inferior epigastric artery for coronary bypass grafting: functional assessment and clinical results. *Eur J Cardiothorac Surg* 1993; **7:** 423–7.
7. Perrault LP, Carrier M, Hebert Y, Cartier R, Leclerc Y, Pelletier LC. Early experience with the inferior epigastric artery in coronary artery bypass grafting. *J Thorac Cardiovasc Surg* 1993; **106:** 928–30.
8. Buche M, Schroeder E, Gurné O *et al.* Coronary artery bypass grafting with the inferior epigastric artery: midterm clinical and angiographic results. *J Thorac Cardiovasc Surg* 1995; **109:** 553–60.
9. Calafiore AM, Di Giammarco G, Luciani N, *et al.* Complex preformed arterial conduits. *Ann Thorac Surg* 1994; **58:** 185–90.
10. Barner HB, Naunheim KS, Fiore AC, Fischer VW, Harris HH. Use of the inferior epigastric artery as a free graft for myocardial revascularization. *Ann Thorac Surg* 1991; **52:** 429–37.
11. Mills NL, Everson CT, Hockmuth DR. Free arterial grafts. *Curr Opin Cardiol* 1991; **6:** 898–903.
12. Seki T, Kitamura S, Kawachi K *et al.* A quantitative study of postoperative luminal narrowing of the internal thoracic artery graft in coronary artery bypass surgery. *J Thorac Cardiovasc Surg* 1992; **104:** 1532–8.
13. Loop FD, Lytle BW, Cosgrove DM, Golding LAR, Taylor PC, Stewart RW. Free aorto-coronary internal mammary artery graft. *J Thorac Cardiovasc Surg* 1986; **92:** 827–31.

Part V
Other arterial conduits

17 Radial artery: surgical techniques and clinical results

Christophe Acar, Victor Jebara, Jean N. Fabiani, Alain Deloche and Alain Carpentier

Compared to the other conduits available for coronary artery revascularization, the radial artery (RA) has the following potential advantages:

- it is an arterial graft adapted to systemic pressure;
- its diameter is slightly greater than that of the internal thoracic artery (ITA) matching that of the coronary arteries;
- the quality of its wall is thicker and more resistant than that of the ITA providing good technical characteristics for anastomosis;
- its superficial position in the forearm allows easy harvesting which can proceed simultaneously with ITA dissection and need not increase the operative time;
- it has sufficient length to reach any target vessel on the heart; moreover in certain instances, two separate grafts can be performed using the same radial artery.

Despite these advantages the use of the RA as a coronary conduit has remained subject to controversy for many years. Due to encouraging results observed in a recent study, there has been a renewal of interest in this graft. However, several years of data collection are still required in order to define the exact place of this conduit in coronary surgery.

Historical background

In 1971, Carpentier used the RA for the first time ever to bypass coronary arteries.[1] A series of thirty patients were then operated upon using the RA at Hospital Broussais. Four years later, at the Annual Meeting of the American Association for Thoracic Surgery in New York, Carpentier reported a 30 per cent occlusion rate of the RA grafts.[2] He suggested that occlusion of this arterial conduit was due to spasm of the denervated vessel and concluded that the RA should not be used as a graft until this physiological problem had been resolved. Shortly after, two other reports from separate centres in the USA confirmed these results and the use of the RA was completely abandoned.[3,4]

In 1989, we received from a referring cardiologist an angiographic control of a patient operated on 14 years earlier using the RA anastomosed to the left anterior descending which at that time was considered to be occluded. The recent control showed a perfectly patent RA graft revascularizing the left anterior descending with no evidence of graft disease (Fig. 17.1). Five additional angiographic controls of patients operated on in the early 1970s using the RA showed perfectly patent radial artery grafts 13–18 years postoperatively.

The technique of preparation of the RA used 20 years earlier was probably the cause of graft failure. The artery was dissected alone, separately from the satellite veins. Moreover, progressive instrumental dilatation of the vessel was performed using metallic probes which might have caused severe intimal damage. At that time, no vasodilating drugs were used.

In view of the recent advances in arterial revascularization and an improved understanding of the vasoreactivity of arterial conduits, we decided to reinvestigate the use of the RA for coronary bypass.[5] Harvesting of the vessel was performed using a perfectly atraumatic technique. The artery was dissected 'en bloc' with the satellite veins in a similar manner to ITA dissection and no instrumental manoeuvre was performed. The artery was dilated using blood and papaverine at low pressure and an

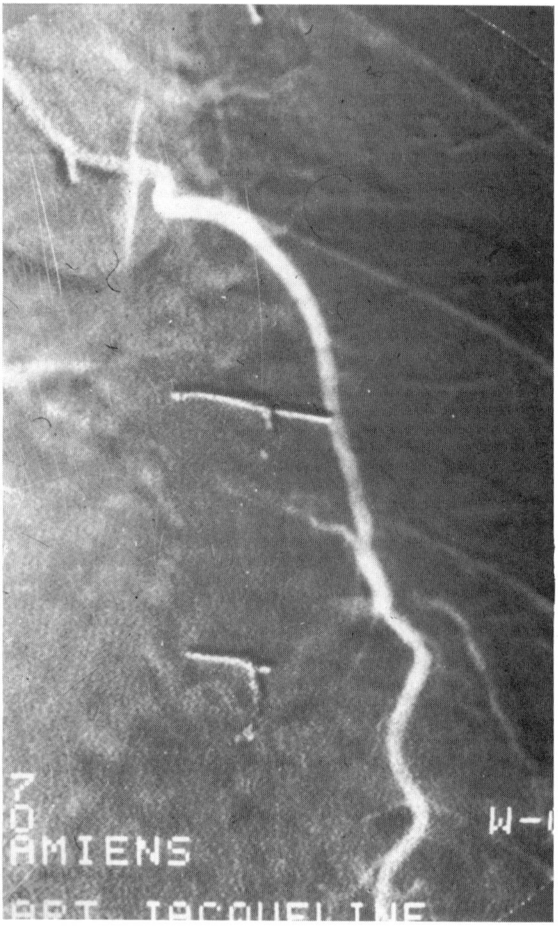

Fig. 17.1 RA graft to left anterior descending coronary artery at 14 years. Reproduced with permission from Acar *et al.*[5]

antispastic drug (diltiazem) was administered topically.

At our institution, indications for the use of the RA were initially restricted to patients with unsuitable saphenous veins. However, due to the encouraging clinical and angiographic results, these indications were extended, and to date (July 1989–July 1994) 324 patients have received the RA graft for coronary revascularization. At the present time this graft is our preferred arterial conduit after the *in situ* ITA. Recently, other groups have reported similar use of this conduit.[6,7]

Histology

The RA is a 'muscular' artery whose wall is significantly thicker than that of the ITA. The intima consists of several layers of endothelial cells, including a small number of myocytes which is a normal finding in ageing arterial walls. The main difference between these vessels resides in the media, which in the case of the radial artery is constituted of multiple tight layers of vascular smooth muscle cells.[8,9] The *vasa vasorum* are exclusively located in the adventitia and do not significantly contribute to blood supply to the RA wall.[9]

Intimal hyperplasia, a well known phenomenon widely studied and documented in both cardiac and vascular surgery as a cause of graft failure,[10–13] has been reported in rare operative samples of occluded RA grafts.[3]

Surgical techniques

The left RA is harvested in right-handed individuals and vice versa. The patient is positioned with the arm at a 90° angle with the longitudinal axis of the body. Arterial blood pressure is monitored using an RA catheter on the opposite side. No intravenous catheters are inserted on the side of RA harvesting because section of the superficial veins would produce a back flow from the infusion line in the operative field. The dissection of the RA is performed simultaneously with that of the ITA.

The incision starts 1 cm above the wrist laterally to the midline of the elbow (Fig. 17.2(a)). The antebrachial fascia is incised above the vascular pedicle. In the upper third of the forearm the RA runs deep underneath the brachioradialis muscle which is retracted laterally without being divided. The numerous collateral branches are secured using metallic clips and the vascular pedicle is harvested 'en bloc' with the artery and both satellite veins (Fig. 17.2(a)).

Anatomical variations of the RA are rare.[14] Occasionally, the distal part of the vessel lies superficially above the antebrachial fascia; however, the operative technique remains unchanged. The RA can be harvested up to the bifurcation of the brachial artery depending upon the number of grafts required and their respective length. The only potential hazard that might be encountered is damage to the ulnar artery. In fact, the bifurcation of the brachial artery is usually located below the elbow and the origin of

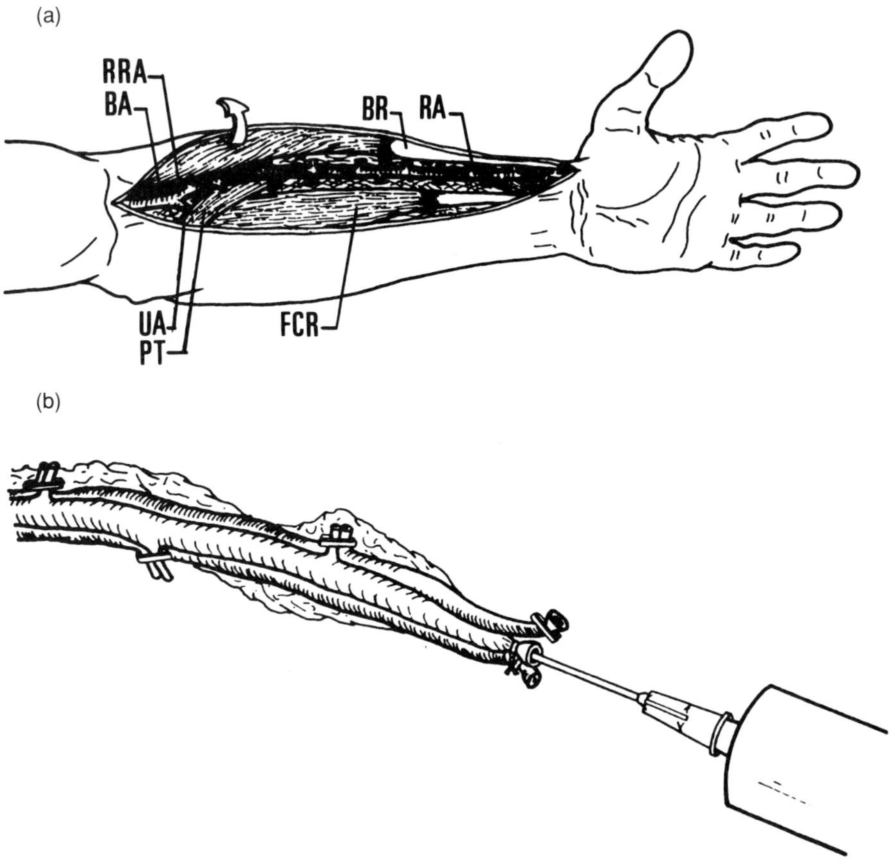

Fig. 17.2 Harvesting technique of the RA. (a) The brachioradialis muscle (BR) is retracted without being divided. (UA: ulnar artery, BA: brachial artery; RRA: recurrent radial artery; FCR: flexor carpi radialis; PT: pronator teres); (b) The RA is harvested together with its satellite veins, and hydrostatic dilatation is performed immediately before implantation.

the ulnar artery lies deep posteriorly hidden by the muscle belly of the pronator teres (Fig. 17.2(a)). Two anatomical landmarks indicate the proximity of the bifurcation of the brachial artery: the emergence of the recurrent RA and dense venous anastomosis around the RA. We recommend staying 1 cm away from the brachial bifurcation.

Following explantation, the RA is usually vasoconstricted and should not be immediately used for bypass. It should first be stored in a solution of blood, heparin and papaverine. The proximal end of the artery is then catheterized using a 16 gauge catheter and hydrostatic dilatation is achieved at a low pressure using the same mixture (Fig. 17.2(b)). Thus, the surgeon can visualize progressive release of the spasm and check haemostasis of small collateral branches. We have demonstrated that this procedure does not damage the vessel wall and in particular the intima.[5]

The blood supply to the hand and forearm is mostly furnished by the ulnar artery. The interosseous artery which arises from the ulnar artery, is embryologically the nutrient artery of the forearm. In case of RA occlusion, distal perfusion of the limb is supplied by collaterals from the ulnar artery.

The Allen test has been proposed to detect insufficient collateral flow from the ulnar artery. However, several studies have shown frequent false positives using this test.[15] In this situation, patency of the ulnar artery should be verified using pulse palpation or doppler study. Finally, the use of plethysmography as suggested by Brodman could be a valuable adjunct that would allow the assessment of peripheral perfusion pressure in the fingers. In our clinical practice, a positive Allen test has never been considered a contraindication to RA use. No signs of acute or chronic ischaemia (claudication) have been observed in our experience. However, in one patient a technical error resulted in a stenosis at the origin of the ulnar artery due to proximal ligation of the RA and required rapid surgical reintervention with no further consequence. Even in patients with manual professions, removal of the RA has been proven to be safe.

Another potential complication is damage to the superficial branch of the radial nerve. This was observed in 8 per cent of our cases and resulted in paraesthesia of the thumb that always resolved within 2 to 3 months.

Haematoma formation at the site of harvesting is a rare complication (five cases in our series). This can be prevented by careful haemostasis at the end of surgery following protamine administration. Meticulous suturing of subcutaneous tissue using absorbable sutures is mandatory. The superficial fascia is not closed, in order to prevent a compartment syndrome. During closure care should also be taken to avoid damage to the superficial branch of the radial nerve.

In case of severe renal insufficiency that may require chronic haemodialysis, it is preferable to preserve the use of the RA for an arteriovenous fistula. In patients with diabetes mellitus, the RA can occasionally be the site of medial calcinosis (non-obstructive calcification of the artery wall). In rare cases of severe multifocal atherosclerosis, atheromatous lesions of the RA may be observed in its distal third; however, the proximal portion of the vessel usually remains normal and can be used for bypass. Finally, focal fibrosis can be observed in patients undergoing reoperation who have had prior catheterization via the brachial artery.

The surgical technique of coronary bypass using the RA presents few particular problems. The distal anastomosis is performed in the usual manner using 7/0 or 8/0 prolene depending on the wall thickness and diameter of the target vessel. When cardioplegia is repeated, care should be taken to clamp the RA in order to avoid steal through the graft which contains no valves. Proximal anastomosis is performed directly on the ascending aorta using a side-biting clamp. When the target vessel is a proximal obtuse marginal, the RA graft is anastomosed to the posterior aspect of the aorta via the transverse sinus. In other cases, the anastomosis is constructed on the anterior aspect of the aorta. A 4-mm circular aperture is created in the aortic wall using a punch and the proximal RA anastomosis is performed using a 7/0 prolene. Rather than a sequential bypass with the RA, a Y graft may be preferred that provides a better route and avoids the risk of kinking.[16] In fact, the RA graft itself constitutes an excellent site for proximal anastomosis of other types of free arterial grafts.

Vasoreactive pharmacological responses

The RA is a muscular artery with important vasoreactive properties. In the clinical setting, we have observed that it is very sensitive to mechanical stimuli and reacts instantaneously by going into spasm. We have conducted studies using organ chamber techniques with various pharmacological agents (KCL, norepinephrine, serotonin and thromboxane A_2) and compared the RA to both the ITA and the right gastroepiploic arteries.[17] We were able to demonstrate that the sensitivity of the three vessels to different vasoconstricting agents was identical (defined as the concentration of the agent required to obtain 50 per cent of maximal contraction). However, the force of contraction of the RA was significantly superior to both the ITA and the right gastroepiploic artery. The propensity to spasm of the RA is probably explained by the high density of smooth muscle cells in its media.

Postoperative angiographic studies of RA coronary bypass grafts confirmed the spastic properties of this conduit. Not infrequently, spasm of the graft

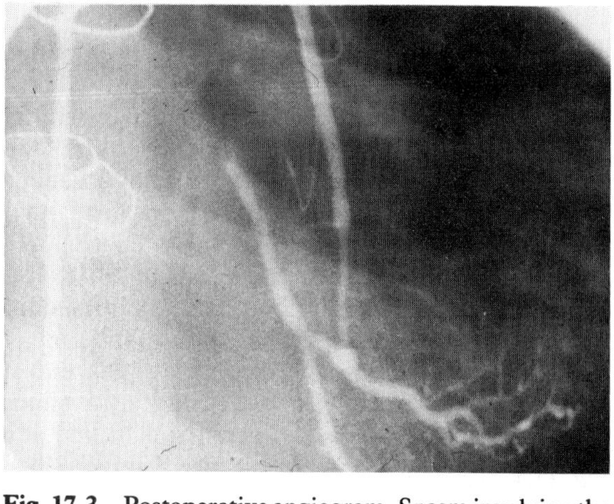

Fig. 17.3 Postoperative angiogram. Spasm involving the distal portion of a RA graft probably secondary to incomplete hydrostatic dilatation during the operation.

could be observed at the point of contact with the tip of the catheter, in particular, in case of selective injection. However, spasm of the RA could occasionally involve the distal part of the conduit (Fig. 17.3). This was probably due to incomplete resolution of the spasm induced during the operation by the harvesting process. *In situ* instillation of vasodilators (nitroglycerin) or a calcium channel blocker (nifedipine) does not always relieve this angiographic spasm. Although spontaneous regression of spasm is possible (Fig. 17.4), it can be responsible for haemodynamic disturbances leading to graft occlusion. It is therefore of utmost importance to dilate the RA carefully and completely (as described earlier) at the time of its removal. In addition, administration of a calcium channel blocker is indicated; we use diltiazem where the vasodilating properties have been well documented (this drug being available both orally and intravenously). Diltiazem is administered systemically following discontinuation of bypass (0.1 mg/kg/hour) and increased to 0.2 mg/kg/hour in the early postoperative period. As soon as possible, diltiazem is prescribed orally (250 mg/day) in conjunction with aspirin (100 mg/day).

(a)

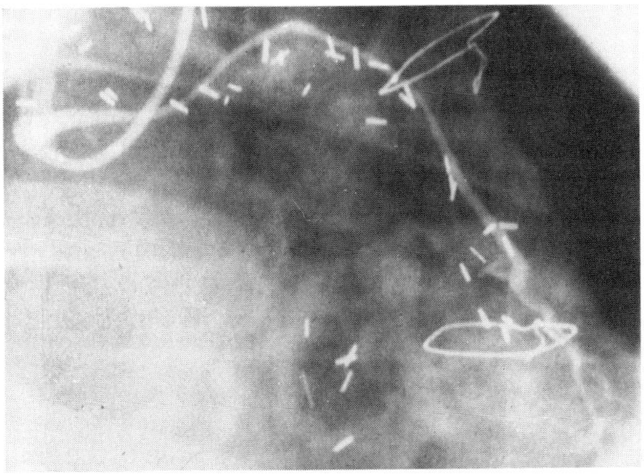

(b)

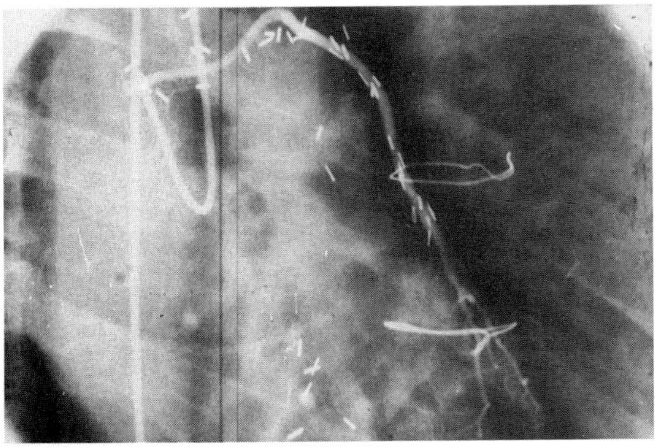

Fig. 17.4 RA graft to diagonal coronary artery: (a) postoperative angiogram showing extensive spasm; (b) one year later: total resolution of the spasm. Reproduced with permission from Acar *et al.*[5]

Clinical and angiographic results

Operative mortality (1.6 per cent) is comparable to that of any similar population of patients undergoing coronary bypass grafting. Similarly, the incidence of perioperative myocardial infarct (2.5 per cent) is not increased with the use of the RA graft. As mentioned above, morbidity associated with RA harvesting is negligible.

Seventy-five patients underwent early angiographic studies with 98 per cent patency of the RA graft (one occlusion). The incidence of RA spasm, defined as a narrowing of the graft unrelated to the anastomostic line, was 15 per cent. This spasm was responsible for a significant stenosis in four cases and could be relieved by *in situ* vasodilators in half of them.

Several studies have demonstrated that the patency of coronary grafts was directly proportional to the diameter and the site of the target vessel. As a rule, the RA was anastomosed to coronary arteries where the diameter was below 2 mm in the following order of frequency: the circumflex (half of the cases), the right coronary artery, the diagonal and rarely the left arterior descending.[18] Consequently, early patency rate of RA grafts (98 per cent) appears superior to that reported for venous grafts constructed to the circumflex or right coronary systems, when compared to a recent Spanish multicentre study.[18]

Fifty-six patients underwent angiographic studies at a mean follow-up of 1 year. Four patients were symptomatic for stable angina and fifty-two were totally asymptomatic. In these patients sixty-one RA grafts were studied and fifty-five were patent (90 per cent). All controlled grafts were angiographically normal but one had a stenosis at the anastomotic site. Interestingly two patients with RA spasm, observed at early postoperative angiography, had normal appearances. (Fig. 17.4(b)) Among the six non-functional grafts, four were totally occluded and two presented a string sign. Two of these grafts had been implanted on coronary arteries with a 50 per cent stenosis of the left main coronary. On the control study performed 14 months later the left main stenosis had substantially resolved and the RA presented a classical string sign probably due to competitive flow. Two patients with occluded RA grafts underwent successful coronary angioplasty.

At 1 year, the patency rate of RA grafts (90 per cent) is significantly superior to that of venous grafts anastomosed to the same target vessels (58 per cent), if one refers to a recent multicentre study from France.[19] Nevertheless, this result remains inferior to that obtained by *in situ* ITA to left anterior descending coronary artery.

Conclusions

At present, one may assert that the RA is an excellent conduit for coronary artery surgery. It offers satisfactory early clinical and angiographic results with minimal morbidity. The use of the RA to the circumflex or to the right coronary artery in conjunction with the pedicled ITA graft to the left anterior descending constitutes a highly efficient combination for total arterial revascularization. Although the early and mid term results are encouraging, further data are required to define the place of this conduit in coronary artery surgery.

References

1. Carpentier A, Guermonprez JL, Deloche A, Frechette C, Dubost C. The aorta-to-coronary radial bypass graft: a technique avoiding pathological changes in grafts. *Ann Thorac Surg* 1973; **16:** 111–21.
2. Carpentier A. Discussion of Geha AS, Krone RJ, McCormick JR, Baue AE. Selection of coronary bypass: anatomic, physiological and angiographic considerations of vein and mammary artery grafts. *J Thorac Cardiovasc Surg* 1975; **70:** 414–31.
3. Curtis JJ, Stoney WS, Alford WC, Burrus GR, Thomas CS. Intimal hyperplasia: a cause of radial artery aortocoronary bypass graft failure. *Ann Thorac Surg* 1975; **20:** 628–35.
4. Fisk RL, Brooks CH, Callaghan JC, Dvorkin J. Experience with the radial artery graft for coronary bypass. *Ann Thorac Surg* 1976; **21:** 513–18.
5. Acar C, Jebara V, Porthogese M *et al.* Revival of the radial artery for coronary bypass grafting. *Ann Thorac Surg* 1992; **54:** 652–60.
6. Calafiore AM, Di Giammarco G, Teodori G, Angelini R. Radial artery for myocardial revascularization. *Eur Heart J* 1994; **95:** 29.
7. Reyes AT, Frame R, Brodman RF. A technique for harvesting the radial artery as a coronary artery bypass graft. *Ann Thorac Surg* (in press).
8. Van Son JA, Smedts F, Vincent JG, Van Lier HJ, Kubat K. Comparative anatomic studies of various arterial conduits for myocardial revascularization. *J Thorac Cardiovasc Surg* 1990; **99:** 703–7.
9. Acar C, Jebara V, Porthogese M *et al.* Comparative anatomy and histology of the radial artery and the internal thoracic artery: implication for coronary bypass. *Surg Radiol Anat* 1991; **13:** 283–8.
10. Echave V, Koornick AR, Haimovici M, Jacobson JH. Intimal hyperplasia as a complication of the use of polytetrafluorethylene graft for femoral-popliteal bypass. *Surgery* 1979; **86:** 791–9.
11. Dardick H, Baier RE, Weinberg S *et al.* Morphologic and biophysical assessment of long term human umbilical cord vein implants used as vascular conduits. *Surg Gynecol Obstet* 1982; **154:** 17–21.
12. Grondin CM, Meere C, Castonguay Y, Lepage G, Grondin P. Progressive and late obstruction of an aorta-coronary venous bypass graft. *Circulation* 1971; **43:** 698–705.
13. Acar C, Bruneval P. Reply to Van Son JA, Smedts F: Revival of the radial artery for coronary artery bypass grafting: l'histoire se répète. *Ann Thorac Surg* 1993; **55:** 1596–8.
14. Hoeber PB. Vessels and nerves of the flexor forearm. In: Hoeber PB. *Anatomy for surgeons: the back and limbs.* Harper & Brothers 1958: 413–19.
15. Kaminski RW, Barnes RW. Critique of the Allen test for continuity of the palmar arch assessed by Doppler ultrasound. *Surg Gynecol Obstet* 1976; **142:** 861–4.
16. Acar C, Farge A, Chardigny C *et al.* Utilisation de l'artère radiale pour les pontages coronaires. Nouvelle expérience 20 ans après. *Arch Malad Coeur* 1993; **86:** 1683–9.
17. Chardigny C, Jebara V, Acar C *et al.* Vasoreactivity of the radial artery. Comparison with the internal mammary and gastroepiploic arteries with implications for coronary artery surgery. *Circulation* 1993; **88** (Suppl. II): II115–27.
18. Paz MA, Lupon J, Bosch X, Pomar JL, Sanz G. Predictors of early saphenous vein aortocoronary bypass graft occlusion. *Ann Thorac Surg* 1993; **56:** 1101–6.
19. Ollivier JP. Etude de la perméabilité des pontages aortocoronaires à 6 mois. Etude multicentrique française. *Arch Malad Coeur* 1991; **84:** 537–42.

18 Use of the subscapular artery for coronary artery bypass

Noel L. Mills, John R. Breaux and Cody L. Leger

The atherosclerotic changes which are progressive in coronary saphenous bypass grafts have resulted in a continuous yearly increase in reoperations for coronary artery disease. Surgeons are faced with problems of obtaining adequate quantity and quality of conduit for use in these reoperations. Once the usual sources of reliable conduit have been exhausted, alternative conduits must be sought. Problems in obtaining conduit coupled with a significant probability of damage to existing functioning grafts at the time of a double, triple or quadruple reoperation have prompted use of the left thoracotomy to bypass certain lesions accessible through that approach. It was this search for adequate conduits using the left thoracotomy approach that led us to consider the subscapular artery as an alternative conduit for coronary bypass.

Latissimus dorsi muscle flaps have been used by our plastic surgeon colleagues for a number of years as composite grafts. The arterial and venous blood supply is re-established with the use of these grafts. The size and length of the subscapular artery was noted to be adequate for its use as a coronary bypass conduit.

Anatomical notes

The subscapular artery arises inferiorly from the third part of the axillary artery. After giving off a circumflex scapular arterial branch the name changes to the dorsal thoracic artery, even though it is essentially a continuation of the same vessel. The subscapular artery is the largest branch of the axillary artery and it has *vena comitantes* which parallel it as it courses inferiorly and medially along the anterior border of the subscapularis muscle and under the latissimus dorsi muscle. The circumflex scapular artery is of variable size and length, being less consistent than the subscapular artery itself (Fig. 18.1).

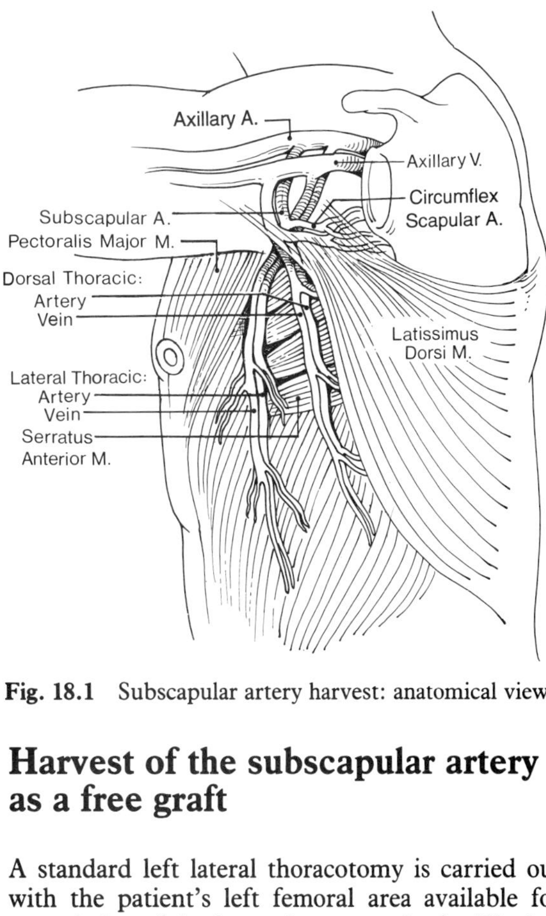

Fig. 18.1 Subscapular artery harvest: anatomical view.

Harvest of the subscapular artery as a free graft

A standard left lateral thoracotomy is carried out with the patient's left femoral area available for cannulation of the femoral artery and vein. The left thoracic cavity is entered by way of the bed of the fifth rib. Prior to the thorax being opened, the latissimus dorsi muscle is identified. Arterial branches with their vena comitantes supplying the latissimus dorsi muscle are identified and traced retrogradely to identify the dorsal thoracic artery as it lies under the cover of the latissimus dorsi muscle. In our early experience we performed an inverted 'T' extension in the mid portion of the lateral thoracotomy incision. We performed the incision from the mid axillary line up to the base of the axillary fascia. In the last three cases, this inverted 'T' incision has not been found necessary as the dorsal thoracic and subscapular artery may be harvested to the axillary artery using a narrow Deaver retractor. Branches of the dorsal thoracic artery are identified and ligated along with the veins with 4–0 silk sutures. The dissection progresses superiorly until the circumflex scapular artery is identified. As much length as possible is taken of the circumflex scapular artery if there is a possibility of it being used as a 'Y' graft from the parent subscapular artery. The subscapular artery is ligated at its origin and divided proximally and distally. It is then dilated with an intraluminal solution of papaverine hydrochloride in normal saline (60 mg in 40 ml of normal saline). Haemostasis is checked and any bleeding points are ligated with 4–0 silk. The lengths of the subscapular arteries harvested range from 12 to 14 cm. The proximal internal diameters range from 3.25 mm to 4.5 mm. Distal internal diameters are invariably 2 mm. After completing the operation a fenestrated suction drain is used to prevent haematoma formation in the space left by harvest of the subscapular artery. The muscles of the chest wall are closed anatomically. The subscapularis is not divided.

Clinical material

We have attempted to use the subscapular artery as a coronary bypass graft in six patients. In one patient, the artery was found to be too small to consider use as a bypass graft as the distal dorsal thoracic artery was less than 1.5 mm internal diameter. The subscapular artery in that patient nearest to its origin was only 2 mm internal diameter. Five patients have had successful revascularization using the subscapular artery. (Table 18.1) Ages ranged from 53 to 66. All patients were male. One patient was undergoing his first reoperation, two patients a second reoperation, one a third reoperation and a final patient was undergoing his 4th reoperation.

In three patients the proximal subscapular artery was directly anastomosed to the descending aorta below the subclavian artery and brought anterior to the hilum of the lung to bypass branches of the circumflex system. (Fig. 18.2(a)) Two patients had atherosclerosis of the descending aorta. In one, the subscapular artery graft was anastomosed to a pericardial patch on the aorta and in the other it was anastomosed to the origin of a new lesser saphenous vein graft. One patient had a large natural Y bifurcation which was used as an inverted 'Y' graft. A second patient had division of the distal subscapular conduit and that was anastomosed to the parent graft to fashion an artificial 'Y' graft (Fig. 18.2(b)). The remainder of the patients had single anastomoses to circumflex marginal branches making a total of seven distal anastomoses using five subscapular arterial conduits. All distal anastomoses used

Table 18.1 Use of subscapular artery as a coronary artery bypass

Case	*Sex*	*Age*	*Indication*	*Follow-up*	*Comment*
1	M	64	Reop. × 4; no available conduit	4 years 2 months	Patent early restudy
2	M	63	Reop. × 2; poor quality SVG	3 years	Refused restudy
3	M	53	Reop. × 2; no available conduit	3 years	Patent late restudy; negative Thallium stress
4	M	57	Reop.; no graft	2 years	Patent late restudy; marked improvement of angina
5	M	66	Reop. × 3; failed PTCA; stents	21 months	Descending aortic athersclerosis

8–0 Prolene (Ethicon Inc., Summerville, New Jersey, USA) and the proximal anastomoses were performed with 6–0 Prolene. Loupe magnification (3.5 power) was used in all cases.

All patients survived the operation with basically uneventful postoperative courses. Follow-up has been from 21 months to 4 years. One patient with incomplete revascularization has occasional postoperative angina that is markedly improved over his preoperative clinical state. Early angiography was performed at 1 week postoperatively in one patient with a natural 'Y' subscapular free arterial graft. A widely patent graft was found to both target vessels.

Conclusion

The subscapular artery was studied in fifty fresh cadavers (mean age 66 years) and 8 per cent were found to have significant atherosclerosis. Occlusive atherosclerosis was found in 0 per cent.[1] A separate origin of the circumflex scapular artery occurs from the axillary artery in approximately 4 per cent of the population. The dorsal thoracic artery bifurcates in its lower portion in approximately 86 per cent of patients which allowed its use in one of our patients as a natural 'Y' graft. This artery offers an alternative arterial conduit when the left thoracic approach is utilized for coronary bypass reoperation. With multiple operations, scarring and adhesions can make a second to fourth reoperation particularly hazardous. Angiography of functioning left internal mammary grafts often reveals that the conduit is intimately stuck to the mid portion of the undersurface of the sternum. Damage to such a functioning internal thoracic artery graft can have catastrophic results and can be conveniently avoided by using a left thoracotomy with cannulation of the left femoral

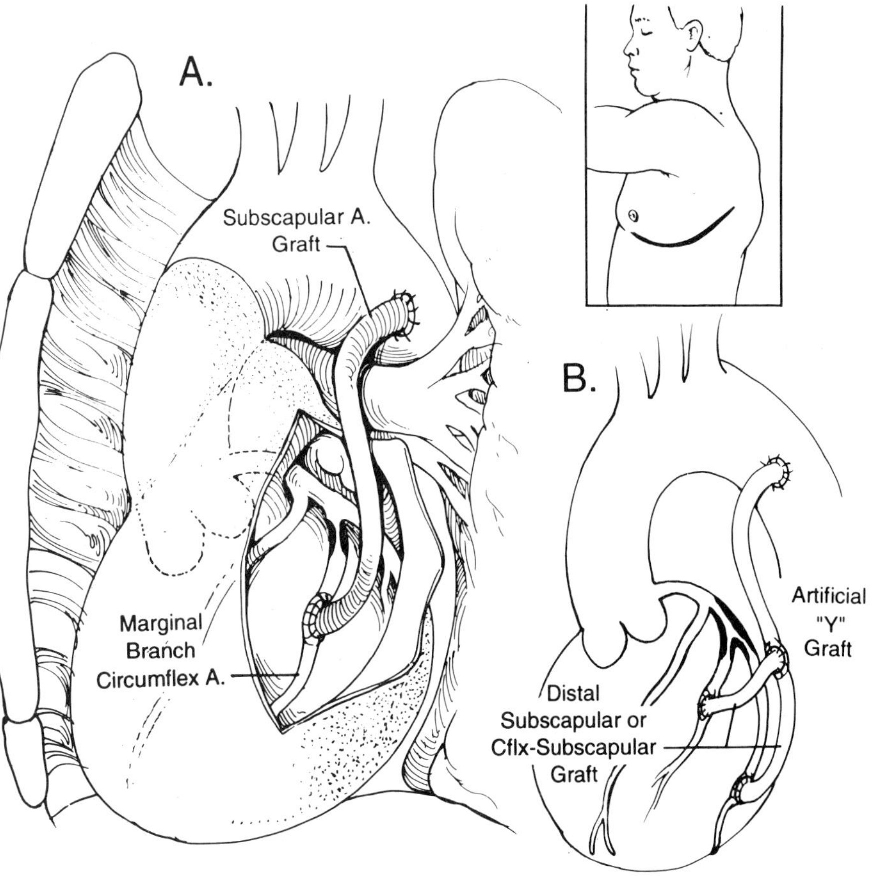

Fig. 18.2 Course of Subscapular artery used as a graft between descending aorta and the coronary circumflex system (a) as a single graft; (b) here, an artificial 'Y' graft has been anastomosed.

artery or descending thoracic aorta and the left common femoral vein.

Mathes and Nahal,[2] have classified the vascular anatomy of muscles and noted that the latissimus dorsi muscle may be classified as the Type V defined as 'one dominant vascular pedicle with secondary segmental vascular pedicles'. In our experience this graft has been utilized to branches of the left coronary system which include the ramus marginalis, the first and second marginal and also to an old functioning distal vein graft.[3] Although atherosclerosis has been reported as mentioned in the subscapular artery, we have not noted any disease in the conduits in these patients. We have not used preoperative angiography to assess this vessel. If a left thoracotomy was being performed with the subscapular as the *only* conduit available with no other choice, then a preoperative angiogram would be wise as one of six of our patients was found to have a subscapular artery that was too small to use as a bypass graft. We have used low flow or circulatory arrest with hypothermia to perform this operation. Although we have been prepared to cannulate the left atrial appendage in lieu of cardiac distention during ventricular fibrillation, we have not had to use any cardiac decompression in this group of patients. External patches which are placed on the chest preoperatively are used to defibrillate the heart. The proximal anastomoses have been performed to the descending aorta from within a partially occluding clamp while rewarming. Drainage of the underlying dead space from the subscapular arterial bed is strongly advised in order to avoid a haematoma or wound problems.

In three of our five patients diltiazem has been administered postoperatively in view of the experience from France which has shown the importance of this drug with free radial artery conduits.[4] This operation is more time consuming and tedious than routine coronary artery bypass yet offers the opportunity for an additional conduit when a left thoracotomy approach is used to revascularize the ramus marginalis or branches of the circumflex coronary artery system. Exposure is adequate for bypass to the diagonal branches of the left anterior descending coronary artery. The long-term results with use of this graft are uncertain at this time. However, our initial experience has been very rewarding as four of five patients have returned to an asymptomatic cardiac state and long-term follow-up has been up to 4 years and 2 months at the time of this report.

References

1. Bartlett SP. The latissimus dorsi muscle: a fresh cadaver study of the primary neurovascular pedicle. *Plast Reconstr Surg* 1981; **67:** 631–6.
2. Mathes SJ, Nahal F. Classification of the vascular anatomy of muscles: Experimental and clinical correlation. *Plast Reconstr Surg* 1981; **67:** 177.
3. Mills NL, Dupin CL, Everson CT, Leger CL. The subscapular artery: An alternative conduit for coronary bypass. *J Card Surg* 1993; **8:** 66–71.
4. Acar C, Jebara VA, Portoghese M *et al*: The radial artery for coronary bypass operations: Revival of an old conduit. *Ann Thorac Surg* 1992; **54:** 652–9.

Part VI
Postoperative management and reoperation

19 Postoperative management

Luc Jacquet, Martin Goenen, Philippe Baele and Robert Dion

The general postoperative care of patients having undergone myocardial revascularization with the use of arterial conduits is not different from the usual care of patients after adult cardiac surgery.[1–3] We will focus here on some aspects that are specifically influenced by the use of arterial conduits.

Ischaemia

Postoperative myocardial ischaemia is an important predictor of adverse cardiac outcome due to its association with low output syndrome, myocardial infarction and even death of the patients.[4,5] However, diagnosis and management of ischaemia remains difficult and necessitates close co-operation between the surgeon and the intensive care staff.

Diagnosis

Electrocardiographic changes

These remain the most widely used indicator of postoperative ischaemia. New ST depression or elevation at the J point are usually considered to suggest oxygen deficit in a myocardial area.[6] However, non-specific ST-segment changes may occur after cardiac surgery, related to changes in electrolyte concentrations, ventilation or pericardial inflammation. Moreover, the association of ST-segment changes and ischaemia during right bundle branch block which is frequent after surgery or during supraventricular arrhythmia is not well characterized.[7]

Transoesophageal echocardiography (TOE)

TOE can be used to detect regional wall motion abnormalities that are an earlier and more sensitive indicator of ischaemia than the ECG.[8–10] This method is useful only if a preoperative comparison is available especially in patients with previous myocardial infarction. Moreover, changes in the loading conditions or in the inotropic support can modify the degree of regional dysfunction and mask ongoing ischaemia.[11,12] Although it has been claimed that routine intraoperative TOE monitoring can improve outcome of patients undergoing myocardial revascularization,[13] its postoperative use, while clearly of value in certain circumstances, is not of proven value for routine monitoring, and the practicalities of implementing such a strategy mean that it cannot currently be recommended.

Other

With severe ischaemia, haemodynamic changes (increased pulmonary capillary wedge pressure, low cardiac output, decreased blood pressure) are expected, but only later after the onset of ischaemia.[14]

Serum enzyme levels will increase only when myocardial damage has taken place. Coronary sinus dosages of lactate and hypoxanthine may help in the diagnosis of ischaemia but are not routinely performed.[15]

Management

Several factors can contribute to postoperative myocardial ischaemia:

- intra-operative factors
  - inadequate protection
  - incomplete revascularization
  - reperfusion injury
- inadequate flow through ITA
- native coronary artery spasm
- increased 0_2 demand.

Therapeutic interventions will be adapted according to the underlying mechanism of ischaemia.

Intraoperative factors

These include inadequate myocardial protection, incomplete revascularization resulting from technical difficulties and reperfusion injury.

The extensive use of pedicled arterial grafts may interfere with myocardial protection, particulary in evolving ischaemia due to the acute occlusion of a coronary vessel, and in a reoperation when an old pedicled arterial graft on a significant coronary vessel has remained patent. The retrograde delivery of cardioplegia through the coronary sinus (and clamping the old patent arterial graft at reoperation) is then needed to achieve a homogenous myocardial protection, as recommended by Lytle.[16]

Incomplete revascularization should never be tolerated and if technical difficulties preclude complete revascularization of a myocardial area with arterial grafts alone, one should not hesitate to add saphenous vein grafts.

Antegrade controlled reperfusion,[17] also becomes impossible after the use of pedicled arterial grafts; here again retrograde delivery of the reperfusion solution before unclamping of these grafts and of the aorta is advocated.

Inadequate flow through arterial grafts

Flemma[18] showed, as early as 1975 that, initially, flow through the ITA is lower than through saphenous vein grafts; flow can even decrease in some haemodynamic conditions or if spasm occurs in the ITA.[19]

ITA spasm has been occasionally described in the postoperative period.[20] Spasm of the GEA is more frequent and is partly due to the greater amount of muscle in the media and partly to a different reaction of its endothelium to mechanical and pharmacological stimuli.[21–23] Spasm also occurs frequently in the inferior epigastric artery[24] and in the radial artery.[25]

Arterial graft spasm is very difficult to diagnose without performing angiography, which is, in its turn, usually not allowed by the patient's condition at the time when problems occur. Spasm must be suspected when acute ischaemia of the corresponding myocardial area occurs without apparent reason, after a period of haemodynamic and electrocardiographic stability.[19,26]

The mechanisms involved in the pathogenesis of vascular spasm include local manipulation of the artery, decreased body temperature, increased release of vasoconstrictive substances by the platelets, increased blood pH, histamine release and impaired release of endothelium-derived relaxing factor.[27] Prophylaxis usually includes wrapping the ITA and other arterial grafts in a papaverine-soaked swab before grafting,[28,29] or topical use of other vasodilators,[30] as well as infusion of vasodilators into the graft.[24,31] Treatment usually consists of topical and intravascular application of vasodilators[29,32] and of systemic administration of nitrates and/or calcium-channel blockers.[20,29,32,33] If no response is observed, additional saphenous vein grafting of the coronary vessel already revascularized with the arterial graft is the treatment of choice.[20,26,28] Even if no spasm occurs, flow can be insufficient to meet metabolic requirements in some circumstances.[19]

Experimental studies have shown a dramatic decrease in ITA flow in association with sudden hypovolaemia and administration of high doses of nitrates. After induced hypovolaemia, administration of epinephrine even decreased the ITA flow.[34] However, under normovolaemic conditions, blood flow clearly paralleled changes in systolic blood pressure and no deleterious effect of systemic vasoconstricting agents was observed (epinephrine, metaraminol, phenylephrine).[34,35]

From these studies, it is clear that restoring normovolaemia and maintaining an adequate driving pressure is of prime importance in maintaining satisfactory ITA flow. We have observed the disappearance of ST-segment changes following the administration of α-adrenergic substances (norepinephrine), their effect on systemic blood pressure being probably more important than the direct vasoconstrictive action on the ITA (Fig. 19.1). In other cases, insertion of an intra-aortic balloon results in a dramatic improvement of the ECG changes: flow may be enhanced both in the native coronary arteries as well as in the arterial grafts. Flow enhancement is mediated by an increase in cardiac output, a raised diastolic pressure (Fig. 19.2) and decreased coronary resistance due to the reduction in myocardial wall stress.

If an intra-aortic balloon is needed, correct positioning of the tip of the balloon is more important than ever, since placement at the level of the left subclavian artery could reduce ITA flow.[36] Once again, if ischaemia persists or the haemodynamic situation deteriorates, adding a saphenous vein graft in parallel to an arterial graft may be necessary.[26,29]

Native coronary artery spasm

Spasm can also occur in the native coronary arteries and, rarely, in saphenous vein grafts.[32,37–39] Segmental ST-segment elevation and absence of atherosclerotic lesions, in previous or subsequent

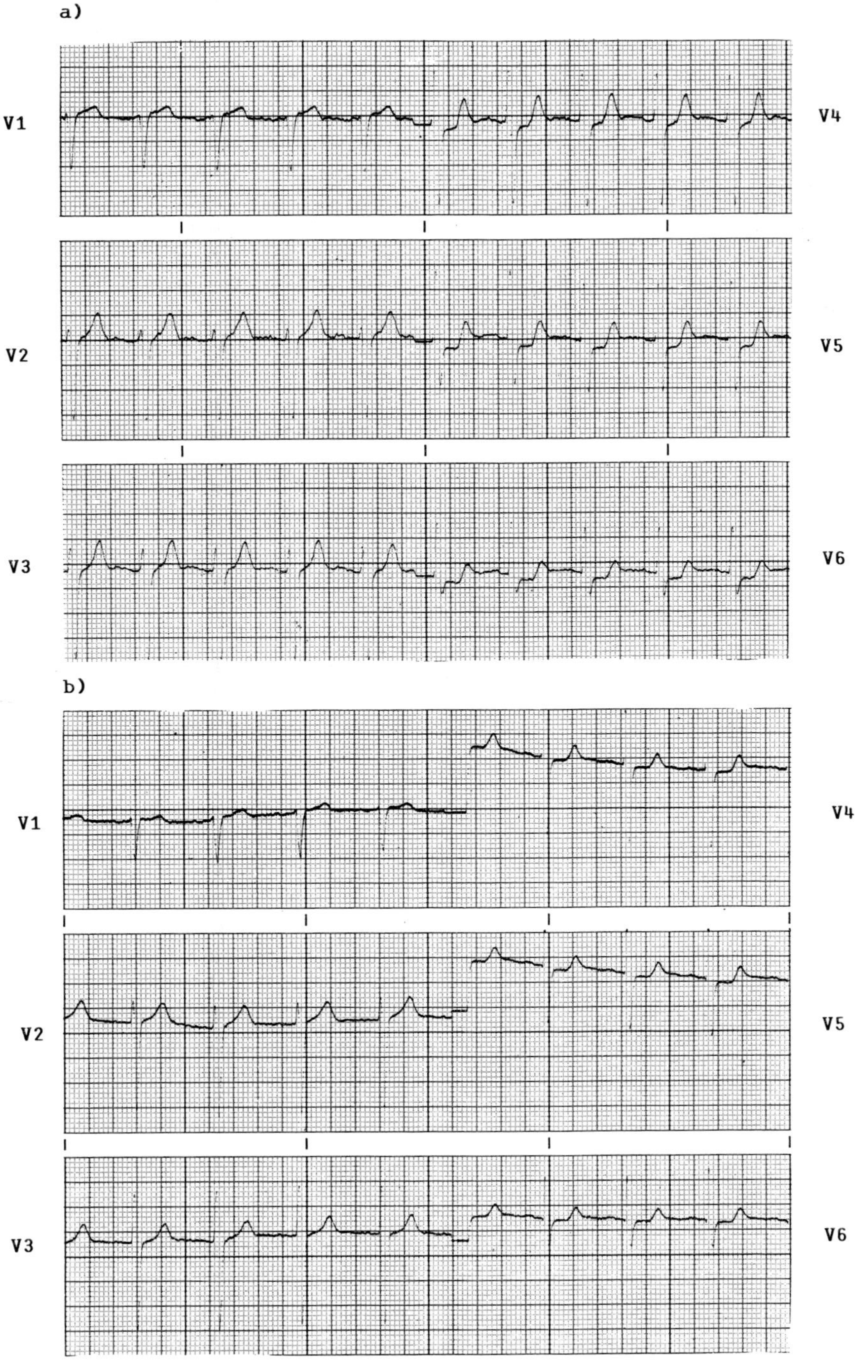

Fig. 19.1 (a) ST segment depression (2 mm) in leads V4, V5, V6 at arrival in ICU; heart rate 98/min; blood pressure 85/50 mmHg; (b) 30 minutes later with norepinephrine infusion (0.1 μ/kg/min), ST segment almost normal; heart rate 88/min; blood pressure 110/65 mmHg.

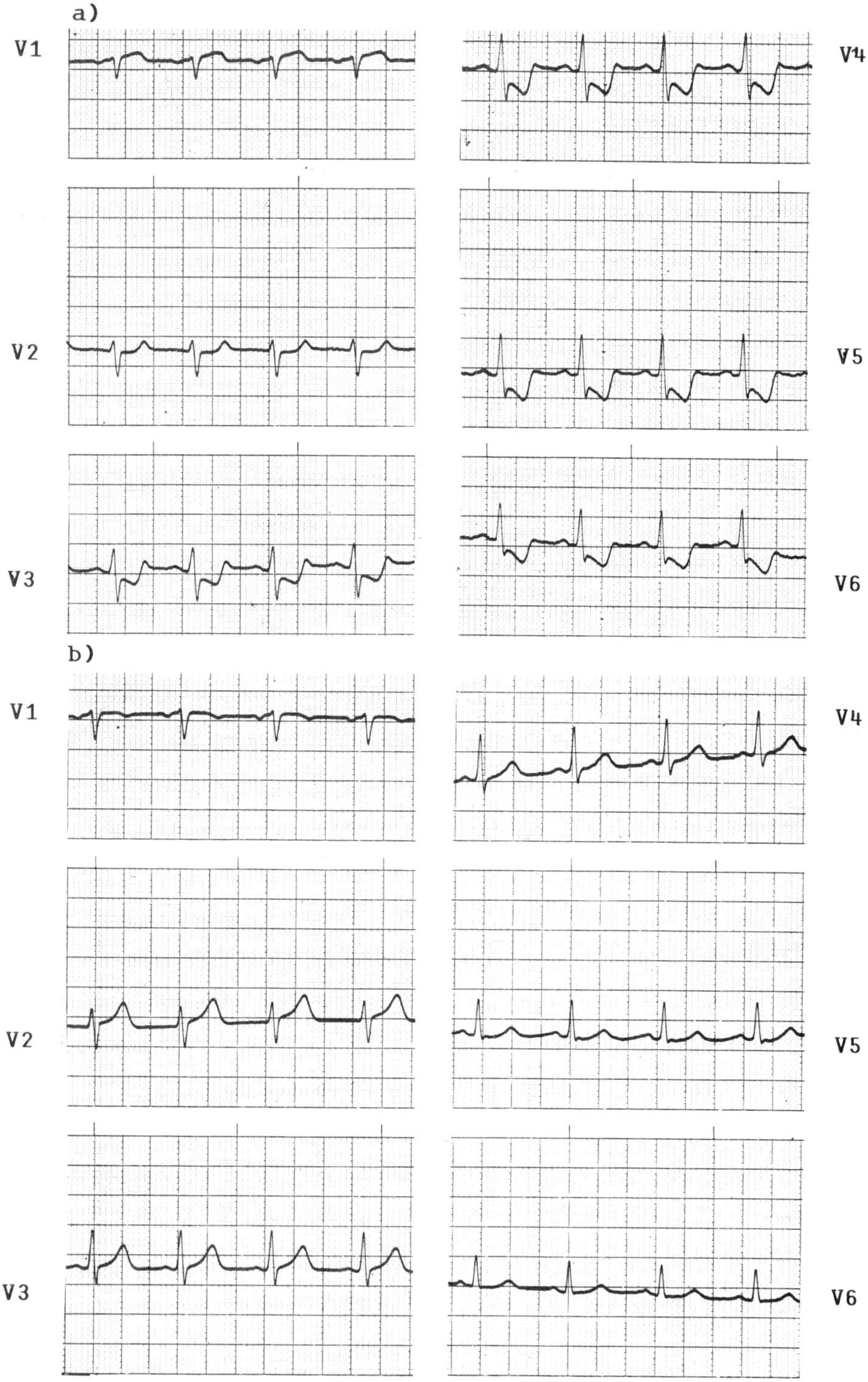

Fig. 19.2 (a) Profound ST segment depression (> 3 mm) from V3 to V6 on intravenous nitroglycerine; heart rate 108/min; blood pressure 100/70 mmHg; (b) 10 minutes after insertion of an intra-aortic balloon, normalization of the ECG.

cineangiograms, beyond the site of anastomoses is suggestive of native coronary spasm.[37] Occasionally this phenomenon has been documented angiographically and has led to perioperative haemodynamic collapse.[39,40] Treatment includes intravenous and, in some refractory cases, direct intracoronary infusion of vasodilators.[32,33] In most cases, native coronary artery spasm cannot be differentiated from graft spasm and identical management is therefore advocated.

Increased oxygen demand

Ischaemia results from imbalance between myocardial oxygen supply and demand. If supply is transiently inadequate as can be the case early after ITA and other arterial grafting,[18] increased demand can cause ischaemia and ECG abnormalities. This is especially true when patients awaken after surgery and are exposed to stress and pain.[41] Mangano *et al.* have demonstrated that prolonged intensive analgesia could significantly decrease ischaemic episodes.[42] In our experience, administration of beta-blockers has been found useful for decreasing catecholamine-induced increases in myocardial oxygen demand (Fig. 19.3).

Respiratory problems

Alterations in pulmonary function have been documented after coronary surgery[43] and more so after the use of ITA graft.[41,44] The causes can be divided into parenchymal or mechanical failure.

Parenchymal failure

Several factors can cause lung damage during cardiac surgery independent of whether arterial conduits have been used for revascularization:[45–48]

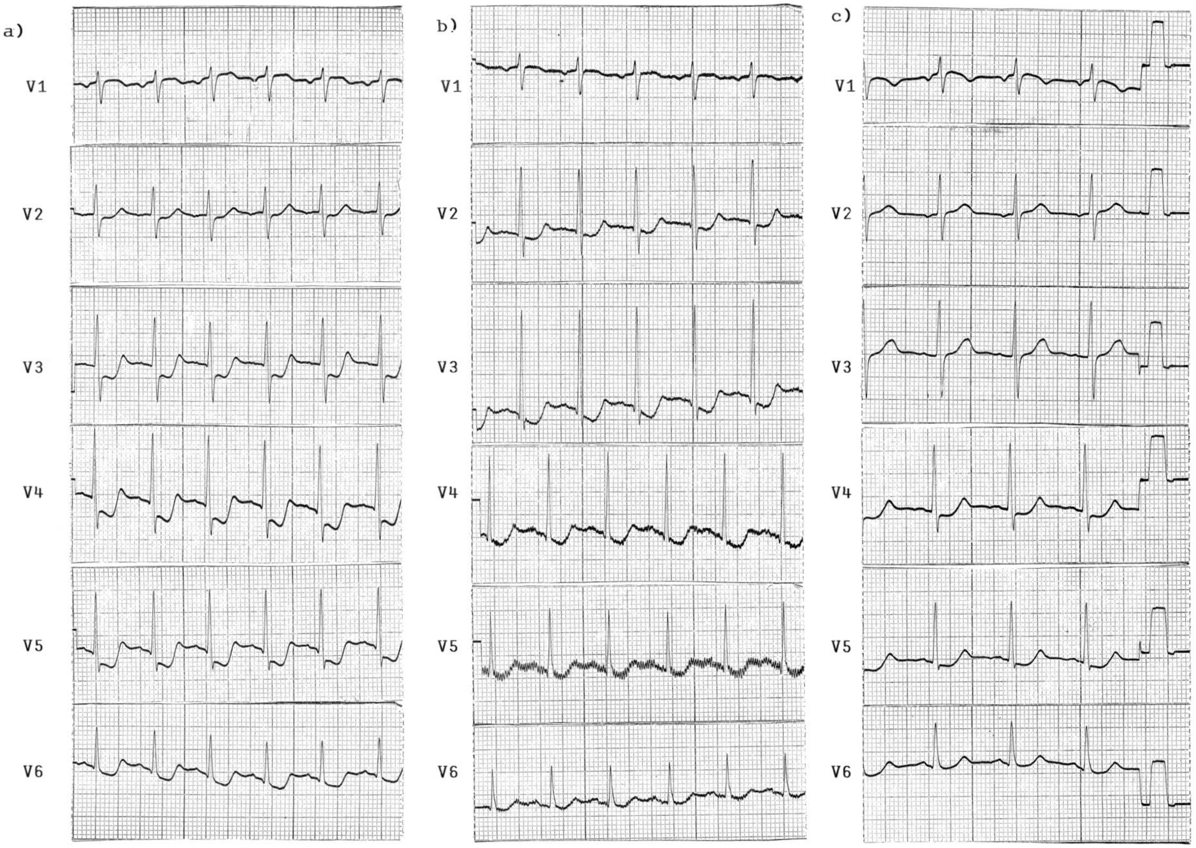

Fig. 19.3 (a) At arrival from the OR, ST segment depression in leads V2 through V6; heart rate 118/min; blood pressure 140/80 mmHg; (b) after 2 mg propranolol iv, heart rate 110/min; blood pressure 120/70 mmHg; (c) after 4 mg propranolol iv, heart rate 90/min; blood pressure 110/65 mmHg.

- trauma to the lung or airways
- pulmonary venous distension
  - vent malfunction
  - left ventricular dysfunction
- loss of surfactant
- hypoxic damage to the lung
- inflammatory reaction to CPB
  - pulmonary microemboli
  - complement activation
  - inflammatory reaction

A correlation also exists between duration of CPB and the degree of lung injury. The extensive use of arterial grafts is usually associated with longer CPB time and may increase the risk of lung damage.

Mechanical failure

These alterations are found more frequently after harvesting of one or both ITAs. They are mostly related to lobar atelectasis, phrenic nerve injury or sternal dehiscence.

Atelectasis

Atelectasis is the most common pulmonary mechanical complication following cardiac surgery. Several factors predispose to this complication:

- preoperative factors
  - chronic pulmonary disease
  - obesity
  - pulmonary oedema
- intraoperative factors
  - passive ventilation (diaphragm paralysed)
  - heart weight on immobile and deflated lower lobe
  - bronchial suctioning leading to mucosal damage
  - open pleural cavity
  - phrenic nerve injury.

Harvesting of the ITA is frequently accompanied by pleural opening. Blood and fluid can compress the adjacent left lower lobe, and pain related to the presence of chest drainage tubes can induce hypoventilation.[49–51] The most effective means of reversing atelectasis is to provide ventilation with positive end-expiratory pressure (PEEP).[52] Care must be taken to avoid excessive distension of the lung that could displace or stretch the ITA graft.

Phrenic nerve paresis

Phrenic nerve injury and subsequent diaphragmatic paresis is reported with an incidence of 10–73 per cent depending on specific surgical procedure and methods of detection.[53,54] Such injuries are associated with atelectasis, pneumonia, pleural effusion and, if bilateral, prolonged mechanical ventilation and hospital stay.[55] Iced slush used as an adjunctive myocardial cooling measure is implicated in phrenic nerve injury.[54] Using a cardiac insulating pad could decrease the incidence of this potentially serious complication.[56] ITA grafting seems to be associated with a higher incidence of phrenic neuropathy that is probably associated with the technique of harvesting.[57] Division of the small proximal pericardiophrenic artery can lead to ischaemia of the phrenic nerve.[58]

Sternal dehiscence

This complication does not affect early pulmonary function and weaning from the ventilator but can, significantly decrease vital capacity after a few days.[51] Once sternal consolidation is achieved, ventilatory parameters return to more normal values. Studies in animals and humans using tomographic scanning or microsphere injections have demonstrated that blood is supplied to the sternum almost exclusively by branches of the ITA.[59] Harvesting one ITA should decrease blood supply to the ipsilateral hemisternum by 90 per cent.[60] The level of ischaemia is influenced by several factors including the technique of harvesting and position of the sternal wires.[61,62]

However, ischaemia is only transient and other factors like diabetes, obesity, advanced age, chronic obstructive pulmonary disease, the need for early resternotomy, end-stage renal failure requiring chronic dialysis and multiorgan failure, contribute to the development of sternal dehiscence and sternal infections. In our institution, the incidence of sternal complications (2.5 per cent) in bilateral ITA grafting is increased three-fold in the presence of insulin-dependent diabetes and six-fold in patients under chronic renal replacement therapy. Some studies suggest that the combination of diabetes and double ITA grafts increases almost fifteen-fold the risk of infection.[63] We believe that any degree of sternal dehiscence after bilateral ITA grafting should be treated aggressively in order to prevent a secondary infection.

Postoperative bleeding

Bilateral ITA grafting has been reported to generate a greater incidence of excessive bleeding (up to 6 per cent) when compared to saphenous vein graft surgery and even to single ITA grafting.[29,64,65] However, technical experience[64,66] and the use of drugs such as epsilon-aminocaproic acid, tranexamic acid or aprotinin[67] may minimize this risk. In our institution, the transfusion requirements (allogeneic blood products) have decreased ten-fold over the last 8 years (Fig 19.4): the median number of exposures decreased from 10 units to 1 unit for the whole hospital stay. These results were achieved thanks to improved and more expeditious surgical technique, intraoperative blood salvage, active intraoperative haemodilution, acceptance of lower haematocrits (21 per cent) on bypass, a shorter extracorporeal circuit, low prime oxygenators,

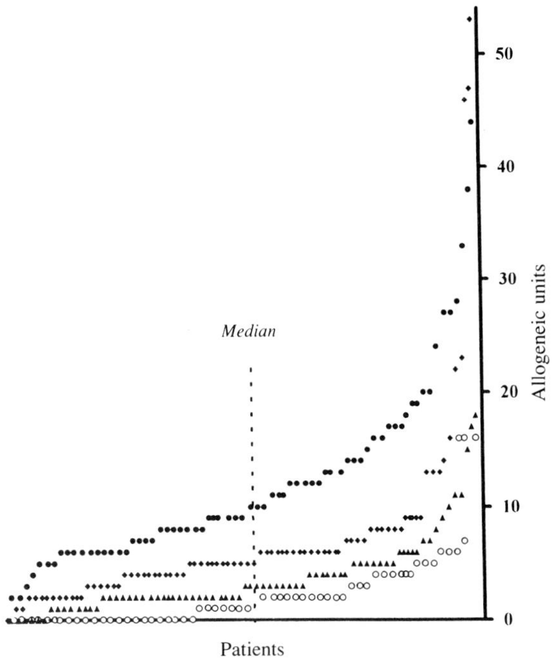

Fig. 19.4 Elective coronary artery bypass grafts: allogeneic exposure. Four series of consecutive patients undergoing coronary artery bypass grafts, spanning an 8-year evolution marked by efforts toward blood conservation. In 1986, sixty-nine patients (●) were operated on during the 2 months prior to the start of a blood conservation programme based on intraoperative blood retrieval; eighty-two patients were operated upon in the two following months (◆). Seventy-five patients were randomized for the Sanguis study[68] in 1990 (▲) and (○) represents our current practice patients in 1994 (n = 60). For each series, one symbol stands for one patient and patients are aligned from left to right according to their increasing exposure to allogeneic blood products (whole blood, red cells, plasma or platelets) expressed in number of donors.

tranexamic acid or aprotinin (1994) and accepting lower haematocrit values in the immediate postoperative period (28 vs 30 per cent) and at discharge (33 vs 36 per cent). These results were obtained despite the fact that, from 1986 to 1994, the mean age of elective CABG patients increased by 7 years, and that the number of arterial grafts rose over the years: 2.2–3.0 distal anastomoses per patient.

Preoperative autologous blood deposit involved only a minority (15 per cent) of elective cases because of the high incidence of concomitant contraindications to predeposit: cerebrovascular disease, aortic valve stenosis, left main stenosis or angina at low levels of exercise (75 watts or less). Postoperative reinfusion of mediastinal blood drainage has not been used in our centre. Normothermic systemic perfusion also seems to decrease the postoperative blood loss.[69]

Peripheral nerve injury

Brachial plexus injury is a relatively common complication of cardiac operation performed with a median sternotomy and is more frequent with ITA harvesting.[70,71] Excessive sternal spreading rotates the first rib upwards thereby stretching the brachial plexus, or can cause fracture of the first rib, leading to nerve compression.[71] ITA harvesting requires both wide and asymmetric sternal spreading. If the surgeon remains aware of this potential complication by accepting some discomfort during harvesting, the incidence should be maintained around 1 per cent.[72]

Miscellaneous

Patients undergoing revascularization using the gastroepiploic artery are expected to have gastroparesis for 2–3 days that necessitates keeping a nasogastric tube in the stomach to avoid gastric distension. No case of postoperative pancreatitis has been reported. In our experience of more than 300 patients, an asymptomatic elevation of lipase enzymes has been noted in a few cases. No gastric bleeding or ulceration has been encountered, confirming the experience of Suma *et al.*.[73] The harvesting of both IEAs may result in significant ischaemia of the abdominal wall and Barner has reported one case of necrosis of the abdominal wall after bilateral ITA and IEA grafting.[74]

References

1. Kaplan JA ed. *Cardiac anesthesia*, 3 edn. Philadelphia: WB Saunders Company, 1993.
2. Moreno-Cabral C, Mitchell RS, Miller DC. *Manual of postoperative management in adult cardiac surgery*. Baltimore: Williams and Wilkins, 1988.
3. Tarhan S ed. *Anesthesia and coronary artery surgery*. Chicago: Year Book Medical Publisher, 1986.
4. Leung J, O' Kelly B, Browner W. *et al*. Prognostic importance of postbypass regional wall-motion abnormalities in patients undergoing coronary artery bypass graft surgery. *Anesthesiology* 1989; **71**: 16–25.
5. Slogoff S, Keats AS. Further observations on perioperative myocardial ischemia. *Anesthesiology* 1986; **65**: 539–42.
6. Smith RC, Leung JM, Mangano DT S.P.I. Research Group: Postoperative myocardial ischemia in patients undergoing coronary artery bypass graft surgery. *Anesthesiology* 1991; **74**: 464–73.
7. Marriott HJL. *Coronary insufficiency and related matters. Practical electrocardiography*, 8th edn. Baltimore: Williams and Wilkins, 1988: 451–77.
8. Smith JS, Cahalan MK, Benefiel DJ *et al*. Intraoperative detection of myocardial ischemia in high-risk patients: Electrocardiography versus two-dimensional transesophageal echocardiography. *Circulation* 1985; **72**: 1015–21.
9. Kerber RE, Marcus ML, Ehrhardt J. *et al*. Correlation between echocardiographically demonstrated segmental dyskinesis and regional myocardial perfusion. *Circulation* 1975; **52**: 1097–104.
10. Hong YW, Orihashi K, Cochran T. *et al*. Detection of myocardial ischemia by transesophageal echocardiography during vein graft repair. *J Cardiothorac Vasc Anesth* 1991; **5**: 498–501.
11. Shah PM, Kyo S, Matsumura M. *et al*. Utility of biplane transesophageal echocardiography in left ventricular wall motion analysis. *J Cardiothorac Vasc Anesth* 1991; **5**: 316–19.
12. Ross J. Assessment of ischemic regional myocardial dysfunction and its reversibility. *Circulation* 1986; **74**: 1186–90.
13. Kato M, Nakashima Y, Levine J, Goldiner PL, Oka Y. Does transesophageal echocardiography improve postoperative outcome in patients undergoing coronary artery bypass surgery? *J Cardiothorac Vasc Anesth* 1993; **7**: 285–9.
14. Hauser AM, Gangadgaran V, Ramos RG *et al*. Sequence of mechanical, electrocardiographic and clinical effects of repeated coronary occlusion in human beings: echocardiographic observation during coronary angioplasty. *J Am Coll Cardiol* 1995; **5**: 193–7.
15. Serruys PW, Suryapranata H, Piscione F. *et al*. Myocardial release of hypoxanthine and lactate during percutaneous transluminal coronary angioplasty. *Am J Cardiol* 1989; **63**: 45E–51E.
16. Lytle BW, McElroy D, McCarthy P. *et al*. Influence of arterial coronary bypass grafts on the mortality in coronary reoperations. *J Thorac Cardiovasc Surg* 1994; **107**: 675–83.
17. Julia PL, Buckberg GD, Acar C, Partington MT, Sherman MP Studies of controlled reperfusion after ischemia. XXI. Reperfusate composition: Superiority of blood cardioplegia over crystalloid cardioplegia in limiting reperfusion damage – importance of endogenous oxygen free radical scavengers in red blood cells. *J Thorac Cardiovasc Surg* 1991; **101**: 303–13.
18. Flemma RJ, Singh HM, Tector AJ, Lepley D, Franzier BL. Comparative hemodynamic properties of vein and mammary artery in coronary bypass operations. *Ann Thorac Surg* 1975; **20**: 619–27.
19. Loop FD, Thomas JD. Hypoperfusion after arterial bypass grafting. *Ann Thorac Surg* 1993; **56**: 812–13.
20. von Segesser L, Simonet F, Meier B, Faidutti L. Inadequate flow after internal mammary-coronary artery anastomoses. *J Thorac Cardiovasc Surg* 1987; **35**: 352–4.
21. Ochiai M, Ohno M, Taguchi J. *et al*. Responses of human gastroepiploic arteries to vasoactive substances: comparison with responses of internal mammary arteries and saphenous vein. *J Thorac Cardiovasc Surg* 1992; **104**: 453–8.
22. Hanet C, Dion R, Wyns W. Coronary bypass grafts vasomotion. In: *Quantitative coronary angiography in clinical practice*. Serruys PW, Foley DP, de Feyter PJ, eds. Dordrecht: Kluwer Academic Publishers, 1994: 355–69.
23. Yang Z, Siebenmann R, Studer M, Egloff L. Lüscher TF. Similar endothelium-dependent relaxation, but enhanced contractility of the right gastroepiploic artery as compared with the internal mammary artery. *J Thorac Cardiovasc Surg* 1992: **104**: 459–64.
24. Buche M, Schoevaerdts JC, Louagie Y *et al*. Use of the inferior epigastric artery for coronary bypass. *J Thorac Cardiovasc Surg* 1992; **103/4**: 665–70.
25. Acar C, Jebara V, Porthogese K *et al*. Revival of the radial artery for coronary bypass grafting. *Ann Thorac Surg* **54**: 652–60.
26. Vajtai P, Ravichandran PS, Fessler CL *et al*. Inadequate internal mammary artery graft as a cause of postoperative ischemia: incidence, diagnosis and management. *Eur J Cardiothorac Surg* 1992; **6**: 603–8.
27. Johns RA, Peach MJ, Flanagan T, Kron IL. Probing of the canine mammary artery damages endothelium and impairs vasodilation resulting from prostacyclin and endothelium-derived relaxing factor. *J Thorac Cardiovasc Surg* 1989; **97**: 252–8.
28. Mills NM, Bringaze WL. Preparation of the internal mammary artery graft: which is the best method ? *J Thorac Cardiovasc Surg* 1989; **98**: 73–9.
29. Dion R, Etienne Y, Verhelst R *et al*. Bilateral mam-

mary grafting. Clinical, functionnal and angiographic assessment in 400 consecutive patients. *Eur J Cardiothorac Surg* 1993; **7:** 287–94.
30. Cooper GJ, Wilkinson GAL, Angelini GD. Overcoming perioperative spasm of the internal mammary artery: which is the best vasodilator? *J Thorac Cardiovasc Surg* 1992; **104:** 465–8.
31. Suma H, Wanibushi Y, Terada Y, Fukuda S, Takayama T, Furuta S. The right gastroepiploic artery graft. *J Thorac Cardiovasc Surg* **105:** 615–23.
32. Nijsen-Karelse M, Dion RAE, Jambroes G. Nifedipine in cardiac operations. *J Thorac Cardiovasc Surg* 1982; **84:** 145.
33. Amrani M, Matta A, Dion RA. Beneficial effect of nicardipine on perioperative myocardial ischemia. *Ann Thorac Surg* 1993; **55:** 813–814.
34. von Segesser LK, Lehman K, Turina M. Deleterious effects of shock in internal mammary artery anastomoses. *Ann Thorac Surg* 1989; **47:** 575–9.
35. Mc Cormick JR, Kaneko M, Barre AE, Geha AS. Blood flow and vasoactive drug effects in internal mammary artery and venous bypass grafts. *Circulation 52* 1975; (Suppl 1, Part 2): 72–80.
36. Rodigas PC, Bridges KG. Occlusion of left internal mammary artery with intra-aortic balloon: clinical implications. *J Thorac Cardiovasc Surg* 1986; **91:** 142–9.
37. Zeff RJ, Iannone LA, Kongtahworn C *et al.* Coronary artery spasm following coronary artery revascularization. *Ann Thorac Surg* 1982; **34:** 196–9.
38. Skarvan K, Graedel E, Hasse J *et al.* Coronary artery spasms after coronary by-pass surgery. *Anesthesiology* 1994; **60:** 323–7.
39. Pichard AD, Ambrose J, Mindich B *et al.* Coronary artery spasm and perioperative cardiac arrest. *J Thorac Cardiovasc Surg* 1980; **80:** 249–54.
40. Dion R, Jambroes G, Nijsen M, Hitchcock JF. Intracoronary nifedipine in patients suspected of perioperative coronary spasm. In: Unger F ed. *Coronary artery surgery*. Berlin: Springer Verlag, 1984: 119–25.
41. Cohen AJ, Moore P, Jones C *et al.* Effect of internal mammary harvest on postoperative pain and pulmonary function. *Ann Thorac Surg* 1993; **56:** 1107–9.
42. Mangano DT, Siciliano D, Hollenberg M *et al.* Postoperative myocardial ischemia. Therapeutic trials using intensive analgesia following surgery. *Anesthesiology* 1992; **76:** 331–3.
43. Estenne M, Desmet JM, Detroyer A, Yernault JC. Effects of coronary artery bypass surgery on respiratory mechanics. *Circulation* 1982; **224:** 66.
44. Hurlbut D, Myers ML, Lefcoe M, Golbach M. Pleuropulmonary morbidity: Internal thoracic artry versus saphenous vein graft. *Ann Thorac Surg* 1990; **50:** 959–64.
45. Byrick RJ, Noble WH. Postperfusion lung syndrome. *J Thorac Cardiovasc Surg* 1978; **76:** 685–93.
46. Howard R, Crain C, Franzini D *et al.*: Effects of cardiopulmonary bypass on pulmonary leukostasis and complement activation. *Archs Surg* 1988; **123:** 1496–501.
47. Balis JU, De Villota D, Avello F *et al.* The role of pulmonary hypoxia in the post perfusion lung syndrome. *Surg Forum* 1969; **20:** 205–6.
48. Pitt B, Gillis N, Hammond G. Depression of pulmonary metabolic function by cardiopulmonary bypass procedures increases levels of circulating norepinephrine. *J Thorac Surg* 1984; **38:** 508–613.
49. Peng MJ, Vargas FS, Cukier A, Terra-Filho M, Teixeira LR, Light RW. Postoperative pleural changes after coronary revascularization: comparison between saphenous vein and internal mammary artery grafting. *Chest* 1992; **101:** 327–30.
50. Vargas FS, Cukier A, Terra-Filho M, Hueb W, Teixeira LR, Light RW. Influence of atelectasis on pulmonary function after coronary artery bypass grafting. *Chest* 1993; **104:** 434–7.
51. Hauters Ph, Delecluse V, Lambermont JY *et al.* Revascularisation myocardique avec greffon mammaire: analyse de la morbidité respiratoire postopératoire immédiate et tardive. *Ann Chir: Chir Thorac Cardiovasc* 1991; **45(2):** 77–81.
52. Dobbinson T, Miller J. Respiratory and cardiovascular responses to PEEP in artificially ventilated patients after cardiopulmonary bypass surgery. *Anaesth Intens Care* 1981; **9:** 307–13.
53. Wilcox P, Baile EM, Hards J. Phrenic nerve function and its relationship to atelectasis after coronary artery bypass surgery. *Chest* 1988; **93:** 693–8.
54. Rousou JA, Parker T, Engelman RM, Breyer RH. Phrenic nerve paresis associated with the use of iced slush and the cooling jacket for topical hypothermia. *J Thorac Cardiovasc Surg* 1985; **89:** 921–5.
55. Kohorst WR, Schonfeld SA, Altman M. Bilateral diaphragmatic paralysis following topical cardiac hypothermia. *Chest* 1984; **85:** 65–8.
56. Esposito RA, Spencer FC. The effect of pericardial insulation on hypothermic phrenic nerve injury during open-heart surgery. *Ann Thorac Surg* 1987; **43:** 303–8.
57. De Vita M, Robinson LR, Rehder J, Hattler B, Cohen C. Incidence and natural history of phrenic neuropathy occuring during open heart surgery. *Chest* 1993; **103:** 850–6.
58. O'Brien JW, Johnson SH, VanSteyn SJ *et al.* Effects of internal mammary artery dissection on phrenic nerve perfusion and function. *Ann Thorac Surg* 1992; **52:** 182–8.
59. Arnold M. The surgical anatomy of sternal blood supply. *J Thorac Cardiovasc Surg* 1972; **64:** 586–610.
60. Seyfer AE, Shriver CD, Miller TR, Graeber GM. Sternal blood flow after median sternotomy and

mobilization of the internal mammary arteries. *Surgery* 1988; **104:** 899–904.
61. Parish MA, Asai T, Grossi EA *et al.* The effects of different techniques of internal mammary artery harvesting on sternal blood flow. *J Thorac Cardiovasc Surg* 1992; **104:** 1303–7.
62. Graeber GM. Harvesting of the internal mammary artery and the healing median sternotomy. *Ann Thorac Surg* 1992; **53:** 7–8.
63. Grossi EA, Esposito R, Harris LJ *et al.* Sternal wound infections and use of internal mammary artery grafts. *J Thorac Cardiovasc Surg* 1991; **102:** 342–7.
64. Kouchoukos NT, Wareing TH, Murphy SF, Pelate C, Marshall WG: Risks of bilateral internal mammary artery bypass grafting. *Ann Thorac Surg* 1990; **49**: 210–19.
65. Cosgrove DM, Lytle BW, Loop FD *et al.* Does bilateral internal mammary grafting increase surgical risk? *J Thorac Cardiovasc Surg* 1988; **95:** 850–6.
66. Accola KA, Jones EL, Craver JM *et al*: Bilateral mammary artery grafting: avoidance of complications with extended use. *Ann Thorac Surg* 1993; **56:** 872–9.
67. Bidstrup BP, Royston D, Sapsford RN, Taylor KM. Reduction in blood loss and blood use after cardiopulmonary bypass with high dose aprotinin (Trasylol). *J Thorac Cardiovasc Surg* 1989; **97:** 364–72.
68. Baele PL, De Bruyère M, Deneys V *et al*: Results of the Sanguis study in Belgium. *Acta Chir Belg, Suppl* **94**: 31–37.
69. Yau TM, Carson S, Weisel RD *et al.* The effect of warm heart surgery on postoperative bleeding. *J Thorac Cardiovasc Surg* 1992; **103:** 1155–63.
70. Vahl CF, Carl I, Müller-Vahl H, Struck E. Brachial plexus injury after cardiac surgery. The role of internal mammary artery preparation: a prospective study of 1000 consecutive patients. *J Thorac Cardiovasc Surg* 1991; **102:** 724–9.
71. Baisden CE, Greenwald LV, Symbas PN. Occult rib fractures and brachial plexus injury following median sternotomy for open heart operations. *Ann Thorac Surg* 1984; **38:** 192–4.
72. Weintraub WS, Jones EL, Craver J, Guyton RA, Cohen CL. Determinants of prolonged length of hospital stay after coronary bypass surgery. *Circulation* 1989; **80:** 276–84.
73. Suma H, Wanibushi Y, Furuta S. Does use of gastroepiploic artery graft increase surgical risk? *J Thorac Cardiovasc Surg* 1991; **101:** 121–5.
74. Barner H, Naunheim K, Fiore A, Fischer V, Harris H. Use of the inferior epigastric artery as a free graft for myocardial revascularization. *Ann Thor Surg* 1991; **52:** 3, 429–37.

20 Angioplasty of arterial conduits

Peter Wilde and Alan J. Bryan

Background

Recurrent ischaemia in patients with previous surgical revascularization is a common and increasing clinical problem. By 10 years after coronary artery surgery, 19 per cent of patients require revascularization by repeat grafting or percutaneous transluminal coronary angioplasty (PTCA).[1] In some centres in North America, up to 20 per cent of coronary artery bypass grafting procedures are reoperations.[2] In this situation the therapeutic options are narrowed, especially as repeat surgical revascularization carries an increased operative risk compared to the primary procedure. Recurrent ischaemia is commonly secondary to diseased or occluded vein grafts and less commonly to the progression of disease in the native coronary circulation. Only rarely is it related to intrinsic disease or a technical problem associated with an arterial conduit. In the current era, patients presenting with recurrent ischaemia are most likely to have a patent ITA graft to the anterior descending coronary artery but occluded or diseased vein grafts to circumflex and right coronary arteries.

Angioplasty of diseased native coronary arteries in the postoperative patient can be effective in providing early symptom relief, but may be challenging and yield suboptimal results due to the frequent occurrence of multiple severe and complex stenoses or complete occlusions, which prompted the original surgery. PTCA of native vessels is still subject to restenosis in at least 30 per cent of cases, for which there is currently no effective treatment.[3] Angioplasty of vein grafts has been extensively evaluated and the results are less satisfactory than for native vessels in the long term, with restenosis rates of 50 per cent or more at 1 year.[4]

Reported experience of angioplasty of arterial conduits is limited because of their more recent introduction and their relative freedom from graft disease. PTCA of arterial grafts themselves, anastomotic sites and native vessels beyond have all been reported.[4] The majority of these reports involve ITA grafts reflecting its frequent use. The scant information relating to other arterial conduits should inevitably increase with more widespread application. A particular problem related to pedicled arterial grafts is that these conduits are subject to the influence of proximal occlusive disease in the major feeding arteries which may compromise graft flow. Angioplasty to the proximal arterial tree thus offers a therapeutic option preoperatively to maximize arterial grafting options or postoperatively to treat 'steal' syndrome secondary to proximal occlusive disease.

In the treatment of ischaemic heart disease, surgery and angioplasty are alternative therapeutic strategies that continue to evolve. They should be considered as complementary rather than adversarial and further development and evaluation of PTCA is required to define its role in the context of the postoperative patient with arterial grafts.

Angioplasty in patients with prior surgical revascularization

The choice of revascularization strategies may be difficult, particularly in the presence of a patent arterial graft. Reoperative coronary artery surgery carries a risk three times that of primary surgery.[5] In the UK in 1992 the mortality for reoperative coronary surgery overall was 9.2 per cent compared to 2.4 per cent in those undergoing primary procedures.[6] The Cleveland Clinic data[7] suggest that the presence of a patent ITA graft does not increase operative risk but this data from a large centre is in contrast to reports from other major centres[2,8] which have identified a patent arterial graft as a risk factor at reoperation. In addition, the risk of reoperation in those with bilateral ITA grafts has been reported to be high even in very experienced hands.[9] These surgical problems must be balanced against the risks and potential benefits of angioplasty of vein grafts or the native circulation.

Vein graft PTCA

The group of patients having PTCA post-cardiac surgery is an increasing one and represents up to 25 per cent of the total angioplasties performed in some centres. Initial reports from the National Heart Lung and Blood Institute PTCA Registry[10] showed an increased risk in patients with prior myocardial revascularization but more recent published results have not supported this.[11,12] Review of the available data suggests that PTCA of vein grafts yield a 90 per cent angiographic success rate, with Q wave infarction in 0–2.5 per cent, emergency coronary artery surgery in 4 per cent and an overall mortality of 1 per cent.[13,14] Balloon angioplasty is particularly effective in the early period up to 1 year after operation, but is less successful and carries more risk in older vein grafts with multiple stenoses or thrombus formation. In occluded vein grafts angioplasty is less likely to achieve any success, even with intracoronary thrombolytic therapy and directional atherectomy[15,16] and there is a real risk of distal embolization in the angioplasty of occluded vein grafts. The advent and application of newer atherectomy devices, while there may have broadened the indications, has been associated with a hospital mortality of 3 per cent and poor late outcome.[17]

Restenosis is common and occurs in at least 50 per cent of vein grafts by 1 year and in a higher percentage of older vein grafts, although early results of intravascular stenting report encouraging low restenosis rates.[18,19] In spite of this, the relatively low risk of attempted PTCA, combined with the reduction in surgical options and the presence of one or more patent arterial conduits frequently favours angioplasty as a first option in the patient with recurrent ischaemia following surgical revascularization.

Angioplasty of ITA grafts

Considering the large number of coronary artery bypass grafting procedures using the left ITA, the reported numbers of angioplasties performed is relatively small. Indeed, in the two largest reported series assessing ITA-related PTCA, only 0.4–0.7 per cent of the total population undergoing PTCA required dilatation of these grafts or lesions beyond such grafts.[20,21]

In these patients recurrent ischaemia usually presents within the first postoperative year and is most commonly related to a stenosis at the site of anastomosis between the ITA and the native coronary artery.[4] In one series of forty-five patients having ITA-related PTCA procedures, twenty lesions were related to the anastomosis, twelve were in the artery itself and twenty-four in the distal native artery (using the ITA graft as an access route).[21] In the second large published series of thirty-one patients, twenty-four lesions were at the anastomosis, three were in the distal vessel and in three patients they were at both sites.[20]

Anastomotic stenoses are inevitably related to the surgical procedure in some way, either as a direct consequence of imperfect surgical technique or because the surgery has encouraged subsequent intimal proliferation at the site of a technically satisfactory anastomosis. Lesions within the ITA itself are of uncertain origin. The incidence of atheroma in the vessel is very low and it has been speculated that at least some of the mid or proximal vessel stenoses may be related to localized dissections occurring at the time of surgical mobilization of the vessel from the chest wall, to the previous diagnostic catheter, or rarely to injury from previous chest wall irradiation.

PTCA of ITA graft lesions can be achieved successfully in a high proportion of cases (Fig. 20.1). In a large recent review of seventeen publications reporting results in 177 patients, an initial success rate of 93 per cent was recorded.[4]

Technical aspects

The usual precautions for normal PTCA (including anticoagulation and antiplatelet therapy) apply for ITA PTCA and the technique should be meticulous in all respects. It should not be attempted by an angioplasty operator without significant experience of native vessel PTCA and of diagnostic catheterization of ITAs. In addition it should be remembered that the procedure is a variant of subclavian and carotid angiography, both of which have a small but significant risk. In cannulating the subclavian artery (left or right) it is possible to inadvertently enter either carotid artery and this should be recognized immediately. It is also possible to cannulate the vertebral artery, either from the subclavian artery or

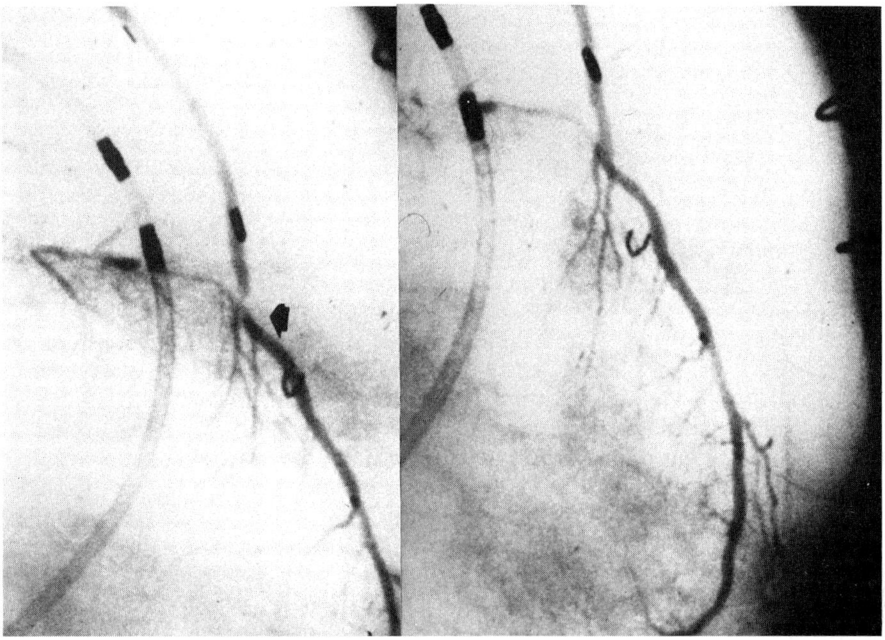

Fig. 20.1 Severe stenosis (left) at the distal anastomosis of a left internal thoracic artery graft with the left anterior descending artery (arrowed); resolution of the stenosis after successful PTCA (right). (Courtesy of Prof. D. Cumberland).

as a common variant directly from the aorta. We recommend the administration of anticoagulation prior to subclavian artery cannulation.

During attempted selection of the ITA ostium, it is frequently necessary to carry out small test injections which may outline muscular branches and for this reason it is probably better to use non-ionic contrast medium to avoid localized pain at these injection sites. This applies also for the ITA itself in some patients who are very sensitive to such injections. The small size of the ITA in some patients and its predisposition to spasm justifies the more liberal use of intracoronary nitrate injection than might be the case for the native coronary arteries.

The anatomical characteristics of the ITA graft represent the major procedural challenges. These include its relatively sharp take-off from the subclavian artery, and its length and tortuosity. The ITA is best located at its origin in the anteroposterior view using the specifically shaped ITA catheter. Initial engagement in the left subclavian artery can sometimes be difficult and an alternative method is to use a right Judkins catheter as this frequently enters the subclavian more easily than the ITA catheter and can often be used successfully to cannulate the ITA origin itself. Occasionally it is necessary to cannulate the subclavian artery with a less suitable catheter (such as a right Judkins catheter or a Cobra catheter) and then use a long exchange wire to introduce the guide catheter into the subclavian artery. Some 8 French ITA guide catheters are designed with a tapered tip to 7.5 French to reduce the possibility of flow obstruction, whilst allowing improved engagement and guiding catheter support. Recently manufacturers have introduced 7 and even 6 French guide catheters with very good performance and these will probably be the choice of most operators.

Caution is always required in the engagement of the guiding catheter in the origin of the ITA since this is the site at which dissection may occur. The tip of the catheter should be well engaged in the ITA origin, lying parallel to the direction of the proximal vessel but without obstructing flow, shown by dampening of the catheter tip pressure trace and slow 'run-off' of contrast from the catheter tip. If there is a tendency to vessel obstruction, the guide catheter should be changed to a smaller size as it is dangerous to carry out a prolonged procedure under this circumstance, particularly when the guide catheter will often be out of the X-ray image at the time of PTCA (due to its distance above the heart). If the ITA has been found but the artery cannot be selectively entered, the lateral view should be used to ensure that the catheter tip faces anteriorly towards the origin of the vessel. Interventional procedures have been carried out predominantly by the femoral route,[25] although the brachial[26] and axillary[20] approaches have also been used successfully. Non-femoral routes should only be used by those experienced in the same approach for diagnostic catheterization.

Present day guide wires are generally very flexible and steerable, both vital attributes for successful passage down the relatively long and tortuous artery. Usually a 0.014 inch wire is appropriate, normally with a soft or floppy tip (ACS Hi-Torque Floppy, ACS UK, Basingstoke, UK), or Bard Hiperflex (Bard Limited, Crawley, UK). In a few cases it may be helpful to use a finer 0.012 inch wire (Bard Silk, Bard Limited, Crawley, UK) but there will be inevitable loss of control as the flexibility and 'trackability' improve. Stiffer or larger wires are to be avoided wherever possible to avoid trauma to the relatively fragile artery.

The length and tortuosity of the ITA, coupled with the acute take-off angle, means that, in general, smaller balloon catheters, often mounted on a 2.7 French shaft should be used. There is some debate as to whether the 'over-the-wire' or the 'monorail' approach is superior but no clear answer has emerged. The 'over-the-wire' balloons allow a steady incremental advance of wire followed by balloon, the latter giving close support. In the 'monorail' technique it is sometimes possible to advance the wire fully past the lesion before advancing the balloon but if support is required, the balloon can still be brought close to the wire tip. In either case it is essential to select equipment with maximal 'trackability' and 'pushability'. Often coated wires and balloons reduce friction in the vessel and on the wire. It is at the stage of advancing the balloon down the ITA that the solid support of an appropriate guide catheter position is required. This is all the more important if the distal lesion is tight and potentially difficult to cross.

Clearly the lowest profile balloons must be used and it is rarely helpful to use specialist variant balloons such as perfusion or long balloons, both of which are bulkier and harder to pass down the vessel. Balloon size is selected as with other PTCA procedures, so 2.5 mm or 3.0 mm are the most commonly used. The distance from the guide catheter tip to the lesion is usually greater than for native vessel PTCA due to the length of the ITA and the operator is advised to estimate from the difference between guide catheter and balloon catheter, which is often no more than 20 cm with standard equipment. If the length of the ITA graft is unusually great, modified equipment may be required.

If it is considered that a stent might be implanted then care must be taken with guide catheter support and assessment of catheter and vessel tortuosity. If there are too many bends, there will come a point when the best equipment will fail to pass and it is most undesirable to be forced to deploy a stent proximally in the ITA (it is generally unwise to attempt to draw a stent back into the guide catheter as it can dislodge from the mounting balloon). Some stents can now be delivered down 6 French catheters under optimal conditions but care should be taken if this approach is selected as it will be technically much more challenging than for a native coronary artery.

At the completion of the procedure care is required in removing the guide catheter from the ITA origin since at this time also dissection may occur. Post-procedural care of such patients is no different to those undergoing conventional PTCA.

Right ITA grafts

Generally techniques are similar to those used for the left ITA with the exception that the cannulation of the vessel origin from the right subclavian artery may be a little more difficult as it is more proximal in the aorta and is generally less familiar to most operators. The graft route to the heart may also be a little longer than for the left side, depending on the site of anastomosis.

Complications

The incidence of complications is difficult to quantify given the small number of reported procedures. The technical difficulty is undoubtedly greater than for PTCA of most native vessels. Access to the origin of the ITA and the satisfactory positioning of the guide catheter in its proximal artery is more difficult than for native arteries, and this vessel is usually longer and more tortuous than a typical native coronoary vessel. This requires better guide catheter support, a more controllable guide wire and a more flexible or 'trackable' balloon catheter.

Dissections of the ITA origin following PTCA have been reported, probably as a consequence of this technical difficulty as well as the recognized frailty of the vessel itself.[20,21] This complication may require emergency or elective reoperative revascularization. Early restenosis has also been reported in a small number of cases.

Successful placement of an intravascular stent with satisfactory early outcome offers a therapeutic alternative in this situation.[22,23] The limited data available does not provide any real basis on which to formulate guidelines for such a strategy. Overall there has been a high degree of symptom relief and, at least in the medium term, minimal risk of restenosis up to 3 years.[20,21]

Coronary 'steal' phenomenon

Recurrent clinical ischaemia has been reported in association with large intercostal or pericardial branches of the ITA not divided at the time of operation, resulting in a 'steal' phenomenon. To avoid further operative intervention, coil embolization of the branches has been reported with early clinical success.[24] However, while individual branches of the ITA seen on postoperative angiography are relatively common, recurrent ischaemia as a result of 'steal' is very rare.

Angioplasty of right GEA grafts

Due to the relatively recent introduction and limited use of this conduit, reported experience has been very small.[27,28] The techniques are demanding and require selective catheterization by the gastroduodenal artery. The group of twelve patients reported recently by Isshiki *et al.* comprised six patients with occluded grafts and six patients with graft stenoses. Not surprisingly, attempts to reopen occluded grafts were almost universally unsuccessful. However, the success rate of 83 per cent for those with stenoses is commendable, given the difficulty of the procedure. No major complications were reported, though spasm was common. In those where the right GEA graft failed, native right coronary angioplasty provided an acceptable alternative in three of the other patients.[29]

Technical considerations

This description is based on that of Isshiki *et al.*[28] The anatomy is complicated and a diagram shows the major branches of the coeliac axis (Fig. 20.2). A femoral approach was used. Selective catheteri-

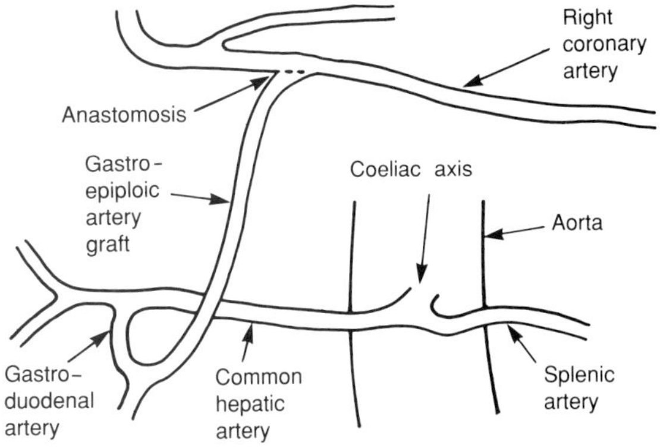

Fig. 20.2 Anatomy of the coeliac axis and its branches (modified after Isshiki).

zation of the coeliac axis was performed with a standard 7 French JR4 guiding catheter which was advanced to the gastroduodenal artery if possible using a 0.025 inch coated guide wire. Isosorbide dinitrate was usually injected directly into the graft to prevent vasospasm. If the guide catheter could be advanced to this position a conventional 'over-the-wire' technique was used, employing the lowest possible profile balloons (e.g. 2.8 French catheter, ACS Ten (ACS UK, Basingstoke, UK) with a conventional PTCA guide wire. If the guide catheter could not be passed far enough along this selective route, an alternative method was employed, using a specially designed 65 cm 7 French J-shaped Teflon sheath (Cook UK Limited, Letchworth, UK) engaged in the coeliac trunk. Through this was advanced a 4 French probing catheter (Bard Limited, Crawley, UK) within which was an angioplasty 'balloon-on-a-wire' system (Bard Probe 1.7 French) or Scimed Ace 1.8 French (Scimed Lifesystems Limited, Sawbridgeworth, UK) which was deployed in the stenosis.

The key technical considerations required are a guide catheter with sufficient back-up force to hold a balloon catheter with low profile and good trackability. The low profile balloon catheter allows better advancement, and in general it is suggested that the over-the-wire system is superior, particularly from the point of view of catheter advancement.

Angioplasty of subclavian artery grafts

Pedicled arterial grafts are dependent on proximal flow. In patients scheduled to undergo myocardial revascularization, PCTA of the subclavian artery has been proposed prior to myocardial revascularization in those with significant subclavian stenoses.[30,31] In addition, it also offers an alternative treatment for coronary–subclavian steal syndrome where previously carotid–subclavian bypass would have been the treatment of choice.[31–34] In both of these situations small numbers of patients with relatively short-term follow-up have been reported. As a preoperative intervention the significance of a subclavian stenosis may be difficult to assess; in addition, the late results of subclavian angioplasty with a 30 per cent restenosis rate at 4 years[35] make this a controversial approach.[36] In the presence of known preoperative disease, free arterial grafts offer a sensible alternative. As a postoperative treatment in those with coronary–subclavian steal balloon, angioplasty offers an excellent alternative to carotid–subclavian bypass with a high degree of early angiographic success, and symptomatic relief with a low incidence of complications.[31–34]

Conclusion

There is limited experience worldwide of angioplasty to arterial conduits. The excellent clinical performance of ITA grafts means that they rarely require any intervention, although distal anastomotic strictures, when they occur, may be treated effectively in almost all cases by balloon angioplasty. Angioplasty of stenosed GEA grafts is rarely necessary and is technically demanding but is successful in the majority of patients.

In the context of recurrent myocardial ischaemia after prior surgical revascularization, the narrowing of therapeutic options and the low relative risk of PTCA make it an attractive option, particularly to the native coronary arteries but also to stenosed vein grafts and particularly in the presence of patent arterial grafts.

Subclavian angioplasty may be used to treat the rare problem of late coronary steal syndromes in those with proximal subclavian stenosis, but its preoperative application to allow use of pedicled ITA grafts is controversial.

Patients suffering recurrent ischaemia require individual assessment by an experienced interventional cardiologist and surgeon together. Awareness of the potential risks and benefits of the complementary therapeutic options available allows determination of the most appropriate treatment strategy.

References

1. Weintraub WS, Jones EL, Craver JM, Guyton RA. Frequency of repeat coronary bypass or coronary angioplasty after coronary artery bypass surgery using saphenous venous grafts. *Am J Cardiol* 1994; **73:** 103–12.
2. Akins CW, Buckley MJ, Daggett WM *et al.* Reoperative coronary grafting: changing patient profiles, operative indications, techniques and results. *Ann Thorac Surg* 1994; **58:** 359–65.
3. McEwan J. Therapeutic approaches to the control of fibrocellular intimal hyperplasia after angioplasty. *Br Heart J* 1993; **70:** 1–3.
4. Douglas JS Jr. Percutaneous approaches to recurrent myocardial ischemia in patients with prior surgical revascularisation. *Sem Thorac Cardiovasc Surg* 1994; **6:** 98–108.
5. Loop F.D., Lytle B.W., Cosgrove D.M. *et al.* Reoperation for coronary atherosclerosis: Changing practice in 2509 consecutive patients. *Ann Surg* 1990; **212:** 378–86.
6. United Kingdom Cardiac Surgical Register 1992, Society of Cardiothoracic Surgeons of Great Britain and Ireland.
7. Lytle BW, McElroy D, McCarthy P *et al.* Influence of arterial coronary bypass grafts on mortality in coronary reoperations. *J Thorac Cardiovasc Surg* 1994; **107:** 675–83.
8. Ivert TSA, Ekestrom S, Peterffy A, Welti R Coronary artery reoperations. *Scand J Thorac Cardiovasc Surg* 1988; **22:** 111–18.
9. Joyce FS, McCarthy PM, Taylor PC, Cosgrove DM, Lytle BW Cardiac reoperation in patients with bilateral internal thoracic artery grafts. *Ann Thorac Surg* 1994; **58:** 80–5.
10. Kent KM, Bentivoglio LG, Block PC *et al.* Percutaneous transluminal coronary angioplasty: report from the Registry of the National Heart Lung and Blood Institute Registry. *Am J Cardiol* 1982; **49:** 2011–20.
11. Detre K, Holubkov R, Kelsey S *et al.* Percutaneous transluminal coronary angioplasty in 1985–1986 and 1977–1981. The National Heart Lung and Blood Institute Registry. *New Engl J Med* 1988; **318;** 265–70. •
12. Douglas JS Jr, Gruentzig AR, King SB III *et al.* Percutaneous transluminal angioplasty in patients with prior coronary bypass surgery. *J Am Coll Cardiol* 1983; **2:** 745–54.
13. Douglas JS Jr Percutaneous approaches to recurrent myocardial ischemia in patients with prior surgical revascularisation. *Sem Thorac Cardiovasc Surg* 1994; **6:** 98–108.
14. Plokker HWT, Meester BH, Serruys PW The Dutch experience in percutaneous transluminal angioplasty of narrowed saphenous veins used for

aortocoronary arterial bypass. *Am J Cardiol* 1991; **67:** 361–7.
15. de Feyter PJ, Serruys P, van den Brand M, Meester H, Beatl K, Suryapramata H Percutaneous transluminal angioplasty of a totally occluded bypass graft: a challenge that should be resisted. *Am J Cardiol* 1989; **64:** 88–90.
16. Hartmann JR, McKeever LS, Stamato NJ *et al.* Recanalisation of chronically occluded aortocoronary saphenous vein bypass grafts by extended infusion of urokinase: initial results and short term clinical follow up. *J Am Coll Cardiol* 1991; **18:** 1517–23.
17. O'Neill WW, Kramer BL, Sketch MH Jr *et al.* Mechanical extraction atherectomy: report of the US transluminal extraction catheter investigation. *Circulation* 1992; **86:** (Suppl. I) 779.
18. Urban P, Sigwart V, Golf S, Kaufmann V, Sadeghi H, Kappenberger I Intravascular stenting for stenosis of aortocoronary venous bypass grafts. *J Am Coll Cardiol* 1989; **13:** 1085–91.
19. de Scheerder IK, Strauss BH, de Feyter PJ *et al.* Stenting of venous bypass grafts: a new treatment modality for patients who are poor candidates for reintervention. *Am Heart J* 1992; **123:** 1046–54.
20. Dimas AP, Arora RR, Whitlow PL *et al.* Percutaneous transluminal angioplasty involving internal mammary artery grafts. *Am Heart J* 1991; **122:** 423–9.
21. Shimshak TM, Giorgi LV, Johnson WL *et al.* Application of percutaneous transluminal coronary angioplasty to the internal mammary artery graft. *J Am Coll Cardiol* 1988; **12:** 1205–14.
22. Bajaj RK, Roubin GS Intravascular stenting of the right internal mammary artery. *Cath Cardiovasc Diag* 1991; **24:** 252–5.
23. Almagor Y, Thomas J, Colombo A Balloon expandable stent implantation of a stenosis at the origin of the left internal mammary artery graft: A case report. *Cath Cardiovasc Diag* 1991; **24:** 256–8.
24. Schmid C, Heublein B, Reichelt S, Borst HG Steal phenomenon caused by a parallel branch of the internal mammary artery. *Ann Thorac Surg* 1990; **50:** 463–4.
25. Pinkerton CA, Slack JD, Orr CM, Van Tassel JW Percutaneous transluminal angioplasty involving internal mammary artery bypass grafts: a femoral approach. *Cath Cardiovasc Diag* 1987; **13:** 414–18.
26. Salinger M, Drummer E, Furey K, Bott-Silverman C, Franco I Percutaneous angioplasty of internal mammary artery graft stenosis using the brachial approach. *Cath Cardiovasc Diag* 1986; **12:** 261–5.
27. Kamiyama N, Nakamishi S, Yanagishita Y *et al.* Percutaneous transluminal coronary angioplasty of gastoepiploic artery graft. *Cath Cardiovasc Diag* 1990; **21:** 177–9.
28. Isshiki T, Yamaguchi T, Tamura T *et al.* Percutaneous angiopleasty of stenosed gastoepiploic artery grafts. *J Am Coll Cardiol* 1993; **21:** 727–32.
29. Isshiki T, Yamaguchi T, Makamura M *et al.* Postoperative angiographic evaluation of gastoepiploic artery grafts: technical considerations and short term patency. *Cath Cardiovasc Diag* 1991; **21:** 233–8.
30. Ernst S, Bal E, Plokker T, Mast G, Tjon M, Ascoop C Percutaneous balloon angioplasty (PBA) of a left subclavian artery stenosis or occlusion to establish adequate flow through the left internal mammary artery for coronary bypass purposes. *Circulation* 1991; **84:** 591.
31. Perrault LP, Carrier M, Hudon G, Lemarbre L, Hebert Y, Pelletier LC Transluminal angioplasty of the subclavian artery in patients with internal mammary grafts. *Ann Thorac Surg* 1993; **56:** 927–30.
32. Shapira S, Braun SD, Puram B, Patel G, Rotman H Percutaneous transluminal angioplasty of proximal subclavian artery stenosis after left internal mammary to left anterior descending artery bypass surgery. *J Am Coll Cardiol* 1991; **18:** 1120–3.
33. Belz M, Marshall JJ, Cowley MJ, Vetrovec GW Subclavian balloon angioplasty in the management of the coronary-subclavian steal syndrome. *Cath Cardiovasc Diag* 1992; **25:** 161–3.
34. Laub GW, Muralidharan S, Naidech H, Fernandez J, Adkins M, McGrath LB Percutaneous transluminal subclavian angioplasty in a patient with postoperative angina. *Ann Thorac Surg* 1991; **52:** 850–1.
35. Helbrang A, Maskovic J, Tomoc B Percutaneous transluminal angioplasty of the subclavian arteries: long term results in 52 patients. *Am J Roentg* 1991; **156:** 1091–4.
36. McGrath LB, Invited commentary to Perrault *et al.*[31] above. *Ann Thorac Surg* 1993; **56:** 930.

21 Arterial grafts and reoperative coronary bypass surgery

Bruce W. Lytle

The success of coronary bypass surgery in prolonging the survival of patients with severe coronary atherosclerosis, combined with the fact that coronary atherosclerosis is a progressive disease, have meant that an increasing number of patients are becoming candidates for coronary reoperations. In part because of the early advent of widespread bypass surgery in the United States, the incidence of reoperation is high, now constituting over 30 per cent of isolated bypass operations at The Cleveland Clinic Foundation.[1–6] However, the need for treatment of patients who have had previous bypass surgery and present with recurrent ischaemia is becoming common at most cardiac surgical centers throughout the world and it will become even more common in the future.

The most distinctive characteristic of reoperative candidates is that they almost always have multiple sources of myocardial blood supply, including the native coronary circulation, stenotic or patent vein grafts, stenotic or patent internal thoracic artery (ITA) grafts, and, at times, significant non-coronary collaterals. These characteristics can make myocardial protection complicated (as opposed to primary operations where delivery of aortic root cardioplegia duplicates the preoperative myocardial perfusion) and it also has important implications related to graft selection at reoperation. Other frequent characteristics of reoperative candidates include diffuse native vessel coronary atherosclerosis, a lack of bypass conduits, extensive epicardial scarring, and diffuse non-cardiac peripheral vascular disease.

The in-hospital risks associated with reoperations are increased over those for primary operations.[3–5] This relationship is not always apparent when small series are analysed but studies of large numbers of patients have consistently shown a higher perioperative mortality and morbidity for reoperative patients when compared with those undergoing primary surgery.

We now know that the use of ITA grafts for coronary bypass grafting produces substantial long-term benefits. The patency rate of left ITA to left anterior descending (LAD) coronary artery bypass grafts is over 90 per cent even more than 10 years after operation and the development of late pathological changes in left ITA to LAD grafts is rare.[7–10] This excellent late patency rate is reflected in superior late clinical results. Studies have shown that patients either with single vessel or multi-vessel disease who received left ITA to LAD grafts have superior late survival, reoperation-free survival and event-free survival when compared to patients receiving only saphenous vein grafts.[10–12] Furthermore, it is also clear that the use of single ITA grafts does not increase the perioperative risk of operations for primary coronary bypass grafting.[13]

Most long-term studies have shown that patency rates of ITA grafts other than the left ITA–LAD graft 'gold standard' are not quite as good, but that those patency rates are superior to the long-term outcome of saphenous vein to coronary grafts. The clinical impact of the effect of a second ITA graft on the clinical outcome of patients undergoing primary surgery has been more difficult to document but there is suggestive evidence that over the first 10 years after operation the incidence of reoperation is decreased for young patients who receive bilateral ITA grafts.[6,14,15]

The purpose of this review is to examine the impact of arterial coronary bypass grafts on coronary reoperations. The issues include the influence of arterial grafts on the indications for reoperation, the technical adjustments surgeons must make when patent arterial grafts are present at a second operation, the use of arterial grafts in reoperative situations, the effect of arterial bypass grafting on perioperative risk and the long-term results of reoperative surgery.

Indications for reoperation

There are few data that pertain to the indications for reoperation for patients with previous bypass surgery and the influence of coronary reoperations on long-term survival. To address these issues we conducted a non-randomized retrospective study of patients who had undergone bypass surgery, then had undergone a postoperative coronary angiogram that documented the presence of at least one stenotic (20–99 per cent) vein graft. Patients who underwent immediate reoperation were compared with those who were initially treated without repeat surgery.[3] The selection of surgical vs medical treatment was not randomized and, in general, the surgical patients were the higher risk group, being older, more symptomatic and having fewer patent bypass grafts. Multivariate analyses showed that for patients with atherosclerotic stenoses in saphenous vein grafts to the LAD long-term survival was better if they underwent immediate operation than if they were treated without surgery, and this was true regardless of the severity of their symptoms. On the other hand, patients with patent ITA to LAD grafts who had stenotic vein grafts to at least one other vessel had equivalent, and very good, survival with both surgical and medical management. It is important to realize that the patients who underwent reoperation were not only much more symptomatic but tended to have larger areas of myocardium in jeopardy than the medically treated patients did. However, it does appear that if patients have a patent ITA–LAD graft and if they are not highly symptomatic and do not have large areas of myocardium jeopardized by atherosclerotic vein grafts, then reoperation may not be mandatory, at least over the short term.

Reoperation with patent ITA–LAD graft

When severe symptoms or the presence of large amounts of myocardium jeopardized by stenotic vein grafts or by stenoses in vein grafts or native coronary vessels indicate a need for reoperation, surgeons must be aware of special problems engendered by the presence of a patent ITA–LAD graft. Those problems are related to the risks of damaging the ITA graft during the repeat sternotomy and dissection, and intraoperative myocardial protection.

The safety of repeat median sternotomy during reoperation for patients with a patent left ITA–LAD graft is very largely established at the time of the primary operation. The only situation where a patent ITA graft is at high risk of being damaged is if it is adherent to the chest wall, particularly if that point of adhesion is near the sternal midline and thus near the repeat median sternotomy. This problem can be prevented by dividing the pericardium posteriorly at the primary operation so that the left ITA–LAD graft lies posteriorly in the pericardial incision, lateral to the pulmonary artery. This manoeuvre will position the graft posterior to the lung, prevent it from being pushed medially and anteriorly by the lung, and prevent its adhesion to the anterior chest wall. Furthermore, the use of metal Haemoclips on the ITA branches during primary operations provide radiopaque markers that allow radiographic visualization of the location of the ITA and provide landmarks during the reoperative dissection. Repeat median sternotomy is accomplished with an oscillating saw and if sternal wires have been used during the previous closure, they are left intact posteriorly. This approach allows the surgeon to detect precisely when the posterior table of the sternum has been divided by both the feel and the grating sound of the teeth of the oscillating saw against the stainless steel sternal wires. Once the posterior table of the sternum has been divided those wires are then completely removed.

Some authors have advocated the initiation of femoral–femoral cardiopulmonary bypass prior to reoperative sternotomy. However, that approach requires that heparinization be undertaken prior to the dissection of the mediastinal structures and prior to the right ITA dissection (if that vessel is to be used as a graft), and the dissection of the left ITA graft that is already in place. In the interest of blood conservation we have rarely employed that strategy.

The left thoracotomy approach has also been used successfully for reoperation, thus avoiding the need for repeat median sternotomy.[16] We have used this approach in small numbers of cases but its disadvantages, including difficult access to the LAD and right coronary artery systems, problems using arterial grafts other than the left ITA, and imperfect myocardial protection, have limited our application of this strategy to anecdotal experience.

Once the sternum is opened, dissection of the mediastinal structures is initiated along the inferior aspect of the incision and is carried laterally in both directions along the diaphragm into both pleural spaces. The pleura on the right side can usually be divided all the way superiorly without much trouble, freeing the entire right half of the sternum from the mediastinal structures. Once the left pleural space has been entered the dissection is also carried superiorly but it must be done carefully in case the left ITA is adherent to the chest wall. It is not necessary to dissect out the left ITA completely at this point of the procedure and if there are difficult adhesions it can be approached later in the operation.

At this point in the operation, if the right ITA is to be used as a graft, it is taken down from the chest wall with the use of electrocautery and clips. During reoperation it can be difficult to establish a good length on the right ITA pedicle because the endothoracic fascia is often scarred. This is particularly a problem during early reoperations (<1 year after previous surgery). Dissection of a thin ITA pedicle and division of the endothoracic fascia at multiple locations will sometimes increase the length of the *in situ* graft, but often the right ITA may need to be used as a free (aorto-to-coronary) graft. Therefore, once the entire pedicle has been dissected, the endothoracic fascia is divided across the pedicle just distal to the take-off of the ITA from the subclavian artery, so if it does need to be divided and used as a free graft, that task is easier during the period of cross-clamping. If the right GEA is going to be used as a graft, that dissection can also be carried out simultaneously with the right ITA dissection and any vein grafts that are going to be used are prepared at this point.

Once the new arterial grafts are prepared, the right atrium and ascending aorta are dissected out so that cannulation is possible and, if the left ITA graft has not been completely freed from the anterior chest wall attention is returned to that task. If the left ITA graft is tightly adherent to the chest wall there are no secrets to its liberation other than using sharp dissection and being extremely careful. Protection of the patent left ITA–LAD graft is critical since it is not common that a reoperation establishes grafts that affect the long-term outcome more than a patent left ITA graft to a good LAD does. Again, precise isolation of the ITA graft is not always necessary. In order to create a pedicle that can be clamped to occlude the graft, the left lung is dissected away from the left side of the mediastinal pleura and the mediastinal fat is dissected away from the left side of the aortic adventitia. The pedicle of tissue that is isolated by this manoeuvre contains the ITA graft and can be clamped even though the left ITA graft is not isolated.

Heparin is given and cannulation is undertaken. Arterial cannulation is usually accomplished via the ascending aorta but if severe ascending aortic atherosclerosis is present we cannulate a femoral artery or the right axillary artery, a vessel that is dissected out through an infraclavicular incision. In many patients arterial cannulation of the axillary artery has advantages over femoral artery cannulation. First, if patients have severe ascending aortic atherosclerosis they will usually also have diseased femoral vessels and descending aortic atherosclerosis as well. Second, retrograde perfusion from the femoral vessels through severe atherosclerosis of the descending aorta and aortic arch may produce retrograde embolization of atherosclerotic debris into the cerebral or coronary vessels.[17] Our standard venous cannulation is a two-stage single atrial cannula. However, at times severely atherosclerotic vein grafts may limit access to the right atrium and in these situations the right femoral vein is dissected out and a long venous cannula threaded through the femoral vein into the right atrium for use as venous cannulation. Cardiopulmonary bypass can be established through this no. 28 or no. 32 cannula and if more effective venous drainage is needed, a second venous cannula can be placed after aortic cross-clamping and control of the atherosclerotic grafts. We also use a transatrial self-inflating coronary sinus cannula (placed through a right atrial pursestring) for delivering retrograde cardioplegia. An aortic cannula (12 French) is used for antegrade cardioplegia delivery and aortic venting.

Myocardial protection

As alluded to previously, myocardial protection is more complicated during coronary reoperations than during primary procedures because the concept of aortic cross-clamping and antegrade cardioplegia delivery down the aortic root is often not sufficient for myocardial protection during reoperation. If the patient has a patent ITA graft, the area subtended by that graft is not protected by aortic root cardioplegia and if atherosclerotic vein grafts are present antegrade cardioplegia creates the danger of embolization of atherosclerotic debris from those vein grafts, a documented cause of myocardial infarction during reoperation.[18,19]

The advent of retrograde (coronary sinus) cardioplegia delivery has been a major step forward in reoperative myocardial protection. Many experimental studies and an increasing volume of clinical work has shown that delivery of cardioplegia retrograde into the coronary venous system through the coronary sinus can produce effective myocardial protection.[20–22] There are specific advantages to retrograde cardioplegia delivery during reoperations. Retrograde cardioplegia can perfuse areas subtended by patent arterial grafts, allowing protection of those areas once the arterial graft is clamped. In addition, retrograde cardioplegia delivery minimizes the need for antegrade cardioplegia and therefore minimizes the risk of atherosclerotic embolization. Furthermore, giving retrograde cardioplegia after a coronary arteriotomy has been performed can treat atherosclerotic embolization by flushing debris out of the microcirculation and retrograde out of the coronary artery.

There are two disadvantages of retrograde cardioplegia. The first is that suboptimal delivery of cardioplegia to the right ventricle is common with retrograde cardioplegia, although the clinical importance of this has been debated.[22] Second, in small numbers of cases cardioplegia delivery to the left ventricle appears to be inconsistent, a problem that may be based on variations in coronary sinus and coronary venous anatomy. Because of these considerations I rarely depend completely on retrograde cardioplegia and instead use a combination of antegrade and retrograde cardioplegia delivery.

The use of warm continuous retrograde cardioplegia has gained some adherents but I have only used intermittent cold cardioplegia.[23] I do not yet have confidence in the consistency of retrograde cardioplegia delivery in all patients and, I usually cannot achieve the visualization and precision needed for difficult reoperative coronary anastomoses when continuous cardioplegia is obscuring the coronary arteriotomy.

The strategy for cardioplegia delivery must be examined in the context of the entire operative plan and the following is a description of the principles of cardioplegia management that I use during reoperations. Once cannulation has been accomplished and the grafts are prepared, cardiopulmonary bypass is initiated, volume is drained into the pump oxygenator reservoir until the heart is emptied and systemic cooling is started. Ultimately systemic cooling is taken to a level of 28–30°C but once the heart begins to become bradycardic the aorta is cross-clamped, patent arterial grafts are also clamped (if possible) and cold blood cardioplegia (Buckberg solution) is infused antegrade through the aortic root for 2–3 min at a rate of 300–400 cc/min.[22,24,25] This initial dose of cardioplegia is given prior to the dissection of the left ventricle and I do not manipulate the heart during cardioplegia induction. We then switch to retrograde cardioplegia and the left ventricle is dissected out while retrograde cardioplegia is delivered through the self-inflating balloon catheter that has been placed into the coronary sinus through a right atrial purse string. This cannula has a side arm for the measurement of coronary sinus pressure.

During retrograde cardioplegia delivery, both during induction and subsequent maintenance doses, the following points are noted to ensure that adequate cardioplegia delivery is being accomplished.

1. The coronary sinus pressure is kept at 25–50 mmHg, usually requiring a delivery rate of 200–300 cc/min.
2. The myocardial veins must be obviously distended with oxygenated blood.
3. The coronary arteries become filled with desaturated blood.
4. The myocardial temperature decreases.
5. Electrical activity is eliminated.

If these criteria are met then I am satisfied with a heavy dependence upon retrograde cardioplegia during the rest of the case. If those criteria are not met I will attempt to reposition the coronary sinus cannula to improve delivery. If that does not correct the situation then I give intermittent doses of antegrade cardioplegia throughout the procedure to make certain that effective protection is accomplished.

While the retrograde cardioplegia induction dose is given, I complete the dissection of the left ventricle. If a patent left ITA–LAD graft is in place, the safest approach is to dissect out the apex of the left ventricle, and at the apex establish a dissection plane lateral to the LAD. Then the pericardium is incised lateral to the LAD back proximally until the graft is identified or it is isolated in a strip of pericardium. During the period of time when the dissection is being carried out close to the left ITA graft, I will often take the bulldog clamp off the left ITA pedicle in order to allow accurate identification of the graft. When diagonal or circumflex grafts are to be done, the patent ITA graft must be dissected off the pulmonary artery to allow the new grafts to pass beneath it. Once this has been accomplished then it is almost always possible to clamp the graft and to give retrograde cardioplegia without it being washed out by antegrade flow down the ITA.

Occasionally when a patent left ITA graft is in place the adhesions are so difficult that the graft cannot be safely dissected out or clamped. In this situation, or if effective retrograde cardioplegia delivery cannot be achieved, the alternative plan for myocardial protection is to use systemic hypothermia down to 18–20°C and allow the patent arterial graft to perfuse the myocardium. Intermittent doses of cold cardioplegia are used as well. That is an effective strategy that we used for myocardial protection before retrograde cardioplegia was available. The disadvantages of that approach are that it takes time for systemic cooling and rewarming and there is some degree of inconvenience as blood is sometimes present in the coronary vessels while the anastomoses are being performed.

During the performance of the rest of the operation I give intermittent 2-min doses of cold cardioplegia (containing less potassium than the induction dose) by either the antegrade or retrograde route every 15–20 min. The choice between the antegrade and the retrograde route depends upon how effectively retrograde cardioplegia appears to be functioning, what we are doing at the time of the operation, and how many patent atherosclerotic vein grafts are present. If patent atherosclerotic vein grafts are present, I try to minimize antegrade cardioplegia in order to minimize embolization of atherosclerotic debris from those grafts. I also make a point of giving retrograde cardioplegia while the coronary arteries have been opened because the retrograde delivery will often flush atherosclerotic debris and air out of those vessels. If retrograde delivery has not been effective then intermittent doses of antegrade delivery are used.

I prefer to use a single period of aortic cross-clamping to perform all distal (graft-to-coronary) and proximal (graft-to-aorta) anastomoses. There are a number of advantages to this approach. First, aortic manipulation is minimized. Many reoperative candidates have a very diffuse systemic atherosclerosis that includes aortic atherosclerosis. Data now exists indicating that aortic manipulation can be a cause of atherosclerotic embolization during cardiac surgery and we wish to minimize that problem.[17] Second, it is often difficult to use a partial occluding clamp on the reoperative aorta due to multiple areas of scarring, the presence of old proximal anastomoses and/or the presence of Teflon felt from the previous procedure. Third, if stenotic grafts have been disconnected, revascularization is not complete until the proximal anastomoses of new grafts have been completed and, fourth, with current cardioplegia techniques the added aortic cross-clamping time needed to complete proximal anastomoses does not constitute a significant risk factor. Once all anastomoses are completed we give a 90-second retrograde dose of warm (37°C) blood cardioplegia (with aspartate and glutamate) as per the Buckberg 'hot shot' protocol, then a 90-second antegrade dose and the cross-clamp is then removed from the aorta.[24,25]

Management of patent or stenotic vein grafts at reoperation

The management of patent or stenotic vein grafts at reoperation is influenced by multiple considerations. First is the possible danger of perioperative complications of those grafts, either embolization of atherosclerotic debris into distal coronary arteries or graft thrombosis.[18,19,26] Second is the risk of development of future stenoses in those vein grafts that are not presently stenotic but that have already been exposed to the patient's atherogenic diathesis since the previous procedure. Third is the assessment of the bypass conduits that are available to replace those old grafts. Fourth, the age and coronary anatomy of the patient are important. Our general approach has been to replace all vein grafts more than 5 years old at any reoperation in order to avoid perioperative atherosclerotic embolization and the subsequent early development of new stenoses in those vein grafts. This is still our general approach but as reoperations have become more complex, exceptions to that policy have become more frequent.

To replace patent vein grafts there must be new grafts to replace them with. As more reoperations are being carried out for patients with multiple previous operations, conduit availability is more commonly an issue. There are some potential difficulties with replacing patent vein grafts with arterial grafts at reoperation, as we will explore in the next section. It is wise to assess carefully the availability of venous bypass grafts prior to a reoperation and currently I perform non-invasive venous Doppler studies of the greater and lesser saphenous vein systems in all patients who are candidates for repeat surgery. Second, it may not be prudent to use a patient's only remaining vein to replace vein grafts that do not have any evidence of stenosis, particularly in young patients. Usually patients that have one atherosclerotic stenotic vein graft also have atherosclerosis in their other grafts even though that atherosclerosis may not be angiographically apparent. On the other hand, data from Campos *et al.* have shown that vein grafts that are angiographically normal or minimally diseased at 5 years after operation had a 53 per cent likelihood of remaining normal or minimally diseased during the next 5–6 years.[27] Those studies were conducted with patients who did not undergo reoperation. In summary, the longer the interval after primary operation the more likely we are to replace patent vein grafts, but, if grafts are without angiographic stenoses and also upon inspection at reoperation appear to be thin walled and without atherosclerosis, we will sometimes individualize and leave those grafts in place.

When patients have had extensive progression of their native vessel disease since their previous operation their stenotic vein grafts may go to very proximal portions of the major coronary vessels and the new grafts may need to be placed quite distally. In that setting, the presence of intervening native vessel stenoses may mean that those distal bypass grafts may not completely revascularize the proximal areas supplied by the old vein grafts. The choices in that situation are to either leave the previously performed vein grafts in place or both to replace the proximal vein grafts and perform distal grafts. Therefore, whereas in the past we have usually replaced old vein grafts with new vein grafts in order to prevent embolization of atherosclerotic debris, because of the more extensive disease present in many of today's reoperative candidates we have more commonly added new vein grafts to old vein grafts and left the old vein grafts in place.

Replacing patent or stenotic vein grafts with ITA grafts

When patients undergoing reoperation have patent or stenotic vein grafts we would like to replace those with arterial grafts. However, the combination of the perioperative dangers of atherosclerotic vein grafts and the risk of hypoperfusion through smaller arterial grafts can put the surgeon in a quandary regarding the details of management.

For example, if a patient has a stenotic vein graft supplying a totally obstructed LAD coronary artery, the surgeon has a number of choices:

1. Replace the old vein graft with a new vein graft. The disadvantage of this approach is that the patient ends up with a vein graft supplying the LAD.
2. Leave the old vein graft in place and add an ITA graft to the LAD. The disadvantages here are, in the short term, the possibility of atherosclerotic embolization from the stenotic vein graft, and, in the long term, the possibility of competition in flow between the old vein graft and the new graft resulting in an ITA 'string sign'.
3. Interrupt the old vein graft, construct a new vein graft to the diagonal branch and also add a new left ITA–LAD graft. The disadvantage here is that a diagonal branch suitable for grafting is not always present.
4. Interrupt the old vein graft and replace it with an left ITA–LAD graft. The disadvantage here is that the new ITA graft, being a smaller calibre vessel, may not provide enough flow acutely to supply the myocardium once the stenotic vein graft is removed.

To examine this issue, we conducted a retrospective study of patients undergoing reoperation from 1985 to 1990 who had the characteristics of a totally obstructed native LAD system supplied by a stenotic (but not totally occluded) vein graft.[28] The clear message from this review was that patients for whom strategy 4 (removing the old vein graft and replacing it with an ITA graft) was employed had a very significant risk of hypoperfusion (18.9 per cent of patients) and a significant increase in their perioperative mortality. The other three strategies were all associated with very low perioperative risk. It appears that the risk of atherosclerotic embolization to the coronary arteries if the old vein graft is left in place is not very high, perhaps because of the extensive use of retrograde cardioplegia and attention to the principle of avoiding manipulation of atherosclerotic grafts. Furthermore, our concerns about competition in flow causing late ITA failure also did not appear to be borne out, as follow-up study showed that twenty of twenty-two ITA grafts that were restudied after reoperation remained patent. The two ITA grafts that became occluded had been grafted to vessels supplied by vein grafts with a less than 50 per cent stenosis.[29] We believe that the axiom 'do not remove a stenotic or patent vein graft and replace it only with an arterial graft' applies to GEA and IEA artery grafts as well as ITA grafts. Jones *et al.* have also noted hypoperfusion when replacing a vein graft with an ITA graft.[30]

The observation that adding an ITA graft to a vessel supplied by a stenotic vein graft does not usually result in a 'string sign' ITA cannot be extended to the situation where the vein graft is patent without stenoses.

Graft selection

There are many advantages of using arterial grafts at reoperation. Reoperative candidates often have very diffuse native vessel disease, situations where the long-term patency advantages of arterial grafts over vein grafts are magnified. In addition, due to total occlusion of coronary branches and previous myocardial infarctions, by the time patients get to reoperation the number of important coronary vessels left to graft may be relatively small in number and if these vessels can be securely revascularized the need for further surgery or invasive procedures can be minimized. Also, patients with previous operations may have limited venous conduits that are available, making the use of arterial grafts a necessity. When patients have limited bypass conduits available I think it is wise to perform ITA angiograms prior to reoperation. The ITAs can be inadvertently damaged during a sternal closure or they may have been dissected previously, not used for a graft and discarded. Before undertaking a reoperation for the purpose of obtaining an ITA graft it is important to be sure an ITA is available for use.

However, many factors also make the use of arterial grafts more difficult at reoperative surgery:

1. By using arterial grafts, the surgeon may be making an already long operation even longer and more complex.
2. Epicardial scarring and the presence of old vein grafts on the surface of the heart can create technical problems involving the length and position of arterial grafts; in particular the use of sequential arterial grafts is often difficult at reoperation.
3. Extension of native coronary artery disease often makes intramyocardial grafting of coronary vessels necessary.
4. When free arterial grafts are used the proximal anastomoses to the reoperative aorta can be difficult.
5. As already discussed, the use of arterial grafts to replace atherosclerotic and stenotic but not totally occluded vein grafts presents the surgeon with difficult choices in terms of whether to remove or leave in place those stenotic vein grafts.

The principle of graft selection and use at reoperation for the arterial grafts we have employed are discussed below.

ITA grafts

During coronary reoperations for patients who received only vein grafts at the first surgery, my goal is to use the left ITA to graft the LAD at their reoperation. Of all the things we know about the long-term results of coronary bypass surgery, the importance of the left ITA–LAD graft is the clearest. If the LAD graft is totally occluded or the LAD was previously ungrafted and is now jeopardized by a native vessel stenosis, the considerations for the use of the ITA are the same as during primary surgery. The exception to this policy is if the LAD is a relatively unimportant vessel and a branch of the circumflex system is more important. In that setting I use the left ITA to graft the most important branch of the left coronary system.

I commonly use the right ITA graft at reoperation, usually as a graft to the circumflex coronary artery. At times *in situ* right ITA to circumflex grafts can be constructed but that is more difficult during a reoperation than during a primary procedure and the use of free (aorta to coronary) right ITA grafts are more common at repeat surgery. This raises the issue of the aortic anastomosis and because the reoperative aorta is often thickened by epicardial scarring, old Teflon felt pledgets and proximal anastomoses, proximal arterial anastomoses can be difficult. Therefore, I usually perform proximal arterial anastomoses not directly to the aorta but rather to the hood of a new or old vein graft. Even if an old vein graft is totally occluded there is usually a small 'bubble' of vein left on the aorta that is thin and without atherosclerosis and it is at that spot that I perform an anastomosis with fine interrupted sutures.

The use of the left ITA as the site of the proximal anastomosis for the right ITA is an option that also should be considered. These 'Y' or 'T' grafts not only can provide a site for a proximal anastomosis for a free graft but they also allow a free graft to reach very posterior circumflex or right coronary branches.[31] The disadvantage of 'Y' grafts are the potential limitations in total flow through the proximal arterial conduit and the danger of atherosclerosis of the proximal graft. When contemplating these types of arterial reconstructions a preoperative angiogram of both ITAs is doubly important.

The right ITA also can be used as a graft to the LAD and the most common use of that strategy is in situations where the left ITA artery has been previously used and is occluded or where it is being used as a circumflex graft. When the right ITA is used to graft the right coronary system it is usually necessary to graft the posterior descending branch since progression of native vessel disease has almost always involved the main right coronary artery. When the heart is lying in the pericardium, the angle at which the *in situ* right ITA inserts into the posterior descending artery is actually better than when it is inserted into the main right coronary artery. Despite that, however, there are times when the *in situ* RITA will just not reach the posterior descending artery.

Right gastroepiploic artery

The GEA is another arterial conduit that has been an effective coronary bypass graft and the majority of cases where I have used the GEA have been during reoperation. The reasons for its use has either been because of a lack of other bypass conduits or the patient has experienced previous vein graft failure and has multiple risk factors for repeat vein graft failure. It is a major advantage to be able to use the GEA as an *in situ* graft because of the opportunity to avoid a proximal anastomosis and also because the patency rate of free GEA grafts has been inferior to that documented for *in situ* grafts. Dissection of the GEA can be undertaken prior to the median sternotomy although it affords somewhat better exposure if the median sternotomy is performed first. Almost always it is used to graft the posterior descending branch of the right coronary artery. Very favourable medium-term patency rates for *in situ* GEA grafts have been established by Suma and colleagues.[32] My most major concern about using the GEA at reoperation relates to the possible negative impact of aortic and coeliac artery atherosclerosis on long-term GEA function.

Inferior epigastric artery

The disadvantages of IEA grafts are that this conduit must be used as a free (aorta-to-coronary) graft and limited data with respect to late patency for this graft are available. In addition, many patients have abdominal incisions that may compromise this vessel.

Although some authors have described use of the IEA as a graft to the right coronary artery we have found that strategy is difficult at reoperation from a graft length standpoint and have usually used this conduit as a free graft to left-sided vessels. If the patient has a patent ITA graft to the LAD and distal native vessel stenoses, the IEA can be anastomosed to the patent ITA graft proximally and the distal LAD where the distal anastomosis is constructed. The proximal anastomosis of the IEA to a patent ITA graft is very straightforward and only a short length is needed, meaning that a very large calibre segment of the IEA can be employed.

Current practice of reoperative coronary surgery

To assess our current practice of reoperative coronary surgery and to examine specifically the influence of arterial grafts at primary operation and at reoperation on the in-hospital risk of repeat surgery, we reviewed the 1663 patients who underwent a first reoperation for isolated bypass grafting at The Cleveland Clinic Foundation during the years 1988 through 1991.[4] Graft selection was not randomized or assigned by policy but was determined by the personal preference of the surgeon combined with the clinical status of the patient. We have been conducting ongoing reviews of reoperative surgery and in comparison with previous time periods those patients reoperated on in the 1988 to 1991 time frame were more likely to be female (15 per cent), were older at reoperation (mean age 63 years, 21 per cent of patients $>$ 70 years of age), and the mean interval between their first and second operation had extended to 116 months. This last figure is important as it signifies that most reoperative patients had primary surgery that was initially successful but that an average of 10 years later they presented for reoperation usually because of a combination of progression of native vessel coronary disease and progressive atherosclerosis in vein grafts.

The number of ITA grafts available to be used at reoperation is obviously dependent upon how frequently they were used at primary surgery. Of the 1088 patients who received no ITA grafts at their first operation, 799 (73 per cent) received at least one ITA graft at reoperation and 126 (12 per cent) received bilateral ITA grafts. For the patients (560) where one ITA had been used at the first operation, the other ITA was used at reoperation in 215 (38 per cent) cases. The right ITA was used at reoperation for 142 patients with patent left ITA grafts with the vessels grafted using the ITA being LAD-diagonal system in twenty-nine (twenty-three *in situ*, six free grafts), circumflex system in fifty-seven (twenty-two *in situ*, thirty-five free grafts) and right coronary system in fifty-six (forty-six *in situ*, ten free grafts). In addition thirty-seven patients received right GEA grafts and in ten patients the IEA was used as a free graft.

For the purposes of analysis of the influence of grafting strategies on in-hospital risk, patients were subgrouped according to the number of ITA grafts used at the primary operation and at the reoperation (Table 21.1). Table 21.1 also contains listings of important patient related variables. There were obvious biases with regard to graft selection. Patients who did not receive an ITA graft at either the first or second operation were more likely to be women, >70 years of age, be undergoing an emergency reoperation, or have had a history of congestive heart failure. Diabetic patients were less likely to receive bilateral ITA grafts.

The overall in-hospital mortality rate was 3.7 per cent with 85 per cent of deaths due primarily to cardiovascular causes. The patient-related descriptors associated with increased risk in multivariate testing, were a history of congestive heart failure, emergency operation, female gender and advancing age. When the graft subgroup was included in the logistic regression analysis model the patients who received no ITA graft at either the first or the second operation were found to have increased mortality. Despite multivariate testing it is difficult to know whether not using ITA grafts was a policy that actually increased risk because all the unfavourable patient-related characteristics were also associated with that subgroup. However, I do think that we can say that with the selection criteria used during these years, that the use of arterial grafts did not appear to increase perioperative mortality.

There was also a trend toward increased morbidity for patients receiving no ITA grafts at either operation, an observation that also could be attributed to patient-related characteristics. Wound complications have been a subject of concern when bilateral ITA grafts have been used for diabetic patients and we have rarely used simultaneous bilateral ITA grafting at reoperation for diabetics.[33] However, it is of interest that when diabetic patients have an ITA graft at primary surgery, and then receive a second ITA graft at reoperation, we have not noted an increased risk of wound complications.

Mortality according to preoperative graft status

Examination of mortality according to preoperative graft status showed that the risk for patients with a

Table 21.1 ITA grafts at primary operation/ITA grafts at reoperation: baseline descriptors and in-hospital mortality

Group	*1*	*2*	*3*	*4*	*5*	*6*	*P value*
ITA at 1st op/ITA at 2nd op	0/0	0/1	0/2	1/0	1/1	2/0	
No. patients	289	673	126	345	215	15	
Mean age	67	63	56	63	59	55	< 0.001
> 70 years (%)	41	20	2	20	11	0	< 0.001
% Female	20	12	6	20	12	33	< 0.001
% Emergency	5	2	1	3	0	13	< 0.001
% CHF	13	11	5	9	7	27	0.017
% Diabetes	19	20	7	20	16	20	0.02
Mortality							
No. patients	23	16	2	16	4	1	
% Patients	8.0	2.4	1.6	4.6	1.9	6.7	

patent ITA – LAD graft was 3.7 per cent and the use of the right ITA for a graft in that setting did not increase risk (2.1 per cent mortality for that subgroup). The risk of damage of a patent left ITA – LAD graft was fourteen of 428 (3.3 per cent), less than half the risk during our early experience, an improvement related almost entirely to increased surgeon experience.[34] We can conclude that at this point in time the presence of a patent left ITA–LAD graft is not even a relative contraindication to reoperation and does not appear to increase risk at all. In fact, such patients have the advantage that their anterior wall function is likely to be well preserved and atherosclerotic embolization from an ITA graft has not been documented.

In addition, the presence of atherosclerotic stenotic vein grafts did not appear to increase risk specifically although there was a non-significant trend toward increased mortality for patients with two or more atherosclerotic vein grafts. In the past, atherosclerotic vein grafts have appeared to increase the risk of reoperation somewhat, both in our experience and in that of Perrault and colleagues.[3,19] The improvement for that patient subset is attributable in part to increased surgeon experience but also to the specific technical advance of retrograde cardioplegia delivery. Twenty-seven patients who died postoperatively after myocardial infarction were examined with autopsy study and in none was atherosclerotic embolization documented.

New myocardial infarction is still the most common cause of in-hospital mortality after reperation. When the twenty-seven patients with perioperative myocardial infarction underwent autopsy, fifteen were found to have vein graft thrombosis associated with distal native coronary artery disease and eight patients had patent graft associated with distal native vessel coronary artery disease in the infarct distribution.

Reoperation following bilateral ITA grafting

One of the major purposes of using both ITAs at a primary operation is to decrease the likelihood of a reoperation. However, despite use of both ITAs, reoperation is sometimes needed due to ITA graft failure, extensive progression of native vessel coronary artery disease, or the need for valvular heart surgery or cardiac transplantation. Review of our experience with reoperation after bilateral ITA grafting up to late 1993 identified thirty-six patients. In six cases reoperation was done for valve surgery or transplantation without bypass grafting and in six cases patients underwent reoperation for combined coronary artery and valve pathology.[35]

In twelve cases, patent *in situ* ITA grafts crossed the mid line. Reoperation was undertaken through a left thoracotomy in one case and by a median sternotomy in the rest although in one of these cases a limited right thoracotomy was employed to allow dissection of the patent left ITA graft from the mid line. Damage to the right ITA graft occurred in one case. When performing *in situ* right ITA grafts at a primary operation we divide the pericardium from the lateral aspect of the aorta posteriorly and then suture that pericardium anterior to the right ITA graft. This manoeuvre usually avoids adhesion of the right ITA to the sternum and that position, combined with extreme care during reoperation and good fortune, will usually allow relatively safe reentry through a median sternotomy.

A thoracotomy approach can be helpful for some kinds of reoperations following bilateral ITA grafting. For patients needing isolated mitral valve surgery, a right thoracotomy is a relatively safe approach and a left thoracotomy can be used when bypass surgery involving the circumflex system is needed. When we have performed reoperations through a thoracotomy we usually use a femoral arterial cannulation (although aortic or axillary cannulation can be employed) and femoral venous cannulation. We do not use aortic cross-clamping and use systemic hypothermia to 20°C to achieve ventricular fibrillation for operative exposure and myocardial protection. Significant aortic insufficiency complicates reoperation through a thoracotomy.

Arterial grafts and the late results of reoperation

The ongoing evolution in the population of patients undergoing reoperation for bypass grafting and the fact that patient-related variables have a major impact on graft selection during reoperation have made it difficult to assess the impact of the use of arterial grafts on long-term survival following repeat surgery. Our last analysis of the 10-year results after reoperation documented an overall 69.3 per cent survival for in-hospital survivors and also showed that moderate-to-poor left ventricular function, age ⩾ 65 years, left main stenosis and a combination of graft failure and progression of native vessel atherosclerosis after primary operation were patient-related factors associated with decreased survival. In addition, patients who did not have any ITA grafts at either their first or second operation had reduced 10-year survival.[2]

Likewise, there are few data that exist regarding graft patency after reoperation. No prospective data are available. We found retrospectively that 684 of our patients had undergone a postoperative angiogram at a mean post-reoperation interval of 58 months, and graft patency rates per vessel were LAD (diagonal) – ITA (308/346) 89 per cent vs SVG (342/481) 71 per cent; circumflex – ITA (44/51) 81 per cent, vs SVG (305/493) 62 per cent; RCA–ITA (11/14) 79 per cent vs SVG (286/464) 62 per cent.[2]

In a retrospective study of seventeen patients who underwent angiography after reoperation, Galbut *et al.* noted 85 per cent patency of twenty left ITA anastomoses, 76.5 per cent patency rate of seventeen right ITA RCA anastomoses, and 66.7 per cent patency of twelve saphenous vein grafts.[9]

Despite the lack of studies specifically relating to late graft patency after reoperation there is no reason to think that the principles of graft patency after reoperation should differ in a major way from the large volume of data concerning primary surgery. In fact, it is intuitive that because of the extensive native vessel disease of many reoperative candidates the relative advantage in terms of patency of arterial grafts over vein grafts would expect to be highlighted during reoperation. To have a positive aspect on a long-term result, a graft must be patent and the chance to obtain increased rates of long-term patency is the best reason to use arterial grafting during reoperation.

References

1. Lytle BW, Loop FD, Cosgrove DM *et al.* Fifteen hundred coronary reoperations: results and determinants of early and late survival. *J Thorac Cardiovasc Surg* 1987; **93:** 847–59.
2. Loop FD, Lytle BW, Cosgrove DM *et al.* Reoperation for coronary atherosclerosis: Changing practice in 2509 consecutive patients. *Ann Surg* 1990; **212:** 378–86.
3. Lytle BW, Loop FD, Taylor PC *et al.* The effect of coronary reoperation on the survival of patients with stenoses in saphenous vein to coronary bypass grafts. *J Thorac Cardiovasc Surg* 1993; **105:** 605–14.
4. Lytle BW, McElroy D, McCarthy PM *et al.* The influence of arterial coronary bypass grafts on the mortality of coronary reoperations. *J Thorac Cardiovascular Surg* 1994; **107:** 675–83.
5. Salomon NW, Page US, Bigelow JC *et al.* Reoperative coronary surgery: comparative analysis of 6591 patients undergoing primary bypass and 508 patients undergoing reoperative coronary bypass. *J Thorac Cardiovasc Surg* 1990; **100:** 250–60.
6. Lytle BW, Cosgrove DM. Coronary artery bypass surgery. In: Wells SA ed. *Current problems in surgery*. Philadelphia: W.B. Saunders Company, 1992; 733–807.
7. Lytle BW, Loop FD, Cosgrove DM, Ratliff NB, Easley K, Taylor PC. Long-term (5 to 12 years) serial studies of internal mammary artery and saphenous vein coronary bypass grafts. *J Thorac Cardiovasc Surg* 1985; **89:** 248–58.
8. Dion R, Verhelst R, Rousseau M *et al.* Sequential mammary grafting. Clinical, functional and angiographic assessment 6 months postoperatively in 231 consecutive patients. *J Thorac Cardiovasc Surg* 1989; **98:** 80.
9. Galbut DL, Traad EA, Dorman MJ *et al.* Bilateral internal mammary artery grafts in reoperative and primary coronary bypass surgery. *Ann Thorac Surg* 1991; **52:** 20–8.
10. Loop FD, Lytle BW, Cosgrove DM *et al.* Influence of the internal-mammary-artery graft on 10-year survival and other cardiac events. *New Engl J Med* 1986; **314:** 1–6.
11. Sargeant P, Lasaffre E, Flameng W *et al.* Internal mammary artery: Methods of use and their effect on survival. *Eur J Cardiothorac Surg* 1990; **4:** 72–8.
12. Boylan MJ, Lytle BW, Loop FD *et al.* Surgical treatment of isolated left anterior descending coronary stenosis: Comparison of left internal mammary artery and venous autograft at 18 to 20 years of follow-up. *J Thorac Cardiovasc Surg* 1994; **107:** 657–62.
13. Cosgrove DM, Loop FD, Lytle BW *et al.* Does mammary artery grafting increase surgical risk? *Circulation* 1985; **72** (Suppl II): 170–4.
14. Galbut DL, Traad EA, Durman MJ *et al.* Seventeen-year experience with bilateral internal mammary artery grafts. *Ann Thor Surg* 1990; **99:** 195.
15. Fiore AC, Naunheim KS, Dean P *et al.* Results of internal thoracic artery grafting over 15 years: single vs double grafts. *Ann Thorac Surg* 1990; **49:** 202.
16. Ungerleider RM, Mills NL, Wechsler AS. Left thoracotomy for reoperative coronary artery bypass procedures. *Ann Thorac Surg* 1985; **40:** 11.
17. Blauth CI, Cosgrove DM, Web BW *et al.* Atheroembolism from the ascending aorta: An emerging problem in cardiac surgery. *J Thorac Cardiovasc Surg* 1992; **103:** 1104–12.
18. Keon WJ, Heggtveit HA, Lecluc J. Perioperative myocardial infarction caused by atheroembolization. *J Thorac Cardiovasc Surg* 1982; **84:** 849–55.

19. Perrault L, Carrier M, Cartier R *et al.* Morbidity and mortality of reoperation for coronary artery bypass grafting: significance of atheromatous vein grafts. *Can J Cardiol* 1991; **7:** 427–30.
20. Menasche P, Kural S, Fanchet M *et al.* Retrograde coronary sinus perfusion: a safe alternative for ensuring cardioplegic delivery in aortic valve surgery. *Ann Thorac Surg* 1982; **34:** 649.
21. Gundry SR, Razzouk AJ, Vigesaa RE *et al.* Optimal delivery of cardioplegic solution for 'redo' operations. *J Thorac Cardiovasc Surg* 1991; **103:** 896–901.
22. Partington MT, Acar C, Buckberg GD *et al.* Studies of retrograde cardioplegia. II. Advantages of antegrade/retrograde cardioplegia to optimize distribution in jeopardized myocardium. *J Thorac Cardiovasc Surg* 1989; **97:** 613.
23. Salerno TA, Houck JP, Barrozo CAM *et al.* Retrograde continuous warm blood cardioplegia: A new concept in myocardial protection. *Ann Thorac Surg* 1991; **51:** 245.
24. Rosenkranz EF, Okamoto F, Buckberg GD *et al.* Safety of prolonged aortic clamping with blood cardioplegia: II. Glutamate enrichment in energy depleted hearts. *J Thorac Cardiovasc Surg* 1984; **88:** 402.
25. Buckberg DG. Strategies and logic of cardioplegic delivery to prevent, avoid and reverse ischemic and reperfusion damage. *J Thorac Cardiovasc Surg* 1987; **93:** 127.
26. Jain U, Sullivan HJ, Pifarre R *et al.* Graft atheroembolism as the probable cause of failure to wean from cardiopulmonary bypass. *J Cardiothoracic Anesth* 1990; **4:** 476–80.
27. Campos EE, Cinderella JA, Farhi ER. Long-term angiographic follow-up of normal and minimally diseased saphenous vein grafts. *JACC* 1993; **21:** 1175–80.
28. Navia D, Cosgrove DM, Lytle BW *et al.* Is the internal thoracic artery the conduit of choice to replace a stenotic vein graft? *Ann Thorac Surg* 1994; **57:** 40–4.
29. Turner E, Lytle B, Navia D. Coronary reoperations: Adding an internal mammary artery to a stenotic vein graft to the left anterior descending coronary artery (in press).
30. Jones EL, Lattouf OM, Weintraub WS. Catastrophic consequences of internal mammary artery hypoperfusion. *J Thorac Cardiovasc Surg* 1989; **98:** 902–7.
31. Tector AJ, Amundsen S, Schmahl TM, Kress DC, Peter M. Total revascularization with T grafts. *Ann Thorac Surg* 1994; **57:** 33–9.
32. Suma H, Wanibuchi Y, Terada Y *et al.* The right gastroepiploic artery graft; clinical and angiographic midterm results in 200 patients. *J Thorac Cardiovasc Surg* 1993; **105:** 615–25.
33. Loop FD, Lytle BW, Cosgrove DM *et al.* Sternal wound complications after isolated coronary artery bypass grafting: early and late mortality, morbidity and cost of care. *Ann Thorac Surg* 1990; **49:** 179–87.
34. Baillot RG, Loop FD, Cosgrove DM, Lytle BW. Reoperation after previous grafting with the internal mammary artery: technique and early results. *Ann Thorac Surg* 1985; **40:** 271–3.
35. Joyce FS, McCarthy PM, Taylor PC, Cosgrove DM, Lytle BW. Cardiac reoperation in patients with bilateral thoracic artery grafts. *Ann Thorac Surg* 1994; **58:** 80–5.

Index